Chapman & Hall/CRC Biostatistics Series

Repeated Measures Design with Generalized Linear Mixed Models for Randomized Controlled Trials

Toshiro Tango
Center for Medical Statistics
Minato-ku Tokyo
Japan

CRC Press
Taylor & Francis Group
Boca Raton London New York

CRC Press is an imprint of the
Taylor & Francis Group, an **informa** business
A CHAPMAN & HALL BOOK

Chapman & Hall/CRC Biostatistics Series

Published Titles

Adaptive Design Methods in Clinical Trials, Second Edition
Shein-Chung Chow and Mark Chang

Adaptive Designs for Sequential Treatment Allocation
Alessandro Baldi Antognini and Alessandra Giovagnoli

Adaptive Design Theory and Implementation Using SAS and R, Second Edition
Mark Chang

Advanced Bayesian Methods for Medical Test Accuracy
Lyle D. Broemeling

Analyzing Longitudinal Clinical Trial Data: A Practical Guide
Craig Mallinckrodt and Ilya Lipkovich

Applied Biclustering Methods for Big and High-Dimensional Data Using R
Adetayo Kasim, Ziv Shkedy, Sebastian Kaiser, Sepp Hochreiter, and Willem Talloen

Applied Meta-Analysis with R
Ding-Geng (Din) Chen and Karl E. Peace

Applied Surrogate Endpoint Evaluation Methods with SAS and R
Ariel Alonso, Theophile Bigirumurame, Tomasz Burzykowski, Marc Buyse, Geert Molenberghs, Leacky Muchene, Nolen Joy Perualila, Ziv Shkedy, and Wim Van der Elst

Basic Statistics and Pharmaceutical Statistical Applications, Second Edition
James E. De Muth

Bayesian Adaptive Methods for Clinical Trials
Scott M. Berry, Bradley P. Carlin, J. Jack Lee, and Peter Muller

Bayesian Analysis Made Simple: An Excel GUI for WinBUGS
Phil Woodward

Bayesian Designs for Phase I–II Clinical Trials
Ying Yuan, Hoang Q. Nguyen, and Peter F. Thall

Bayesian Methods for Measures of Agreement
Lyle D. Broemeling

Bayesian Methods for Repeated Measures
Lyle D. Broemeling

Bayesian Methods in Epidemiology
Lyle D. Broemeling

Bayesian Methods in Health Economics
Gianluca Baio

Bayesian Missing Data Problems: EM, Data Augmentation and Noniterative Computation
Ming T. Tan, Guo-Liang Tian, and Kai Wang Ng

Published Titles

Bayesian Modeling in Bioinformatics
Dipak K. Dey, Samiran Ghosh, and Bani K. Mallick

Benefit-Risk Assessment in Pharmaceutical Research and Development
Andreas Sashegyi, James Felli, and Rebecca Noel

Benefit-Risk Assessment Methods in Medical Product Development: Bridging Qualitative and Quantitative Assessments
Qi Jiang and Weili He

Bioequivalence and Statistics in Clinical Pharmacology, Second Edition
Scott Patterson and Byron Jones

Biosimilar Clinical Development: Scientific Considerations and New Methodologies
Kerry B. Barker, Sandeep M. Menon, Ralph B. D'Agostino, Sr., Siyan Xu, and Bo Jin

Biosimilars: Design and Analysis of Follow-on Biologics
Shein-Chung Chow

Biostatistics: A Computing Approach
Stewart J. Anderson

Cancer Clinical Trials: Current and Controversial Issues in Design and Analysis
Stephen L. George, Xiaofei Wang, and Herbert Pang

Causal Analysis in Biomedicine and Epidemiology: Based on Minimal Sufficient Causation
Mikel Aickin

Clinical and Statistical Considerations in Personalized Medicine
Claudio Carini, Sandeep Menon, and Mark Chang

Clinical Trial Data Analysis using R
Ding-Geng (Din) Chen and Karl E. Peace

Clinical Trial Methodology
Karl E. Peace and Ding-Geng (Din) Chen

Computational Methods in Biomedical Research
Ravindra Khattree and Dayanand N. Naik

Computational Pharmacokinetics
Anders Källén

Confidence Intervals for Proportions and Related Measures of Effect Size
Robert G. Newcombe

Controversial Statistical Issues in Clinical Trials
Shein-Chung Chow

Data Analysis with Competing Risks and Intermediate States
Ronald B. Geskus

Data and Safety Monitoring Committees in Clinical Trials, Second Edition
Jay Herson

Design and Analysis of Animal Studies in Pharmaceutical Development
Shein-Chung Chow and Jen-pei Liu

Design and Analysis of Bioavailability and Bioequivalence Studies, Third Edition
Shein-Chung Chow and Jen-pei Liu

Design and Analysis of Bridging Studies
Jen-pei Liu, Shein-Chung Chow, and Chin-Fu Hsiao

Design & Analysis of Clinical Trials for Economic Evaluation & Reimbursement: An Applied Approach Using SAS & STATA
Iftekhar Khan

Design and Analysis of Clinical Trials for Predictive Medicine
Shigeyuki Matsui, Marc Buyse, and Richard Simon

Design and Analysis of Clinical Trials with Time-to-Event Endpoints
Karl E. Peace

Design and Analysis of Non-Inferiority Trials
Mark D. Rothmann, Brian L. Wiens, and Ivan S. F. Chan

Difference Equations with Public Health Applications
Lemuel A. Moyé and Asha Seth Kapadia

DNA Methylation Microarrays: Experimental Design and Statistical Analysis
Sun-Chong Wang and Arturas Petronis

Published Titles

DNA Microarrays and Related Genomics Techniques: Design, Analysis, and Interpretation of Experiments
David B. Allison, Grier P. Page, T. Mark Beasley, and Jode W. Edwards

Dose Finding by the Continual Reassessment Method
Ying Kuen Cheung

Dynamical Biostatistical Models
Daniel Commenges and Hélène Jacqmin-Gadda

Elementary Bayesian Biostatistics
Lemuel A. Moyé

Emerging Non-Clinical Biostatistics in Biopharmaceutical Development and Manufacturing
Harry Yang

Empirical Likelihood Method in Survival Analysis
Mai Zhou

Essentials of a Successful Biostatistical Collaboration
Arul Earnest

Exposure–Response Modeling: Methods and Practical Implementation
Jixian Wang

Frailty Models in Survival Analysis
Andreas Wienke

Fundamental Concepts for New Clinical Trialists
Scott Evans and Naitee Ting

Generalized Linear Models: A Bayesian Perspective
Dipak K. Dey, Sujit K. Ghosh, and Bani K. Mallick

Handbook of Regression and Modeling: Applications for the Clinical and Pharmaceutical Industries
Daryl S. Paulson

Inference Principles for Biostatisticians
Ian C. Marschner

Interval-Censored Time-to-Event Data: Methods and Applications
Ding-Geng (Din) Chen, Jianguo Sun, and Karl E. Peace

Introductory Adaptive Trial Designs: A Practical Guide with R
Mark Chang

Joint Models for Longitudinal and Time-to-Event Data: With Applications in R
Dimitris Rizopoulos

Measures of Interobserver Agreement and Reliability, Second Edition
Mohamed M. Shoukri

Medical Biostatistics, Third Edition
A. Indrayan

Meta-Analysis in Medicine and Health Policy
Dalene Stangl and Donald A. Berry

Methods in Comparative Effectiveness Research
Constantine Gatsonis and Sally C. Morton

Mixed Effects Models for the Population Approach: Models, Tasks, Methods and Tools
Marc Lavielle

Modeling to Inform Infectious Disease Control
Niels G. Becker

Modern Adaptive Randomized Clinical Trials: Statistical and Practical Aspects
Oleksandr Sverdlov

Monte Carlo Simulation for the Pharmaceutical Industry: Concepts, Algorithms, and Case Studies
Mark Chang

Multiregional Clinical Trials for Simultaneous Global New Drug Development
Joshua Chen and Hui Quan

Multiple Testing Problems in Pharmaceutical Statistics
Alex Dmitrienko, Ajit C. Tamhane, and Frank Bretz

Noninferiority Testing in Clinical Trials: Issues and Challenges
Tie-Hua Ng

Optimal Design for Nonlinear Response Models
Valerii V. Fedorov and Sergei L. Leonov

Published Titles

Patient-Reported Outcomes: Measurement, Implementation and Interpretation
Joseph C. Cappelleri, Kelly H. Zou, Andrew G. Bushmakin, Jose Ma. J. Alvir, Demissie Alemayehu, and Tara Symonds

Quantitative Evaluation of Safety in Drug Development: Design, Analysis and Reporting
Qi Jiang and H. Amy Xia

Quantitative Methods for Traditional Chinese Medicine Development
Shein-Chung Chow

Randomized Clinical Trials of Nonpharmacological Treatments
Isabelle Boutron, Philippe Ravaud, and David Moher

Randomized Phase II Cancer Clinical Trials
Sin-Ho Jung

Repeated Measures Design with Generalized Linear Mixed Models for Randomized Controlled Trials
Toshiro Tango

Sample Size Calculations for Clustered and Longitudinal Outcomes in Clinical Research
Chul Ahn, Moonseong Heo, and Song Zhang

Sample Size Calculations in Clinical Research, Second Edition
Shein-Chung Chow, Jun Shao, and Hansheng Wang

Statistical Analysis of Human Growth and Development
Yin Bun Cheung

Statistical Design and Analysis of Clinical Trials: Principles and Methods
Weichung Joe Shih and Joseph Aisner

Statistical Design and Analysis of Stability Studies
Shein-Chung Chow

Statistical Evaluation of Diagnostic Performance: Topics in ROC Analysis
Kelly H. Zou, Aiyi Liu, Andriy Bandos, Lucila Ohno-Machado, and Howard Rockette

Statistical Methods for Clinical Trials
Mark X. Norleans

Statistical Methods for Drug Safety
Robert D. Gibbons and Anup K. Amatya

Statistical Methods for Healthcare Performance Monitoring
Alex Bottle and Paul Aylin

Statistical Methods for Immunogenicity Assessment
Harry Yang, Jianchun Zhang, Binbing Yu, and Wei Zhao

Statistical Methods in Drug Combination Studies
Wei Zhao and Harry Yang

Statistical Testing Strategies in the Health Sciences
Albert Vexler, Alan D. Hutson, and Xiwei Chen

Statistics in Drug Research: Methodologies and Recent Developments
Shein-Chung Chow and Jun Shao

Statistics in the Pharmaceutical Industry, Third Edition
Ralph Buncher and Jia-Yeong Tsay

Survival Analysis in Medicine and Genetics
Jialiang Li and Shuangge Ma

Theory of Drug Development
Eric B. Holmgren

Translational Medicine: Strategies and Statistical Methods
Dennis Cosmatos and Shein-Chung Chow

CRC Press
Taylor & Francis Group
6000 Broken Sound Parkway NW, Suite 300
Boca Raton, FL 33487-2742

Printed on acid-free paper
Version Date: 20170125

International Standard Book Number-13: 978-1-4987-4789-9 (Hardback)

Visit the Taylor & Francis Web site at
http://www.taylorandfrancis.com

and the CRC Press Web site at
http://www.crcpress.com

Contents

Preface

One of the basic and important ideas about the design of randomized controlled trials (RCT) and the analysis of the data will be that a group of patients to which a new drug was administered is never homogeneous in terms of response to the drug. In response to the drug, some patients improve, some patients experience no change and other patients even worsen contrary to patients' expectation. These phenomena can be observed even in patients assigned to the placebo group. Namely, nobody knows whether or not these changes are really caused by the drug administered. To deal with these unpredictable heterogeneities of the subject-specific response, the generalized linear mixed (or mixed-effects) models are known to provide a flexible and powerful tool where the unpredictable subject-specific responses are assumed to be unobserved random-effects variables.

The primary focus of this book is, as a practical framework of RCT design, to provide a new repeated measures design called *S:T repeated measures design* (S and T denote the number of repeated measures data before and after randomization, respectively) combined with the generalized linear mixed models that is proposed by Tango (2016a). Until recently the use of generalized linear mixed models has been limited by heavy computational burden and a lack of generally available software. However, as of today, the computational burden is much less of a restriction with the introduction of good procedures into the well-known statistical software SAS. The main advantages of the *S:T repeated measures design* combined with the generalized linear mixed models are (1) it can easily handle missing data by applying the likelihood-based ignorable analyses under the missing at random assumption and (2) it may lead to a reduction in sample size, compared with the conventional repeated measures design.

This book presents several types of generalized linear mixed models tailored for randomized controlled trials depending on the primary interest of the trial but emphasizes practical, rather than theoretical, aspects of mixed models and the interpretation of results. Almost all of the models presented in this book are illustrated with real data arising from randomized controlled trials using SAS (version 9.3) as a main software. This book will be of interest to trial statisticians, clinical trial designers, clinical researchers, and biostatisticians in the pharmaceutical industry, contract research organizations, hospitals and academia. It is also of relevance to graduate students of biostatistics and epidemiology. Prerequisites are introductory biostatistics including the design and analysis of clinical trials.

While there are many excellent books on the generalized linear mixed models and the analysis of repeated measures data, there seem to be few books focusing on the generalized linear mixed models for the design and analysis of repeated measures in randomized controlled trials.

This book is organized as follows. In this book, I mainly consider a parallel group randomized controlled trial of two treatment groups where the primary response variable is either a continuous, count or binary response. Chapter 1 provides an introduction to a new repeated measures design and some typical generalized linear mixed models for randomized controlled trials within the framework of *S:T repeated measures design*. This chapter also introduces the important concepts in clinical trials, *superiority and non-inferiority* and discusses the difference. Chapter 2 introduces three typical examples of standard or non-sophisticated statistical analysis for repeated measures data in an animal experiment. These types of analysis are often observed in papers published in many medical journals. This chapter points out statistical problems encountered in each of the analysis plans. Chapter 3 presents several ANOVA models and ANCOVA-type models for repeated measures data with various covariance structures over time and compares their results with those obtained in naive analyses in Chapter 2 using SAS. Chapter 4 discusses the distinction between the ANOVA model and the mixed-effects repeated measures model. Emphasis is placed on the fact that newly introduced *random-effects* variables reflecting *inter-subject heterogeneity* in the mixed-effects repeated measures models determine the covariance structure over time. Chapter 5 illustrates the linear mixed models with real data in more detail to understand the mixed models intuitively and visually. Chapter 6 illustrates a good property of the mixed models for handling missing data, which can allow for the so-called *likelihood-based ignorable analysis* under the relatively weak MAR assumption. Chapter 7 presents several linear mixed-effects models, called "normal linear regression models" in this book, for a continuous response variable with normal error distributions. Chapter 8 presents several mixed-effects logistic regression models for a binary response variable. Chapter 9 presents several mixed-effects Poisson regression models for a count response variable. Chapters 7, 8 and 9 try to emphasize the detailed explanations of the model, illustrating with data arising from real randomized controlled trials, and the interpretation of results. Chapter 7, 8 and 9 also have the section of sample size which provides sample size formula or sample size calculations via Monte Carlo simulations. Detailed calculations based on example data are also given. Chapter 10 presents Bayesian models with non-informative prior using WinBUGS or OpenBUGS for some of the generalized linear mixed models described in previous chapters and discusses the similarity of both estimates. The reason why Bayesian alternatives are presented here is the preparation for the situation where frequentist approaches including the generalized linear mixed models face difficulty in estimation. Chapter 11 introduces some latent class or profile models as a competitor to the mixed models. As mentioned above, the generalized linear mixed models have been developed for dealing with heterogeneity or variability among subject responses. It seems to me, however, that they are still based upon the "homogeneous" assumption in the sense that the fixed-effects mean response profile within each treatment group is meaningful and thus the treatment effect is usually evaluated by the difference in mean response profiles during the pre-specified evaluation period. So, if the subject by time interaction within each treatment group were not negligible, the mean response profiles could be inappropriate measures for treatment effects. To cope with these *substantial heterogeneity*, this chapter introduces some latent class or profile models and illustrates these latent models with real data using R and WinBUGS or OpenBUGS. Chapter 12 considers some generalized linear mixed models for other trial designs including three-arm non-inferiority trials including placebo and cluster randomized trials. Appendix A presents some statistical background for the sample size calculations within the framework of $S{:}T$ repeated measures design. Appendix B presents some statistical background for the maximum likelihood estimator for the generalized linear mixed models within the framework of $S{:}T$ repeated measures design and the computational methods for the numerical integration to evaluate the integral included in the likelihood.

I hope that readers will find this book useful and interesting as an introduction to the subject.

The view of randomized controlled trials embodied in this book is, of course, my own. This has been formed over many years through a lot of experience involved with randomized controlled trials conducted by pharmaceutical companies and collaboration with many medical researchers. Finally I would like to thank John Kimmel of Chapman & Hall/CRC Press Executive editor, statistics, for inviting me to write this book and providing continual support and encouragement.

Toshiro Tango
Tokyo

1

Introduction

In clinical medicine, drugs are usually administered to control some response variable within a specified range reflecting the patient's disease state directly or indirectly. In most randomized controlled trials (RCTs) and randomized animal experiments, to evaluate the efficacy of a new treatment or the toxicity of a new treatment, the primary response variable on the same subject (e.g., a patient, an animal, a laboratory sample) is scheduled to be measured over a period of time, consisting of a baseline period before randomization, treatment period after randomization and, if necessary, a follow-up period after the end of treatment period. These subject-specific **repeated measures** or **subject-specific response profiles** are analyzed for assessing difference in changes from baseline among treatment groups, leading to a treatment effect.

1.1 Repeated measures design

Let y_{ij} denote the primary response variable for the ith subject at the jth time t_{ij}. An ordinary situation of **repeated measures design** adopted in RCTs or animal experiments is when the primary response variable is measured once at baseline period (before randomization) and T times during the treatment period (after randomization) where measurements are scheduled to be made at the same times for all subjects $t_{ij} = t_j$ in the sampling design. We call this design the ***Basic* 1 : *T repeated measures design*** throughout the book, where the response profile vector $\boldsymbol{y}_i$ for the ith subject is expressed as

$$\boldsymbol{y}_i = (\underbrace{y_{i0}}_{\text{baseline data}} , \underbrace{y_{i1}, ..., y_{iT}}_{\text{data after randomization}})^t. \tag{1.1}$$

In exploratory trials in the early phases of drug development, statistical analyses of interest will be to estimate the time-dependent mean profile for each treatment group and to test whether there is any treatment-by-time interaction. In confirmatory trials in the later phases of drug development, on the other hand, we need a simple and clinically meaningful effect size of the new treatment. So, many RCTs tend to try to narrow the evaluation period down to one time point (ex., the last Tth measurement), leading to the so-called *pre-post* design or the ***1:1* design**:

$$\boldsymbol{y}_i = (\underbrace{y_{i0}}_{\text{baseline data}}, y_{i1}, ..., y_{i(T-1)}, \underbrace{y_{iT}}_{\text{data to be analyzed}})^t. \quad (1.2)$$

Some other RCTs define a summary statistic such as the mean $\bar{y}_i$ of repeated measures during the evaluation period (ex., mean of $y_{i(T-1)}$ and y_{iT}), which also leads to a *1:1* design. In these simple *1:1* designs, traditional analysis methods such as analysis of covariance (ANCOVA) have been used to analyze data where the baseline measurement is used as a covariate. In the *1:1 design*, ANCOVA is preferred over the mixed-effects model when the covariance matrix over time is homogeneous across groups (Winkens et al., 2007; Crager, 1987; Chen, 2006) although the difference is small in practice. However, ANCOVA cannot be applied when the covariance matrices over time are heterogeneous across groups. Since the ANCOVA-type method is easily influenced by missing data, some kind of imputation method such as LOCF (last observation carried forward) are inevitably needed for ITT (intention-to-treat) analysis (Winkens et al., 2007; Crager, 1987; Chen, 2006).

In this book, we shall introduce a new $S:T$ ***repeated measures design*** (Tango, 2016) as an extension of the *1:1 design* combined with the generalized linear mixed models and as a formal confirmatory trial design for randomized controlled trials shown below:

$$\begin{aligned} \boldsymbol{y}_i &= (\underbrace{y_{i(-S+1)}, ..., y_{i0}}_{\text{data before randomization}}, \underbrace{y_{i1}, ..., y_{ik}, y_{i(k+1)}, ..., y_{i(k+T)}}_{\text{data after randomization}})^t \\ &= (\underbrace{y_{i(-S+1)}, ..., y_{i0}}_{\text{baseline data to be analyzed}}, y_{i1}, ..., y_{ik}, \underbrace{y_{i(k+1)}, ..., y_{i(k+T)}}_{\text{data to be analyzed}})^t. \end{aligned} \quad (1.3)$$

However, to avoid a notational cumbersome procedure, we shall omit $(y_{i1}, ..., y_{ik})$ and replace $(y_{i(k+1)}, ..., y_{i(k+T)})$ with $(y_{i1}, ..., y_{iT})$ such that

$$\boldsymbol{y}_i = (\underbrace{y_{i(-S+1)}, ..., y_{i0}}_{\text{baseline period}}, \underbrace{y_{i1}, ..., y_{iT}}_{\text{evaluation period}})^t. \quad (1.4)$$

Namely, throughout the book, the ***S:T* design** implies that the repeated measures $(y_{i(-S+1)}, ..., y_{i0})$ denote the data sequence measured during the **baseline period** and the repeated measures $(y_{i1}, ..., y_{iT})$ denote the data sequence measured during the **evaluation period**, defined in the study protocol. Especially, the primary interest of this design in confirmatory trials in the later phases of drug development is to estimate the overall or average treatment effect during the evaluation period. So, in such trial protocols, it is important to select the evaluation period during which the treatment effect could be expected to be stable to a certain extent. As an example of RCTs adopting this type of repeated measures design, I shall introduce one by Schwartz et al. (1998) that studied the effect of troglitazone (two doses) or placebo in patients with poorly controlled non-insulin-dependent diabetes mellitus. They adopted a *5:2* repeat measures design, but changed to *1:1* design in their ANCOVA-type analysis in that the mean of five measurements during baseline period (at -8, -6, -4, -2, 0 weeks before randomization) was used as the baseline value and the mean of two measurements during the evaluation period (at 24, 26 weeks after randomization) was used as the endpoint.

Recently, Takada and Tango (2014) proposed the application of mixed-effects logistic regression models for estimating the treatment effect of eliminating symptoms based on the patient's daily symptoms (0 for no symptoms, 1 for some symptoms) diary (**7:7 design** : seven days before randomization and seven days after randomization) in the area of gastrointestinal disease. They showed, via a Monte Carlo simulation, a better performance of a mixed-effects logistic regression model over the ordinary ANCOVA-type regression models where the primary endpoint is the presence of perfect symptom elimination during the evaluation week, the number of days with some symptoms in the baseline week are used as a covariate, and several imputation methods are utilized when missing data are present. In Section 8.8, a *hypothetical* daily record of patient's symptoms will be analyzed.

On the other hand, there are other study designs where the primary interest is not the average treatment effect but a sort of treatment-by-time interaction (Diggle et al., 2002; Fitzmaurice et al., 2011). For example, in the National Institute of Mental Health Schizophrenia Collaboratory Study, the primary interest is testing the drug by *linear* time interaction, i.e., testing whether the differences between treatment groups are *linearly* increasing over time (Hedeker and Gibbons, 2006; Roy et al., 2007; Bhumik et al., 2008).

Unfortunately, I do not know of any real data on randomized controlled trials adopting an *S:T* design with $S > 1$. So, in the analysis of real data, I shall mainly introduce generalized linear mixed models and its related models assuming the following *1:T* design

$$\boldsymbol{y}_i = (\underbrace{y_{i0}}_{\text{baseline data}}, \underbrace{y_{i1}, ..., y_{i(T-1)}, y_{iT}}_{\text{data during the evaluation period}})^t. \tag{1.5}$$

In Chapter 3, before going into detail of mixed-effects models for randomized controlled trials, I shall introduce traditional analysis of variance (ANOVA) models and analysis of covariance (ANCOVA) models that have been used for the analysis of repeated measures. It should be noted, however, that in Chapter 3, we express the repeated measures by a *triply subscripted array*

$$\{ \ y_{kij} : k = 1, ..., G \ ; i = 1, ..., n_k \ ; j = 0, 1, ..., T \ \}$$

where G denotes the number of treatment groups, and n_k denotes the number of subjects within the kth treatment group. The subscript j indicates the same measurement time as that of y_{ij} expressed in the above-stated repeated measures design.

1.2 Generalized linear mixed models

In this book, we shall consider mainly a parallel group randomized controlled trial or an animal experiment of two treatment groups where the primary response variable is either a continuous, count or binary response and that the first n_1 subjects belong to the control treatment (group 1) and the latter n_2 subjects to the new treatment (group 2). Needless to say, the following arguments are applicable when multiple treatment groups are compared. To a $S{:}T$ repeated measures design, we shall introduce here the following practical and important three types of statistical analysis plans or statistical models that you frequently encounter in many randomized controlled trials:

◇ Model for the treatment effect at each scheduled visit
◇ Model for the average treatment effect
◇ Model for the treatment by linear time interaction

All of these models are based on the *repeated measures models* or *generalized linear mixed models* (GLMM), which are also called *generalized linear mixed-effects models*

1.2.1 Model for the treatment effect at each scheduled visit

Let us consider here the situation where we would like to **estimate the time-dependent mean profile** for each treatment group and to test whether there is any treatment-by-time interaction. One typical model is a so-called *random intercept model*, which will be formulated as

$$
\begin{aligned}
g\{E(y_{ij} \mid b_{0i})\} &= g\{\mu_{ij} \mid b_{0i}\} \\
&= \begin{cases} \beta_0 + \beta_1 x_{1i} + b_{0i} + \boldsymbol{w}_i^t \boldsymbol{\xi} & \text{for } j \le 0 \\ \beta_0 + \beta_1 x_{1i} + b_{0i} + \beta_{2j} + \beta_{3j} x_{1i} + \boldsymbol{w}_i^t \boldsymbol{\xi} & \text{for } j \ge 1 \end{cases} \qquad (1.6) \\
b_{0i} &\sim N(0, \sigma_{B0}^2), \\
i &= 1, ..., n_1 \text{ (control group)}, \\
&= n_1 + 1, ..., n_1 + n_2 \text{ (new treatment group)} \\
j &= -(S-1), -(S-2), ..., 0,\ 1, ..., T
\end{aligned}
$$

where $E(y_{ij} \mid b_{0i})$ are assumed to be constant during the baseline period; the random-effects b_{0i}, called the *random intercept*, may reflect inter-subject variability due to possibly many unobserved prognostic factors for the baseline period and are assumed to be independently normally distributed with mean 0 and variance σ_{B0}^2;

$$
x_{1i} = \begin{cases} 1, & \text{if the } i\text{th subject belongs to the new treatment group} \\ 0, & \text{if the } i\text{th subject belongs to the control group;} \end{cases} \qquad (1.7)
$$

$\boldsymbol{w}_i^t = (w_{1i}, ..., w_{qi})$ is a vector of covariates; and $\boldsymbol{\xi}^t = (\xi_1, ..., \xi_q)$ is a vector of coefficients for covariates. Furthermore, $g(.)$ is the following canonical link function corresponding to the distribution type of y:

$$
g(\mu) = \begin{cases} \mu, & \text{for } y \sim N(\mu, \sigma_E^2) \\ \log\{\mu/(1-\mu)\}, & \text{for } y \sim \text{Bernoulli}(\mu) \\ \log \mu, & \text{for } y \sim \text{Poisson}(\mu). \end{cases} \qquad (1.8)
$$

Regarding the fixed-effects parameters β, we have the following interpretations:

- β_0 denotes the mean response in units of $g(\mu)$ during the baseline period in the control group.
- $\beta_0 + \beta_1$ denotes the mean response in units of $g(\mu)$ during the baseline period in the new treatment group.
- β_{2j} denotes the mean change from baseline in units of $g(\mu)$ at the $j(= 1, ..., T)$th measurement time point in the control group.
- $\beta_{2j} + \beta_{3j}$ denotes the mean change from baseline in units of $g(\mu)$ at the $j(= 1, ..., T)$th measurement time point in the new treatment group.

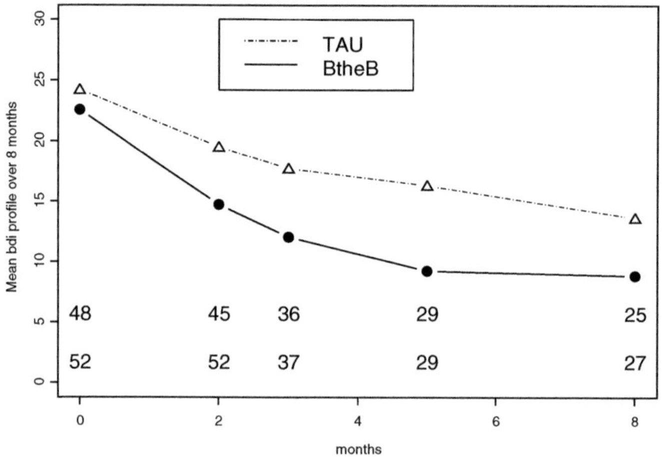

FIGURE 1.1
Mean response profile of BDI (Beck Depression Inventory II) score by treatment group (BtheB,TAU) in a randomized controlled trial evaluating the effects of treatment called "Beat the Blues" (BtheB) in comparison with treatment as usual (TAU) for depression. Sample size at each visit by treatment group is also shown within the figure (upper=TAU group, lower=BtheB group). For details, see Chapter 7.

Therefore, β_{3j} denotes the difference in these two mean changes from baseline at the jth measurement time point or an effect for treatment-by-time interaction at the jth time point. In other words, it actually denotes the **treatment effect of the new treatment at the jth time point** compared with the control treatment. Then, according to the data type, the interpretation of the effect size β_{3j} at the jth time point is as follows:

$$\begin{cases} \text{difference in means of change from baseline,} & \text{for } y \sim N(\mu, \sigma_E^2) \\ \text{difference in log odds ratios of change from baseline,} & \text{for } y \sim \text{Bernoulli}(\mu) \\ \text{difference in log rate ratios of change from baseline,} & \text{for } y \sim \text{Poisson}(\mu) \end{cases}$$

Let us introduce three examples of RCTs, each of whose primary response variables y has a different distribution type:

- Normal distribution:

  Figure 1.1 shows an example of the mean response profile by treatment group over time of the primary response variable BDI (Beck Depression Inventory II score) assumed to be normally distributed in a randomized controlled trial evaluating the effects of treatment called "Beat the Blues" (BtheB) in comparison with treatment as usual (TAU)

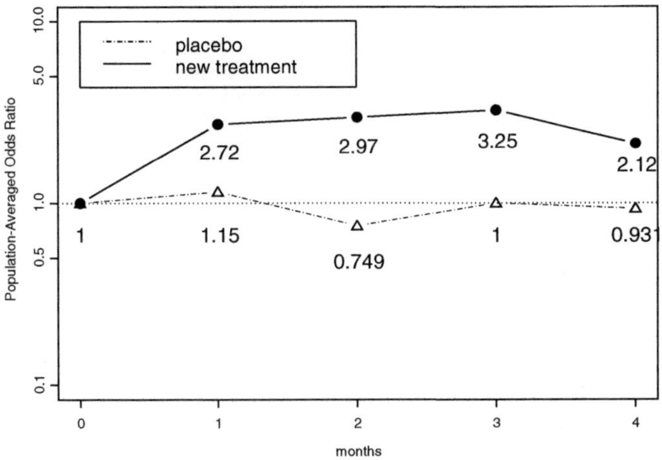

FIGURE 1.2
Mean changes from baseline by treatment group in terms of the odds ratios of being "good" at each visit versus the baseline in a randomized controlled trial evaluating the new treatment for a respiratory illness (for details, see Chapter 8).

for patients suffering from depression. In this example, conditional on the value of the random-effects b_{0i}, the repeated measurements of BDI $(y_{i0}, y_{i1}, ..., y_{i4})$ are assumed to be independent of each other (for details, see Chapter 7).

- Bernoulli distribution:

  Figure 1.2 shows an example of the mean changes from baseline by treatment group in terms of the odds ratios of being "good" at each visit versus the baseline in a randomized controlled trial evaluating a new treatment compared with placebo for patients suffering from respiratory illness. In this example, conditional on the value of the random-effects b_{0i}, the repeated measurements of the respiratory status $(y_{i0}, y_{i1}, ..., y_{i4})$ are assumed to be independent of each other and to have a Bernoulli distribution (for details, see Chapter 8).

- Poisson distribution:

  Figure 1.3 shows an example of the mean response profiles by treatment group based on the mean rates of seizures (per week) in a randomized controlled trial evaluating an anti-epileptic drug "progabide" in comparison with "placebo" for patients suffering from epilepsy. In this example, conditional on the value of the random-effects b_{0i}, the repeated measurements of the number of seizures $(y_{i0}, y_{i1}, ..., y_{i4})$ are assumed to be

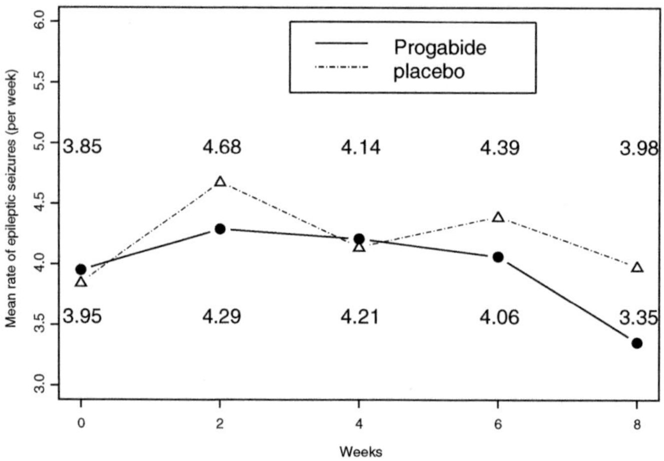

FIGURE 1.3
Mean response profiles by treatment group based on the mean rates of seizures (per week) in a randomized controlled trial evaluating an anti-epileptic drug “progabide” in comparison with “placebo” for patients suffering from epilepsy. The mean rate of seizures at each visit by treatment group are also shown within the figure (upper=placebo, lower=progabide) (for details, see Chapter 9).

independent of each other and to have Poisson distribution (for details, see Chapter 9).

In addition to the *random intercept* model, we can consider the following *random intercept plus slope* model:

$$
\begin{aligned}
g\{E(y_{ij} \mid b_{0i})\} &= g\{\mu_{ij} \mid b_{0i}\} \\
&= \begin{cases} \beta_0 + \beta_1 x_{1i} + b_{0i} + \boldsymbol{w}_i^t \boldsymbol{\xi} & \text{for } j \le 0 \\ \beta_0 + \beta_1 x_{1i} + b_{0i} + \boldsymbol{w}_i^t \boldsymbol{\xi} & \\ \quad + b_{1i} + \beta_{2j} + \beta_{3j} x_{1i} & \text{for } j \ge 1 \end{cases} \\
\boldsymbol{b}_i &= (b_{0i}, b_{1i})^t \sim N(\boldsymbol{0}, \Phi), \\
i &= 1, ..., n_1 \text{ (control group)}, \\
&= n_1 + 1, ..., n_1 + n_2 \text{ (new treatment group)} \\
j &= -(S-1), -(S-2), ..., 0,\ 1, ..., T,
\end{aligned} \tag{1.9}
$$

where the random-effects b_{1i}, called *random slope*, may reflect inter-subject variability of the response to the treatment assumed to be constant in the period after randomization and

$$\mathbf{\Phi} = \begin{pmatrix} \sigma_{B0}^2 & \rho_B \sigma_{B0} \sigma_{B1} \\ \rho_B \sigma_{B0} \sigma_{B1} & \sigma_{B1}^2 \end{pmatrix}. \tag{1.10}$$

It should be noted that the *random slope* introduced in the above model does not mean the *slope* on the time or a linear time trend, which will be considered in section 1.2.3.

1.2.2 Model for the average treatment effect

As mentioned in Section 1.1, the primary interest of *S:T* design, especially in confirmatory trials in the later phases of drug development, is to estimate the overall or average treatment effect during the evaluation period, leading to sample size calculation in the design stage (see Chapter 12 for details). So, let us consider here the case where we would like to estimate the average treatment effect during the evaluation period even though the treatment effect is not always expected to be constant over the evaluation period. However, in such a situation, it is important to select the evaluation period during which the treatment effect could be expected to be stable to a certain extent.

Here also, let us introduce two models, a *random intercept* model and a *random intercept plus slope* model. The former model is

$$\begin{aligned} g\{E(y_{ij} \mid b_{0i})\} &= g\{\mu_{ij} \mid b_{0i}\} \\ &= \begin{cases} \beta_0 + \beta_1 x_{1i} + b_{0i} + \boldsymbol{w}_i^t \boldsymbol{\xi} & \text{for } j \le 0 \\ \beta_0 + \beta_1 x_{1i} + b_{0i} + \beta_2 + \beta_3 x_{1i} + \boldsymbol{w}_i^t \boldsymbol{\xi} & \text{for } j \ge 1 \end{cases} \end{aligned} \tag{1.11}$$

$$\begin{aligned} b_{0i} &\sim N(0, \sigma_{B0}^2), \\ i &= 1, ..., n_1 \text{ (control group)}, \\ &= n_1 + 1, ..., n_1 + n_2 \text{ (new treatment group)}, \\ j &= -(S-1), -(S-2), ..., 0,\ 1, ..., T, \end{aligned}$$

and the latter is

$$g\{E(y_{ij} \mid \boldsymbol{b}_i)\} = \begin{cases} \beta_0 + \beta_1 x_{1i} + b_{0i} + \boldsymbol{w}_i^t \boldsymbol{\xi} & \text{for } j \le 0 \\ \beta_0 + \beta_1 x_{1i} + b_{0i} + b_{1i} + \beta_2 + \beta_3 x_{1i} + \boldsymbol{w}_i^t \boldsymbol{\xi} & \text{for } j \ge 1 \end{cases} \tag{1.12}$$

$$\boldsymbol{b}_i = (b_{0i}, b_{1i})^t \sim N(\mathbf{0}, \Phi), \tag{1.13}$$

where both a random intercept b_{0i} and a random slope b_{1i} denote the same meanings as those introduced in the previous section. It should be noted here also that the *random slope* introduced in the above model does not mean the *slope* on the time or a linear time trend, which will be considered in the next section. Interpretations of the newly introduced fixed-effects parameters β are as follows:

- $\beta_0 + \beta_2$ denotes the mean response in units of $g(\mu)$ during the evaluation period in the control group.
- $\beta_0 + \beta_1 + \beta_2 + \beta_3$ denotes the mean response in units of $g(\mu)$ during the evaluation period in the new treatment group.
- β_2 denotes the mean change from the baseline period to the evaluation period in units of $g(\mu)$ in the control group.
- $\beta_2 + \beta_3$ denotes the same quantity in the new treatment group.

Therefore, β_3 denotes the difference in these two mean changes from the baseline period to the evaluation period, i.e., or the effect for treatment-by-time interaction. In other words, it denotes the **average treatment effect of the new treatment** compared with the control.

1.2.3 Model for the treatment by linear time interaction

In the previous subsection, we focused on the generalized linear mixed models where we are primarily interested in comparing the average treatment effect during the evaluation period. However, there are other study designs where the primary interest is not the average treatment effect but the treatment-by-time interaction (Diggle et al., 2002; Fitzmaurice et al., 2011). For example, in the National Institute of Mental Health Schizophrenia Collaboratory Study, the primary interest is testing the drug by *linear* time interaction, i.e., testing whether the differences between treatment groups are *linearly* increasing over time (Hedeker and Gibbons, 2006; Roy et al., 2007; Bhumik et al., 2008).

So, let us consider here a *random intercept* and a *random intercept plus slope* model **with a random slope on the time** (a linear time trend model) for testing the null hypothesis that the rates of change or improvement over time are the same in the new treatment group compared with the control group. The former model is

$$
\begin{aligned}
g\{E(y_{ij} \mid b_{0i})\} &= g\{\mu_{ij} \mid b_{0i}\} \\
&= \beta_0 + b_{0i} + \beta_1 x_{1i} + (\beta_2 + \beta_3 x_{1i})t_j + \boldsymbol{w}_i^t \boldsymbol{\xi} \qquad (1.14) \\
b_{0i} &\sim N(0, \sigma_{B0}^2), \\
i &= 1, ..., n_1 \text{ (control group)}, \\
&= n_1 + 1, ..., n_1 + n_2 \text{ (new treatment group)}, \\
j &= -(S-1), -(S-2), ..., 0,\ 1, ..., T,
\end{aligned}
$$

where t_j denotes the jth measurement time and we have

$$t_{-S+1} = t_{-S+2} = \cdots = t_0 = 0.$$

Interpretation of the fixed-effects parameters $\boldsymbol{\beta}$ of interest are as follows:

1. β_2 denotes the rate of change over time in the control group.
2. $\beta_2 + \beta_3$ denotes the same quantity in the new treatment group.
3. β_3 denotes the difference in these two rates of change over time, i.e., the **treatment effect of the new treatment** compared with the control treatment.

The *random intercept plus slope* model is given by

$$\begin{aligned} g\{E(y_{ij} \mid \boldsymbol{b}_i)\} &= \beta_0 + b_{0i} + \beta_1 x_{1i} + (\beta_2 + \beta_3 x_{1i} + b_{1i})t_j \\ &\quad + \boldsymbol{w}_i^t \boldsymbol{\xi} \\ \boldsymbol{b}_i &= (b_{0i}, b_{1i})^t \sim N(\boldsymbol{0}, \Phi). \end{aligned} \tag{1.15}$$

Interpretations of the fixed-effects parameters $\boldsymbol{\beta}$ are the same as the above.

1.3 Superiority and non-inferiority

In all the application of the generalized linear mixed models and their related models, we mainly use the statistical analysis system called `SAS`. In any outputs of SAS programs you can see several p-values (two-tailed) for fixed-effects parameters of interest. It should be noted, however, that any p-value (two-tailed) for the parameter $\beta_3 (= \mu_2 - \mu_1)$ of the primary interest shown in the SAS outputs is implicitly the result of a test for a set of hypotheses

$$H_0 \; : \; \beta_3 = 0, \text{ versus } H_1 : \beta_3 \neq 0, \tag{1.16}$$

which is also called a *test for superiority.* In more detail, the definition of superiority hypotheses is as follows:

Test for *superiority*

If a negative β_3 indicates benefits, the superiority hypotheses are interpreted as

$$H_0 \quad : \quad \beta_3 \geq 0, \text{ versus } \; H_1 : \beta_3 < 0. \tag{1.17}$$

If a positive β_3 indicates benefits, then they are

$$H_0 \quad : \quad \beta_3 \leq 0, \text{ versus } \; H_1 : \beta_3 > 0. \tag{1.18}$$

These hypotheses imply that investigators are interested in establishing whether there is evidence of *a statistical difference* in the comparison of interest between two treatment groups. However, it is debatable whether the terminology *superiority* can be used or not in this situation. Although the set of hypotheses defined in (1.16) was adopted as those for *superiority tests* in regulatory guidelines such as FDA draft guidance (2010), I do not think this is appropriate.

The non-inferiority hypotheses of the new treatment over the control treatment, on the other hand, take the following form:

Test for *non-inferiority*

If a positive β_3 indicates benefits, the hypotheses are

$$H_0 \quad : \quad \beta_3 \leq -\Delta, \text{ versus } \; H_1 : \beta_3 > -\Delta, \tag{1.19}$$

where $\Delta (> 0)$ denotes the so-called *non-inferiority margin.* If a negative β_3 indicates benefits, the hypotheses should be

$$H_0 \quad : \quad \beta_3 \geq \Delta, \text{ versus } \; H_1 : \beta_3 < \Delta. \tag{1.20}$$

In other words, *non-inferiority* can be claimed if the 95%CI (confidence interval) for β_3 lies entirely above $-\Delta$ for the former case and lies entirely below Δ for the latter. It should be noted that for the generalized linear mixed model with a logit link $\log\{\mu/(1-\mu)\}$ for a logistic regression model or a log link $\log \mu$ for a Poisson regression model, the *non-inferiority margin* $\Delta^*(> 0)$ must be defined in the unit of *ratio of two odds ratios* (or odds ratio ratio, ORR) or *ratio of two rate ratios* (or rate ratio ratio, RRR). Namely, if a negative β_3 indicates benefits, the non-inferiority hypotheses are given by

$$H_0 \quad : \quad e^{\beta_3} \geq 1 + \Delta^*, \text{ versus } \; H_1 : e^{\beta_3} < 1 + \Delta^*.$$

If a positive β_3 indicates benefits, then they are

$$H_0 \quad : \quad e^{\beta_3} \leq 1 - \Delta^*, \text{ versus } H_1 : e^{\beta_3} > 1 - \Delta^*.$$

Therefore, the definition of non-inferiority hypotheses in terms of β_3 should take the following form:

Non-inferiority hypotheses for a logistic or Poisson model

If a negative β_3 indicates benefits, the hypotheses are

$$H_0 \quad : \quad \beta_3 \geq \log(1 + \Delta^*), \text{ versus } H_1 : \beta_3 < \log(1 + \Delta^*). \quad (1.21)$$

If a positive β_3 indicates benefits, then they are

$$H_0 \quad : \quad \beta_3 \leq \log(1 - \Delta^*), \text{ versus } H_1 : \beta_3 > \log(1 - \Delta^*). \quad (1.22)$$

While *superiority* of the new treatment over the control treatment is defined as $\beta_3 = \mu_2 - \mu_1 > 0$, the *inferiority* of the new treatment over the control treatment can be defined as $\beta_3 = \mu_2 - \mu_1 < -\Delta$, not as $\beta_3 = \mu_2 - \mu_1 < 0$. I think that readers who are not familiar with clinical trials may not see a rationale behind the asymmetry in these requirements. This seems to be obviously due to a bad definition of "superiority" adopted in regulatory guidelines. Namely, the current definition of superiority seems to be biased toward the interests of pharmaceutical companies.

Concerning this issue, we shall highlight two pertinent passages excerpted from two regulatory guidelines. The first passage is excerpted from European Agency for the Evaluation of Medicinal Products, *Points to Consider on Switching between Superiority and Non-inferiority* (2000, p. 5):

If the 95% confidence interval for the treatment effect not only lies entirely above $-\Delta$ but also above zero then there is evidence of superiority in terms of statistical significance at the 5% level ($p < 0.05$) ... There is no multiplicity argument that affects this interpretation because, in statistical terms, it corresponds to a simple closed test procedure.

However, Δ is defined as the maximum clinically irrelevant difference between treatments. So, we statisticians and also even general people not familiar with statistics will naturally think that we cannot say that there is evidence of superiority unless the 95% confidence interval for the treatment effect lies entirely above Δ. The second example is excerpted from US Food and Drug Administration, *FDA Guidance for Industry Non-Inferiority Clinical Trials* (2011, Case 6, Figure 2):

Point estimate of $C - T$ favors C (active reference treatment) and C is

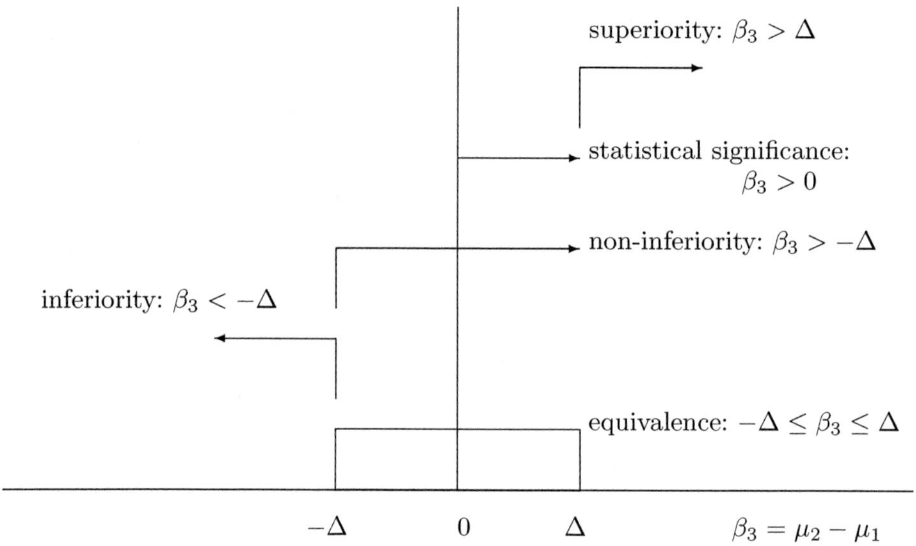

FIGURE 1.4
Statistically sound and impartial definitions of superiority, non-inferiority and equivalence (when a positive β_3 indicates benefits) based on the margin Δ which is defined as the maximum clinically irrelevant difference between treatments (Tango, 2003).

statistically significantly superior to T (experimental treatment).
Nonetheless, upper bound of the 95% CI for $C - T < 2$ $(= M_1 = \Delta)$, so that NI (of T over C) is also demonstrated for the NI margin M_1 (This outcome would be unusual and could present interpretive problems).

This example shows an obvious flaw of the current definition of superiority. As the upper bound of the 95% CI for the difference $C - T$ is less than the maximum clinically irrelevant difference between treatments, there is no way that the difference is statistically significant.

In my personal opinion, just after the appearance of non-inferiority trials with a pre-fixed margin Δ, the regulatory agency should have changed the definition of superiority to $\beta_3 = \mu_2 - \mu_1 > \Delta$ from $\beta_3 = \mu_2 - \mu_1 > 0$ by introducing the *superiority margin* Δ like the *non-inferiority* margin adopted in non-inferiority trials. In Figure 1.3 excerpted from Tango (2003), we show statistically sound and "impartial" definitions of superiority, non-inferiority and equivalence between the new treatment (μ_2) and the control treatment

(μ_1) where the superiority margin is identical to the non-inferiority margin. So, I think that real *superiority* should be defined as $\beta_3 = \mu_2 - \mu_1 > \Delta$ when a positive β_3 indicates benefits.

However, in this book, I will not change the definition as it is, i.e., $\beta_3 = \mu_2 - \mu_1 > 0$, to avoid needless confusion that might occur among readers. Instead, I shall define a new term, *substantial superiority*, as $\beta_3 = \mu_2 - \mu_1 > \Delta$. If you really insist the *superiority* of the new treatment over to the control treatment, you have to, at first, determine the *superiority* margin $\Delta(> 0)$ and the null and alternative hypotheses should take the following form:

Test for *substantial superiority*

If a positive β_3 indicates benefits,

$$H_0 \quad : \quad \beta_3 \leq \Delta, \text{ versus } H_1 : \beta_3 > \Delta. \tag{1.23}$$

If a negative β_3 indicates benefits, the hypotheses should be

$$H_0 \quad : \quad \beta_3 \geq -\Delta, \text{ versus } H_1 : \beta_3 < -\Delta. \tag{1.24}$$

In other words, *substantial superiority* can be claimed if the 95%CI for β_3 lies entirely above Δ for the former case and lies entirely below $-\Delta$ for the latter. In a similar manner, for a logistic or Poisson regression model, the definition of substantial superiority hypotheses in terms of β_3 should take the following form:

Substantial superiority hypotheses for a logistic or Poisson model

If a negative β_3 indicates benefits, the hypotheses are

$$H_0 \quad : \quad \beta_3 \geq \log(1 - \Delta^*), \text{ versus } H_1 : \beta_3 < \log(1 - \Delta^*). \tag{1.25}$$

If a positive β_3 indicates benefits, then they are

$$H_0 \quad : \quad \beta_3 \leq \log(1 + \Delta^*), \text{ versus } H_1 : \beta_3 > \log(1 + \Delta^*). \tag{1.26}$$

where Δ_3^* denotes the *superiority margin* defined in units of the ratio of two odds ratios or the ratio of two rate ratios.

2

Naive analysis of animal experiment data

2.1 Introduction

Table 2.1 shows the data set called *Rat Data* from an animal experiment with a *1:3* repeated measures design on the primary response variable (some laboratory data) comparing two drugs (an experimental drug and a control drug). Twelve rats were randomly assigned to either the experimental drug ($n_1 = 6$) or the control drug ($n_2 = 6$). Measurements of this response variable were made on four occasions, once at baseline, and three time points (1, 2 and 3 weeks) during the 3-week treatment period. The experimental drug is expected to reduce the value of the response variable more than the control drug. Figure 2.1 shows the subject-specific response profiles over time. In this chapter, we introduce three examples of standard or unsophisticated statistical analysis for this type of repeated measurement data in an experiment. These are often observed in papers published in many medical journals, and we shall point out statistical problems encountered in each of analysis plans.

TABLE 2.1
Rat Data: Some laboratory data measured in an animal experiment comparing two drugs with six rats randomly assigned to each of two treatment groups.

	Experimental group Weeks after treatment					Control group Weeks after treatment			
No.	0	1	2	3	No.	0	1	2	3
1	7.5	8.6	6.9	0.8	7	13.3	13.3	12.9	11.1
2	10.6	11.7	8.8	1.6	8	10.7	10.8	10.7	9.3
3	12.4	13.0	11.0	5.6	9	12.5	12.7	12.0	10.1
4	11.5	12.6	11.1	7.5	10	8.4	8.7	8.1	5.7
5	8.3	8.9	6.8	0.5	11	9.4	9.6	8.0	3.8
6	9.2	10.1	8.6	3.8	12	11.3	11.7	10.0	8.5

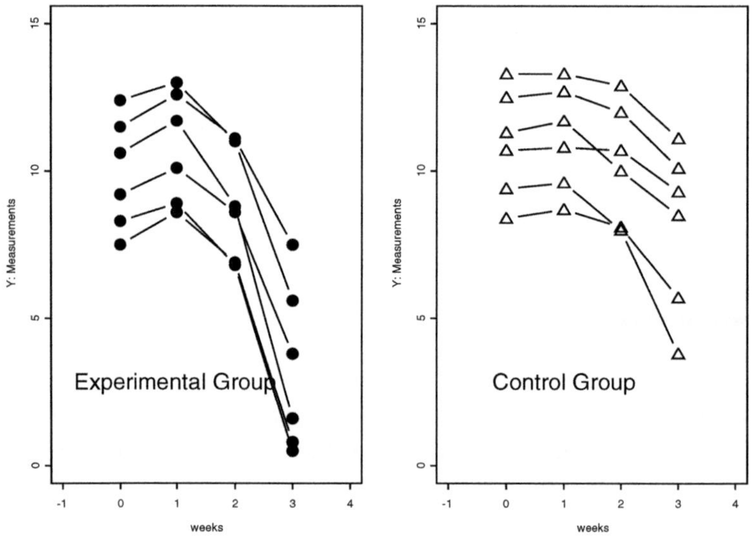

FIGURE 2.1
Rat Data. Subject-specific response profiles over time in an animal experiment comparing two drugs.

2.2 Analysis plan I: Difference in means at each time point

This analysis plan declares the repeated use of Student's two-sample t-test for the null hypothesis of no difference in means between two groups at each measurement time point without any adjustment for multiple testing. The results are shown in Table 2.2 and Figure 2.2. The difference was statistically significant (two-tailed $p = 0.0146$) only at week 3. In this analysis, Student's t-test was also applied to the baseline data (week 0), which raises the question "What does the difference in means at baseline?" However, as far as I know, this type of *naive-analysis* has often been observed in some medical journals.

2.3 Analysis plan II: Difference in mean changes from baseline at each time point

Analysis plan II considers the change from baseline (CFB), $y_{ij} - y_{i0}$, as the primary response variable that may reflect the efficacy of the drug, and repeats the use of Student's two-sample t-test for the difference in mean changes from

TABLE 2.2
Rat Data. Results of the repeated application of Student's two-sample t-test for the null hypothesis of no difference in means between two groups at each measurement time point.

	Time	0	1	2	3
Experimental group	mean	9.92	10.82	8.87	3.30
	S.D.	0.78	0.77	0.77	1.16
Control group	mean	10.93	11.13	10.28	8.08
	S.D.	0.75	0.73	0.82	1.14
Difference	mean	-1.02	-0.32	-1.42	-4.78
(Exp. Control)	S.E.	1.08	1.06	1.12	1.62
	t-value (d.f. 10)	-0.94	-0.30	-1.26	-2.95
	two-tailed p value	0.370	0.771	0.236	0.0146

baseline between two groups at each measurement time point. Furthermore, to adjust for multiple testing, the Bonferroni corrected significance level, i.e., $\alpha = 0.05/3 = 0.0167$, is used at each measurement time point. The results are shown in Table 2.3 and Figure 2.3. Statistically significant differences were observed at weeks 1 and 3 after the start of treatment. However, the problem is the interpretation of the results. As compared with the baseline, the mean CFB increased by 0.90 ± 0.09 (mean $\pm$ SE) in the experimental group at week 1, which is significantly larger than the increase 0.20 ± 0.06 in the control group. At week 3, on the other hand, the mean CFB decreased by -6.62 ± 0.72 in the experimental group; this decrease is significantly larger than -3.77 ± 0.93 in the control group. Furthermore, the two-tailed p-value $p < 0.0001$ at week 1 is less than $p = 0.0023$ at week 3, although the mean difference 0.7 ± 0.11 at week 1 is quite small as compared with -3.77 ± 0.93 at week 3. This is a good example where larger mean differences does not automatically result in smaller p values because of the variability in a particular group. In any case, judging from these time-dependent conflicting results, we cannot simply conclude that there was significantly more decrease in the experimental group than in the control group.

2.4 Analysis plan III: Analysis of covariance at the last time point

In analysis plan III the primary response variable is the CFB at week 3 and analysis of covariance (ANCOVA) is applied for comparison between groups

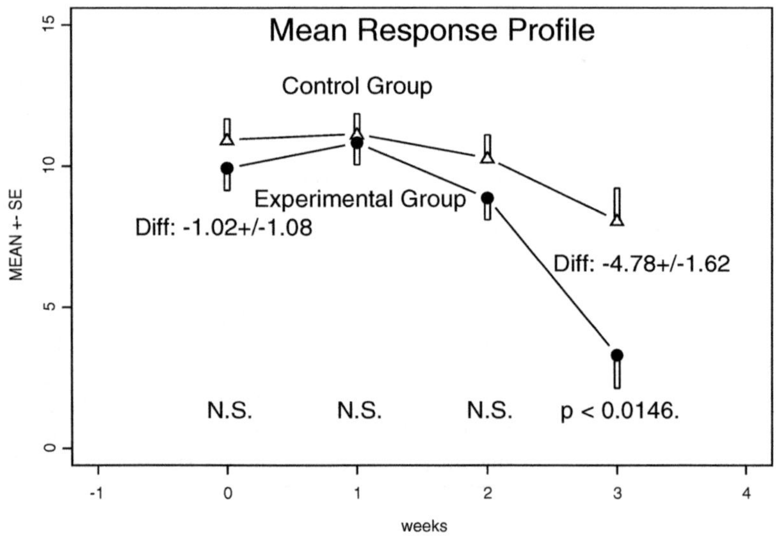

FIGURE 2.2
Rat Data. Mean response profiles by treatment group and the results of repeated application of Student's two-sample t-test at each measurement time point.

adjusting for the difference in means at baseline. A flow of analysis of covariance is shown below:

Step 1. Figure 2.4 shows a scatter plot of measurements at week 3 (y) and measurements at baseline (x) with their correlation coefficient and estimated regression lines by treatment group. A high positive correlation coefficient 0.782 was observed.

Step 2. Then, consider the linear regression line of y on x by group

$$y = \alpha_k + \beta_k x + \epsilon \quad \text{for treatment group } k = 1, 2$$

where ϵ is an error term. The error terms are assumed to be independent random variables having normal distribution with mean zero and variance σ^2 common to both treatment groups. To check whether those two regression lines are parallel, we applied the following linear model including the interaction term between baseline measurements and treatment group using the SAS procedure `PROC GLM`:

```
model y = group + base + group * base
```

TABLE 2.3
Rat Data. Results of the repeated application of Student's t-test for the difference in means changes from baseline between two groups at each measurement time with Bonferroni corrected significance level, i.e.,$\alpha = 0.05/3 = 0.0167$.

	Time	1	2	3
Experimental group	mean	0.90	-1.05	-6.62
	SE	0.09	0.24	0.72
Control group	mean	0.20	-0.65	-2.85
	SE	0.06	0.23	0.59
Difference	mean	0.7	-0.4	-3.77
(Experimental Control)	SE	0.115	0.33	0.93
	t-value (df = 10)	6.06	-1.20	-4.06
	two-tailed p-value	< 0.0001	0.258	0.0023

where the variable `group` is a classification variable or numeric factor (= 1 for the control group; = 2 for the experimental group) and the variable `base` indicates the baseline measurements x. The results appear in Program and Output 2.1.

Program and Output 2.1: SAS procedure `PROC GLM` for ANCOVA with interaction term

```
<SAS program>
data d0;
  infile 'c:\book\RepeatedMeasure\experimentRat3.dat' missover;
  input id group base y;

proc glm; class group/ref=first;
  model y  =  group base group*base  /solution clparm;
run;

<SAS output>
parameter        estimates          s.e.       t-value  Pr > |t|
Intercept       -6.551567398 B 4.56828269    -1.43    0.1894
group       2   -1.873191000 B 6.09174346    -0.31    0.7663
group       1    0.000000000 B . . .
base             1.338557994 B 0.41296151     3.24    0.0119
base*group 2    -0.156229416 B 0.57511924    -0.27    0.7928
base*group 1     0.000000000 B
```

The estimated regression line was $y = -(6.55 + 1.87) + (1.338 - 0.156)x = -8.42 + 1.18x$ for the experimental group and $y = -6.55 + 1.34x$ for the control group, respectively. The resultant two-tailed p-value for the interaction term `base*group` is 0.79, indicating that there is no statistically significant

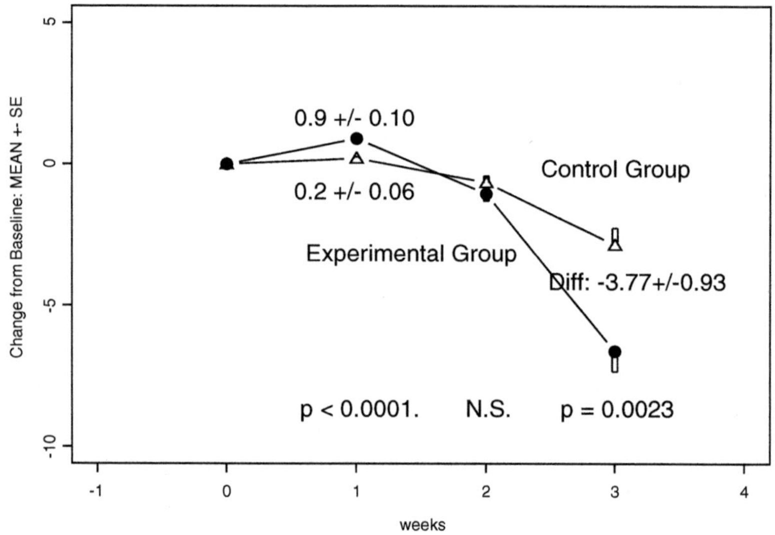

FIGURE 2.3
Rat Data. Mean changes from baseline by treatment group.

evidence for denying the parallelism of the two regression lines.

Step 3. Then, to estimate these two parallel regression lines with the same slope β, we applied the linear model excluding the interaction term using SAS procedure PROC GLM and the results are shown in Program and Output 2.2 and in Figure 2.5.

Program and Output 2.2: SAS procedure PROC GLM for ANCOVA without interaction term

```
<SAS program>
proc glm; class group/ref=first;
model y  =  group base  /solution clparm;
run;

<SAS output>
parameter        estimates         s.e.     t-value  Pr > |t|
Intercept      -5.670886126 B 3.04837299  -1.86  0.0958
group      2   -3.504358658 B 0.97170216  -3.61  0.0057
group      1    0.000000000 B . . . . .
base            1.258007877   0.27222891   4.62  0.0013
```

The estimated regression line is $y = -(5.67 + 3.50) + 1.26x = -9.17 + 1.26x$ for the experimental group and $y = -5.67 + 1.26x$ for the control group, respectively. Table 2.2 shows that the difference in means at baseline $(\bar{x}_2 - \bar{x}_1)$

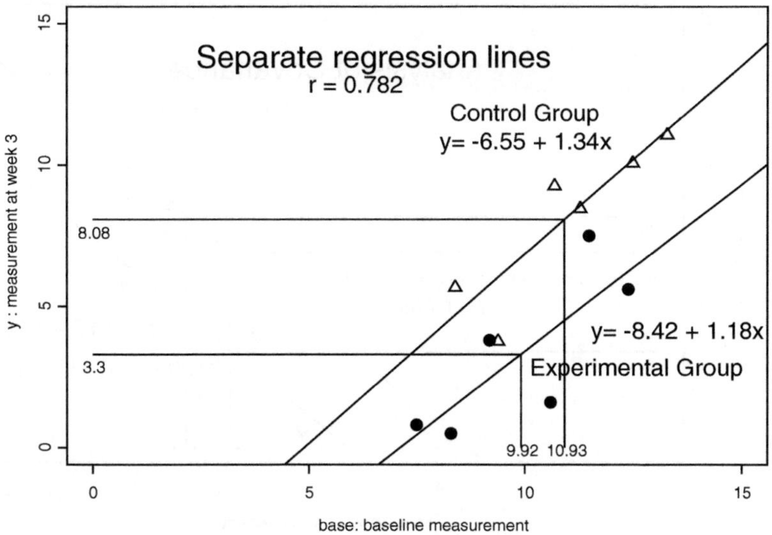

FIGURE 2.4
Rat Data. Scatter plot of data at week 3 (y) and data at baseline (x) with the correlation coefficient and estimated regression lines by treatment group.

is -1.02 and that at week 3 ($\bar{y}_2 - \bar{y}_1$) is -4.87. Then, the analysis of covariance adjusted difference in means at week 3 is estimated as

$$\begin{aligned} \hat{\alpha}_2 - \hat{\alpha}_1 &= (\bar{y}_2 - \bar{y}_1) - \beta(\bar{x}_2 - \bar{x}_1) \\ &= -4.78 - 1.258 \times -1.02 = -3.50 \ (\pm 0.97). \end{aligned}$$

The result of the t-test is highly statistically significant ($t = -3.61$ with degrees of freedom 9 and $p = 0.0057$).

2.5 Discussion

According to the result of analysis of covariance, which was defined as the primary analysis in the study protocol, we can conclude that that there was significantly more decrease in the experimental group than in the control group. However, as is often the case in randomized trials and experiments, the difference in means adjusted for baseline measurements by analysis of covariance, -3.50 ± 0.97 ($p = 0.0057$), is quite similar to the difference in mean changes

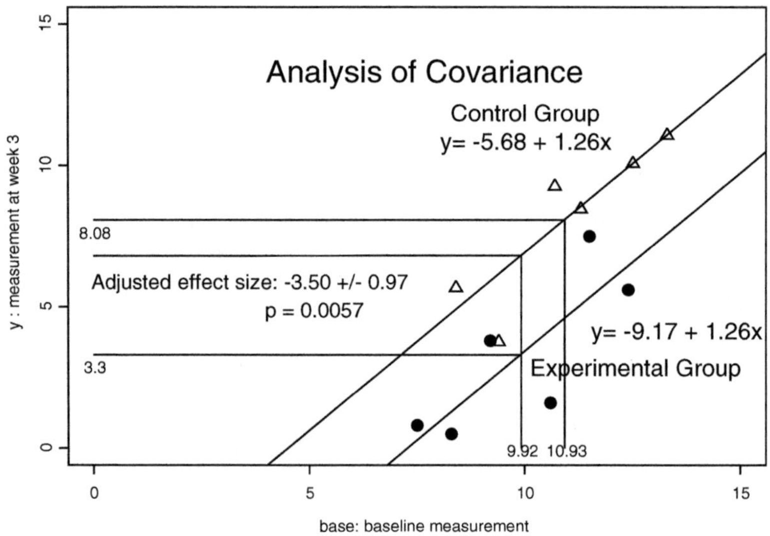

FIGURE 2.5
Rat Data. Scatter plot of measurements at week 3 (y) and measurements at baseline (x), estimated regression lines with equal slope by treatment group, and the analysis of covariance adjusted differences in means at week 3.

from baseline, -3.77 ± 0.93 ($p = 0.002$), shown in Table 2.3. Furthermore, it should be emphasized that, based on these results only, **we cannot judge whether the results from the analysis of covariance adjusted difference in means is better than a simple difference in mean changes from baseline.** For more detail, see Sections 3.7 and 4.4.

3

Analysis of variance models

3.1 Introduction

Analysis of variance (ANOVA) is a generic term used to refer to statistical methods for analyzing data or measurements arising originally from agricultural experiments. Nowadays, ANOVA includes a lot of statistical methods devised depending on the way how the experiment should be planned or the measurements should be taken, i.e., experimental design. Until recently, among other things, ANOVA for *split-plot design* (described in Section 3.3) has been used for analyzing repeated measurements, in which a suitable adjustment is made to take correlations among repeated measurements into account. Therefore, a split-plot ANOVA model for this purpose is sometimes called a *repeated measures* ANOVA model.

However, due to a recent rapid development of (generalized) linear mixed-effects models that are capable of dealing with incomplete data and also of taking account of correlations among repeated measurements, repeated measures ANOVA has recently been used very rarely. Notwithstanding the foregoing, the analysis of variance model includes fundamental and important points for understanding the treatment effect. So, in this chapter, we shall consider the analysis of variance model.

3.2 Analysis of variance model

Consider a clinical trial or an animal experiment to evaluate a treatment effect, such as data shown in Table 2.1, where subjects are randomly assigned to one treatment group, and measurements are made at equally spaced times on each subject. Then, the basic design will be the following:

1. **Purpose**: Comparison of G treatment groups including the control group.

2. **Trial design**: Parallel group randomized controlled trial and suppose that n_k subjects are allocated to treatment group $k(= 1, 2, ..., G), n_1 +$

$n_2 + \cdots n_G = N$, where the first treatment group ($k = 1$) is defined as the control group.

3. **Repeated Measure Design**: Basic *1:T* repeated measures design described in Chapter 1.

A typical statistical model or *analysis of variance model* for the basic design will be

$$\begin{aligned} \text{Response} &= \text{Grand mean} + \text{Treatment group} + \text{time} + \\ &\quad + \text{treatment group} \times \text{time} + \text{error}. \end{aligned} \tag{3.1}$$

However, the prerequisite for the analysis of variance model is the homogeneity assumption for the subject-specific response profile over time within each treatment group so that the mean response profile within each treatment group is meaningful and thus the treatment effect can be evaluated by the difference in mean response profiles. If **the subject by time interaction** within each treatment group is not negligible, the mean response profile within each group could be inappropriate measures for treatment effect. To deal with this type of heterogeneity, see Chapter 11.

In this chapter, we shall use the notation "*triply subscripted array*", which is frequently used in *analysis of variance models*, which is different from the *repeated measures design* described in Chapter 1. For the ith subject ($i = 1, ..., n_k$) nested in each treatment group k, let y_{kij} denote the primary response variable at the jth measurement time t_j. Then, the response profile vector for the ith subject in the kth treatment group is expressed as

$$\boldsymbol{y}_{ki} = (y_{ki0}, y_{ki1}, ..., y_{kiT})^t \tag{3.2}$$

and the analysis of variance model is expressed as

$$\begin{aligned} y_{kij} &= \mu + \alpha_k + \beta_j + \gamma_{kj} + \epsilon_{kij}, \\ &\quad k = 1, ..., G;\ i = 1, ..., n_k;\ j = 0\ (\text{baseline}), 1, 2, ..., T, \end{aligned} \tag{3.3}$$

where

α_k : the fixed effects of the kth treatment group
β_j : the fixed effects of the jth measurement time
γ_{kj} : the fixed effects of the interaction between the kth group and jth time

and $\boldsymbol{\epsilon}_{ki} = (\epsilon_{ki0}, \epsilon_{ki1}, ..., \epsilon_{kiT})^t$ are mutually independent random error terms following the multivariate normal distribution with mean $\mathbf{0}$ and covariance (or variance covariance) matrix $\boldsymbol{\Sigma}_k$, i.e.,

$$\boldsymbol{\epsilon}_{ki} = (\epsilon_{ki0}, \epsilon_{ki1}, ..., \epsilon_{kiT})^t \quad \sim \quad N(\mathbf{0}, \boldsymbol{\Sigma}_k). \tag{3.4}$$

However, the model (3.3) is said to be *over-parameterized* because the number of parameters included in the model are larger than the number of estimable parameters. So, to obtain the unique solution or the unique sets of estimable parameters $(\alpha_k, \beta_j, \gamma_{kj})$, the following constraints are imposed in this book:

$$\begin{cases} \alpha_1 = 0 \\ \beta_0 = 0 \\ \gamma_{10} = \gamma_{11} = \cdots = \gamma_{1T} = 0 \\ \gamma_{10} = \gamma_{20} = \cdots = \gamma_{G0} = 0. \end{cases} \tag{3.5}$$

Namely, the first category of each factor, the first row and column of each two-factor interaction term, are set to zero. In this sense, the first category is sometimes called the *reference category* because the estimated effects of each parameter are relative estimates in comparison with the first category. For example, $\hat{\alpha}_2 = \hat{\alpha}_2 - \hat{\alpha}_1$. This constraint has been used in much of the literature especially for easy interpretation of the results. However, the analysis of variance model generally adopts the following so-called *sum-to-zero constraint*:

$$\sum_{k=1}^{G} \alpha_k = 0, \sum_{j=0}^{T} \beta_j = 0, \sum_{k=1}^{G} \gamma_{kj} = \sum_{j=0}^{T} \gamma_{kj} = 0.$$

The SAS procedures, on the other hand, such as `GLM, MIXED,` and `GLIMMIX`, use the constraint that the last category is set to zero as the default. So, to set the first category to be zero in these procedures, the SAS statement `CLASS` needs to specify the option `/ref=first`. Interpretation of the parameter estimates of the analysis of variance model (3.3) requires the following attention:

1. $\hat{\alpha}_k$: $\hat{\alpha}_k$ denotes the differences in means at time 0 (baseline in *1:T* repeated measures design) for the treatment group k compared with the control group 1, which is expected to be 0 when randomization is done. It should be noted that the hypothesis testing $H_0 : \alpha_1 = \cdots = \alpha_G$ has nothing to do with the treatment effect.

2. $\hat{\beta}_j : (\hat{\beta}_0, \hat{\beta}_1, ..., \hat{\beta}_T)$ represents the overall mean response profile over time. However, the purpose of the trial (experiment) is to evaluate the difference in mean response profiles among treatment groups and so the hypothesis testing $H_0 : \beta_0 = \cdots = \beta_T$ also has nothing to do with the treatment effect of primary interest.

3. $\hat{\gamma}_{kj}$: The null hypothesis on the interaction term

$$H_0 \quad : \quad \gamma_{kj} = 0, \text{ for all } (k, j) \tag{3.6}$$

indicates that there is no statistical evidence for any differences in mean profiles among treatment groups. Therefore, rejection of the null hypothesis indicates *some* differences in mean response profiles among treatment groups. However, testing the null hypothesis (3.6) is an overall *omnibus test* with degrees of freedom $G(T-1)$. Therefore, an estimator reflecting the treatment effect should be devised as a function of some interaction terms γ_{kj}.

In the next section, we shall introduce the so-called *change from baseline* CFB, which is associated with the estimation of the treatment effect.

3.3 Change from baseline

Let CFB_{kij} denote the *change from baseline* at time j for the ith subject in the kth treatment group; then we have

$$C\hat{F}B_{kij} \quad = \quad y_{kij} - y_{ki0} = (\hat{\beta}_j - \hat{\beta}_0) + (\hat{\gamma}_{kj} - \hat{\gamma}_{k0}). \tag{3.7}$$

Namely, the mean change from baseline at time j in the kth treatment group is

$$\frac{1}{n_k}\sum_{i=1}^{n_k} CFB_{kij} \quad = \quad \bar{y}_{k+j} - \bar{y}_{k+0} = (\hat{\beta}_j - \hat{\beta}_0) + (\hat{\gamma}_{kj} - \hat{\gamma}_{k0}). \tag{3.8}$$

Therefore, the difference in mean changes from baseline at time j of the kth treatment group compared with the mth treatment group is expressed as

$$\begin{aligned} \hat{\tau}_{km}^{(j)} &= \left(\frac{1}{n_k}\sum_{i=1}^{n_k} CFB_{kij} - \frac{1}{n_m}\sum_{i=1}^{n_m} CFB_{mij} \right) \\ &= (\hat{\gamma}_{kj} - \hat{\gamma}_{k0}) - (\hat{\gamma}_{mj} - \hat{\gamma}_{m0}) = \hat{\gamma}_{kj} - \hat{\gamma}_{mj}. \end{aligned} \tag{3.9}$$

When the trial consists of two treatment groups, the experimental group and the control group, the difference in mean changes from baseline at time j of the experimental group ($k = 2$) compared with the control group ($k = 1$) is

$$\hat{\tau}_{21}^{(j)} = \hat{\gamma}_{2j} - \hat{\gamma}_{1j} = \hat{\gamma}_{2j} \ (j = 1, ..., T). \tag{3.10}$$

Namely, $\hat{\gamma}_{kj} - \hat{\gamma}_{mj}$ denotes the estimate of the effect size of the kth treatment compared with the mth treatment at time j.

The overall estimate of the relative effect size of the kth treatment compared with the mth treatment over the measurement period ($1 \leq j \leq T$) is

$$\begin{aligned} \hat{\tau}_{km} &= \frac{1}{T} \sum_{j=1}^{T} \hat{\tau}_{km}^{(j)} \\ &= \frac{1}{T} \sum_{j=1}^{T} \left(\frac{1}{n_k} \sum_{i=1}^{n_k} CFB_{kij} - \frac{1}{n_m} \sum_{i=1}^{n_m} CFB_{mij} \right) \\ &= \frac{1}{T} \sum_{j=1}^{T} \{ (\hat{\gamma}_{kj} - \hat{\gamma}_{k0}) - (\hat{\gamma}_{mj} - \hat{\gamma}_{m0}) \}. \end{aligned} \tag{3.11}$$

For example, consider the hypothetical example of the mean change from baseline by treatment group ($T = 3, G = 2$) shown in Figure 3.1, which looks like Figure 2.3. In this case, the overall treatment effect of the experimental group compared with the control group is estimated by the following *linear contrast*:

$$\begin{aligned} \hat{\tau}_{21} &= \frac{1}{3}(\hat{\tau}_{21}^{(1)} + \hat{\tau}_{21}^{(2)} + \hat{\tau}_{21}^{(3)}) = \frac{1}{3} \sum_{j=1}^{3} \{ (\hat{\gamma}_{2j} - \hat{\gamma}_{20}) - (\hat{\gamma}_{1j} - \hat{\gamma}_{10}) \} \\ &= \frac{1}{3}(3, -1, -1, -1, -3, 1, 1, 1)(\hat{\gamma}_{10}, \hat{\gamma}_{11}, \hat{\gamma}_{12}, \hat{\gamma}_{13}, \hat{\gamma}_{20}, \hat{\gamma}_{21}, \hat{\gamma}_{22}, \hat{\gamma}_{23})^t. \end{aligned} \tag{3.12}$$

When we want to evaluate the treatment effect over the period $[j_s \leq j \leq j_e]$, the linear contrast of interest will be

$$\hat{\tau}_{km}(j_s, j_e) = \frac{1}{j_e - j_s + 1} \sum_{j=j_s}^{j_e} \{ (\hat{\gamma}_{kj} - \hat{\gamma}_{k0}) - (\hat{\gamma}_{mj} - \hat{\gamma}_{m0}) \}, \tag{3.13}$$

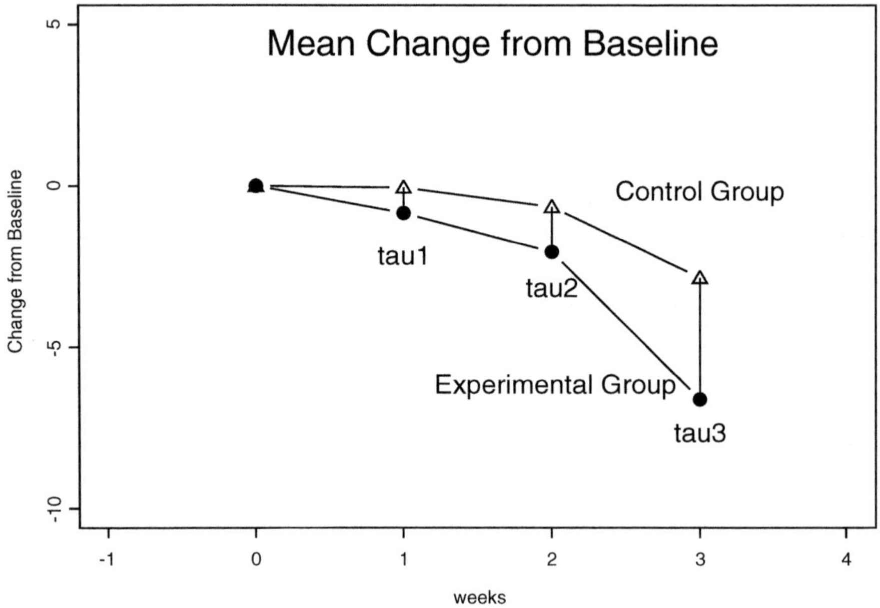

FIGURE 3.1
A hypothetical example of the mean change from baseline by treatment group $(T = 3, G = 2)$.

which is estimated by CFBs

$$\hat{\tau}_{km}(j_s, j_e) \quad = \quad \frac{1}{j_e - j_s + 1} \sum_{j=j_s}^{j_e} \left\{ \frac{1}{n_k} \sum_{i=1}^{n_k} CFB_{kij} - \frac{1}{n_m} \sum_{i=1}^{n_m} CFB_{mij} \right\}. \tag{3.14}$$

The next thing to determine is how to estimate the standard errors of treatment effects such as $\hat{\tau}_{km}^{(j)}, \hat{\tau}_{km}$ and $\hat{\tau}_{km}(j_s, j_e)$. In other words,

1. whether we should utilize only data necessary for evaluation or
2. utilize all the data.

Many researchers in the field of medical and health science tend to choose the former. For example, when we want to estimate the treatment effect based on the estimate (3.14), we can modify the form as

TABLE 3.1
Rat Data (Table 2.1): Estimates of treatment effect based on (3.15) with ($j_s = 1, j_e = 3$) and the results of Student's two-sample t-test for the null hypothesis of no difference.

	Mean	S.E.	
Experimental group (2)	-2.25	0.32	
Control group (1)	-1.1	0.26	
Difference(group 2- group 1)	-1.16	0.41	
t-value (d.f. =10)			2.81
two-tailed p-value			0.019

$$\hat{\tau}_{km}(j_s, j_e) = \frac{1}{n_k}\sum_{i=1}^{n_k}\left(\frac{1}{j_e - j_s + 1}\sum_{j=j_s}^{j_e} CFB_{kij}\right) - \frac{1}{n_m}\sum_{i=1}^{n_m}\left(\frac{1}{j_e - j_s + 1}\sum_{j=j_s}^{j_e} CFB_{mij}\right). \quad (3.15)$$

Then, we can use Student's two-sample t-test for testing the null hypothesis

$$H_0 : \tau_{km}(j_s, j_e) = 0, \quad (3.16)$$

where "sample" $\{x_{ki}; i = 1, ..., n_k\}$ of the kth treatment group is expressed as

$$x_{ki} = \frac{1}{j_e - j_s + 1}\sum_{j=j_s}^{j_e} CFB_{kij}.$$

Table 3.1 shows the estimates of the treatment effect over the study period based on (3.15) with ($j_s = 1, j_e = 3$) and the results of Student's two-sample t-test for the null hypothesis of no difference between groups. The treatment effect over the study period is estimated as $\hat{\tau}_{12} = -1.16,\ t = 2.81,\ d.f. = 10$ and the two-tailed $p = 0.019$.

However, as introduced in what follows, if we apply ANOVA models or linear mixed models using statistical packages such as `SAS` or `R`, it is possible to obtain a good/best result both for estimation and hypothesis testing utilizing all the data, which can flexibly take account of possible modeling for the covariance structure among repeated measurements.

3.4 Split-plot design

The principle of the *split-plot design* is as follows. Let us consider some agricultural field experiment where the field is divided into $N = Gn$ "main plots" to compare the levels of one factor A such as the addition of different ameliorants by allocating them at random to the main plots. Then, each main plot is divided into $T+1$ "subplots" to compare the levels of the other factor, B, such as, the addition of different dressing, by allocating them at random to subplots within a main plot. A naive ANOVA model for this design will be

$$\begin{aligned} y_{kij} &= \mu + \alpha_k + \beta_j + \gamma_{kj} + \epsilon_{kij}, \\ & \epsilon_{kij} \sim N(0, \sigma_E^2) \\ & k = 1, ..., G; \; i = 1, ..., n; \; j = 0, 1, 2, ..., T, \end{aligned} \tag{3.17}$$

where y_{kij} denotes the yield of the jth level of factor B within the ith main plot allocated to the kth level of factor A, α_k denotes the fixed effects of the kth level of factor A, β_j denotes the fixed effects of the jth level of factor B, γ_{kj} denotes the fixed effects of the interaction between the kth level of factor A and the jth level of factor B, and ϵ_{kij} is an random error assumed to be distributed with normal distribution with mean 0 and variance σ_E^2. It should be noted that the subscript j starts from 0, not from 1, because the split-plot design is due to extend to the repeated measures design.

However, the ANOVA model (3.17) assumes that there is no difference in fertilities between the original main plots, which is unlikely in practice. So, to take this variability into account, the following ANOVA model must be considered:

$$\begin{aligned} y_{kij} &= \mu + \alpha_k + \beta_j + \gamma_{kj} + b_{ki} + \epsilon_{kij} \\ & \epsilon_{kij} \sim N(0, \sigma_E^2), \; b_{ki} \sim N(0, \sigma_B^2) \\ & k = 1, ..., G; \; i = 1, ..., n; \; j = 0, 1, 2, ..., T, \end{aligned} \tag{3.18}$$

where a newly introduced term b_{ki} denotes the *unobserved* random effects for the ith main plot allocated to the kth level of factor A reflecting the between-main-plot variability of the original fertility and is assumed to be distributed with normal distribution with mean 0 and variance σ_B^2. The b_{0i} and ϵ_{ij} are assumed to be independent of each other. In this model, the covariance matrix $\boldsymbol{\Sigma}_k$ of $\boldsymbol{y}_{ki} = (y_{ki0}, ..., y_{kiT})^t$ is

$$(\boldsymbol{\Sigma}_k)_{jj'} = Cov(y_{kij}, y_{kij'}) = \sigma_B^2 + \sigma_E^2 \delta_{jj'}, \tag{3.19}$$

TABLE 3.2
Analysis of variance for the split-plot design.

Source	Sum of squares	d.f.	Mean square	F
Between main plots				
Factor A	SS_G	$G-1$	V_G	$F_G = \frac{V_G}{V_{BE}}$
Residuals	SS_{BE}	$N-G$	V_{BE}	
Within main plots				
Factor B	SS_T	T	V_T	$F_T = \frac{V_T}{V_{WE}}$
B × A	$SS_{T\times G}$	$(G-1)T$	$V_{T\times G}$	$F_{T\times G} = \frac{V_{T\times G}}{V_{WE}}$
Within residuals	SS_{WE}	$(N-G)T$	V_{WE}	

where $\delta_{jj'} = 1(j = j'); = 0(j \neq j')$. In other words,

$$\mathbf{\Sigma}_k = \begin{pmatrix} \sigma_E^2+\sigma_B^2 & \sigma_B^2 & \sigma_B^2 & \cdots & \sigma_B^2 \\ \sigma_B^2 & \sigma_E^2+\sigma_B^2 & \sigma_B^2 & \cdots & \sigma_B^2 \\ \sigma_B^2 & \sigma_B^2 & \sigma_E^2+\sigma_B^2 & \cdots & \sigma_B^2 \\ \vdots & \vdots & \vdots & & \vdots \\ \sigma_B^2 & \sigma_B^2 & \sigma_B^2 & \cdots & \sigma_E^2+\sigma_B^2 \end{pmatrix}. \quad (3.20)$$

This implies a constant correlation ρ between any two levels of factor B within the same subplot:

$$\rho = \frac{\sigma_B^2}{\sigma_E^2+\sigma_B^2}, \quad (3.21)$$

which is called *intra-class correlation* or *intra-cluster correlation* where the same subplot is called a *class* or *cluster.* This structure of covariance matrix is called *compound symmetry* or *exchangeable.* Statistical inference for data from the split-plot design can be made based on the split-plot ANOVA shown in Table 3.2.

Application of the split-plot design to the analysis of repeated measurements in clinical trials or animal experiments is mainly due to similar (but not identical) situations involved in the design. The "main plot" corresponds to "human subject" or "animal," the "main plot factor (A)" corresponds to the treatment group and the "subplot factor (B)" corresponds to the different point of "time" within the same subject. However, there is a big difference between these two designs. Because levels of subplot factor B are randomly allocated to subplots, the yields from different subplots in the same main plot are equally correlated with each other as shown in (3.21). However, "different times" cannot be allocated randomly to times within the same subject; responses from points close in time are usually more highly correlated than responses from points far apart in time.

Nevertheless, as far as the structure of the covariance matrix $\mathbf{\Sigma}$ satisfy *compound symmetry*, statistical inference can be made using the same split-plot ANOVA table (Table 3.3) for repeated measurements. For example, to test the null hypothesis of no differences among treatment groups

$$H_0 : \alpha_1 = \cdots = \alpha_G,$$

the following F test can be applied:

$$F = \frac{V_G}{V_{BE}} \sim F_{(G-1,N-G)} \text{ distribution,} \tag{3.22}$$

where

$$\begin{aligned} V_{TG} &= \sum_{kij} (\bar{y}_{k\cdot\cdot} - \bar{y}_{\cdots})^2/(G-1) \\ V_{BE} &= \{\sum_{kij} (\bar{y}_{ki\cdot} - \bar{y}_{\cdots})^2 - \sum_{kij} (\bar{y}_{k\cdot\cdot} - \bar{y}_{\cdots})^2\}/(N-G). \end{aligned}$$

To test the important null hypothesis on the interaction term *time* × *treatment group* (3.6) the following F test can be applied:

$$F = \frac{V_{T\times G}}{V_{WE}} \sim F_{(G-1)T,(N-G)T} \text{ distribution,} \tag{3.23}$$

where

$$\begin{aligned} V_{T\times G} &= \sum_{kij} (\bar{y}_{k\cdot j} - \bar{y}_{k\cdot\cdot} - \bar{y}_{\cdot\cdot j} + \bar{y}_{\cdots})^2/(T(G-1)) \\ V_{WE} &= \sum_{kij} (\bar{y}_{kij} - \bar{y}_{ki\cdot} - \bar{y}_{k\cdot j} + \bar{y}_{k\cdot\cdot})^2/(T(N-G)). \end{aligned}$$

However, when the covariance matrix does not satisfy *compound symmetry*, then we cannot assume F distribution for testing the null hypothesis on the interaction term (3.23). If the compound symmetry assumption is not valid, then the F test becomes too liberal, i.e., the proportion of rejections of the null

TABLE 3.3
Analysis of variance for split-plot design for repeated measurements.

Source	Sum of squares	d.f.	Mean square	F
Between subjects				
Treatment group	SS_G	$G-1$	V_G	$F_G = \frac{V_G}{V_{BE}}$
Residuals	SS_{BE}	$N-G$	V_{BE}	
Within subjects				
Time	SS_T	T	V_T	$F_T = \frac{V_T}{V_{WE}}$
Time × Group	$SS_{T\times G}$	$(G-1)T$	$V_{T\times G}$	$F_{T\times G} = \frac{V_{T\times G}}{V_{WE}}$
Within residuals	SS_{WE}	$(N-G)T$	V_{WE}	

TABLE 3.4
ANOVA for split-plot design applied to the *Rat Data*. GG and FF denote p values based on Greenhouse–Geisser correction and Huyhn–Feldt correction, respectively.

Source	SS	df	MS	F	p	GG p	HF p
Between subjects							
Treatment group	42.56	1	42.56	2.54	0.142		
Residuals	167.54	10	16.75				
Within subjects							
Time (omitted)	...	...	...	...			
Time × Group	35.50	3	11.83	19.67	0.0000	0.0008	0.0004
Within residuals	18.05	30	0.60				

hypothesis is larger than the nominal significance level when the null hypothesis is true. Until recently, as a method for correcting the degrees of freedom of F distribution, which make it possible to conduct an approximate F test, Greenhouse–Geisser correction (1959) and Huyhn–Feldt correction (1976) have been used. The approximate F test is given by

$$F = \frac{V_{T\times G}}{V_{WE}} \sim F_{(G-1)T\epsilon,(N-G)T\epsilon} \text{ distribution,} \tag{3.24}$$

where ϵ denotes the correction term proposed by Greenhouse and Geisser or Huyhn and Feldt.

In Table 3.4, the result of the split-plot design applied to data from the rat experiment (Table 2.1) is shown, where in addition to the p value by the unadjusted F test (3.23) for interaction term, two kinds of p values are shown, which are adjusted for degrees of freedom by using Greenhouse–Geisser correction and Huynh–Feldt correction, respectively. All the F tests are highly significant. It should be noted that the test for the null hypothesis of no difference in groups at baseline is not affected by covariance structure among repeated measurements.

3.5 Selecting a good fit covariance structure using SAS

Recently, it has been possible to fit an analysis of variance model (3.3) based on the restricted maximum likelihood estimation (REML, see Appendix B, Section B.2.1 for the reason why the REML is used) and also select a model for covariance structure that is a good fit to the repeated measurements using some information criterion such as AIC (Akaike information criterion, 1974) or BIC (Schwarz's Bayesian information criterion, 1981),

$$AIC(\text{REML}) = -2 \text{ Res Log Likelihood } + 2p \quad (3.25)$$

$$BIC(\text{REML}) = -2 \text{ Res Log Likelihood } + p \log N \quad (3.26)$$

where "Res Log Likelihood" (shown in SAS outputs) denotes the value of the restricted log-likelihood function and p denotes the number of parameters in the covariance structure model. The model that minimizes AIC or BIC is preferred. If AIC or BIC is close, then the simpler model is usually considered preferable.

It should be noted that, if the REML estimator has been used, the above AIC and BIC can be used for comparing models with different covariance structure only if both models have the same set of fixed effects parameters. For comparing models with different sets of fixed effects parameters, one should consider the following AIC and BIC based on the maximum likelihood (ML) estimation,

$$AIC(\text{ML}) = -2 \text{ Log Likelihood } + 2(p+q) \quad (3.27)$$

$$BIC(\text{ML}) = -2 \text{ Log Likelihood } + (p+q) \log N \quad (3.28)$$

where "Log Likelihood" denotes the value of the log-likelihood function and q denotes the number of fixed-effects parameters to be estimated.

The `SAS` procedure `PROC MIXED` allows you to choose from many candidate covariance models. The following four models for covariance structure (here

4 × 4 matrix) are frequently used in the literature.

(1) CS: compound symmetry model (or exchangeable model)

$$\Sigma = \sigma^2 \times \begin{pmatrix} 1 & \rho & \rho & \rho \\ \rho & 1 & \rho & \rho \\ \rho & \rho & 1 & \rho \\ \rho & \rho & \rho & 1 \end{pmatrix} \quad (3.29)$$

(2) AR(1): First-order autoregressive model

$$\Sigma = \sigma^2 \times \begin{pmatrix} 1 & \rho & \rho^2 & \rho^3 \\ \rho & 1 & \rho & \rho^2 \\ \rho^2 & \rho & 1 & \rho \\ \rho^3 & \rho^2 & \rho & 1 \end{pmatrix} \quad (3.30)$$

(3) TOEP: General autoregressive model (or Toeplitz model)

$$\Sigma = \sigma^2 \times \begin{pmatrix} 1 & \rho_1 & \rho_2 & \rho_3 \\ \rho_1 & 1 & \rho_1 & \rho_2 \\ \rho_2 & \rho_1 & 1 & \rho_1 \\ \rho_3 & \rho_2 & \rho_1 & 1 \end{pmatrix} \quad (3.31)$$

(4) UN: Unstructured model

$$\Sigma = \begin{pmatrix} \sigma_1^2 & \sigma_1\sigma_2\rho_1 & \sigma_1\sigma_3\rho_2 & \sigma_1\sigma_4\rho_3 \\ \sigma_2\sigma_1\rho_1 & \sigma_2^2 & \sigma_2\sigma_3\rho_4 & \sigma_2\sigma_4\rho_5 \\ \sigma_3\sigma_1\rho_2 & \sigma_3\sigma_2\rho_4 & \sigma_3^2 & \sigma_3\sigma_4\rho_6 \\ \sigma_4\sigma_1\rho_3 & \sigma_4\sigma_2\rho_5 & \sigma_4\sigma_3\rho_6 & \sigma_4^2 \end{pmatrix} \quad (3.32)$$

In the first-order autoregressive model and the general autoregressive model, correlation between measurements is a function of their lag in time, indicating that adjacent measurements may tend to be more correlated than those farther apart in time.

Now, let us apply an analysis of variance model (3.3) to the *Rat Data* using `PROC MIXED`. The first step is to rearrange the data structure from the wide format shown in Table 2.1 into the long format structure in which each separate repeated measurement and the associated values of covariates appear as a separate row in the data set. The rearranged data set is shown in Table 3.5 which includes four variables; the variable `id` indicating the rat id is a numeric factor, the variable `group` indicating the treatment group is also a numeric factor (2 = experimental group, 1 = control group), the variable `week` denotes the measurement time point (0, 1, 2, 3 in weeks), and the variable `y` is the response or laboratory data (continuous variable). In this application,

TABLE 3.5
The *Rat Data* with "long format" structure rearranged from the 'wide format' structure shown in Table 2.1 (only the data for the first three rats are shown).

	rat id	treatment group	time	response
variable in SAS	`id`	`group`	`week`	`y`
	1	2	0	7.50
	1	2	1	8.60
	1	2	2	6.90
	1	2	3	0.80
	2	2	0	10.60
	2	2	1	11.70
	2	2	2	8.80
	2	2	3	1.60
	3	2	0	12.40
	3	2	1	13.00
	3	2	2	11.00
	3	2	3	5.60

as the effects of the experimental treatment are compared with the control treatment, we shall estimate the effects at different times j, $\hat{\tau}_{21}^{(j)}$ (3.10) and the overall effects over the measurement period, $\hat{\tau}_{21}$ (3.12) as follows:

1. Treatment effect at week 1: $\tau_{21}^{(1)} = (\gamma_{21} - \gamma_{20}) - (\gamma_{11} - \gamma_{10}) = \gamma_{21}$
2. Treatment effect at week 2: $\tau_{21}^{(2)} = \gamma_{22}$
3. Treatment effect at week 3: $\tau_{21}^{(3)} = \gamma_{23}$
4. Overall treatment effect: τ_{21}: use the following linear contrast

$$\frac{1}{3}(3, -1, -1, -1, -3, 1, 1, 1)(\gamma_{10}, \gamma_{11}, \gamma_{12}, \gamma_{13}, \gamma_{20}, \gamma_{21}, \gamma_{22}, \gamma_{23})^t$$

Now, to estimate the interaction term γ_{ik}, we can use the corresponding linear contrast. But the degrees of freedom of $\{\gamma_{ik}\}$ are $(G-1)T = 3$ and so let us here output these three parameter estimates $\gamma_{21}, \gamma_{22}, \gamma_{23}$ directly. However, as `PROC MIXED` uses the default option that the last category of the ordered categorical variable is set to be zero, the following considerations are required for coding the SAS program:

1. The `CLASS` statement needs the option `/ref=first` to specify the first category be the reference category.
2. The basic order of the elements $\{\gamma_{kj}\}$ of the `group` $\times$ `week` interaction is

$$(\gamma_{10}, \gamma_{11}, \gamma_{12}, \gamma_{13}, \gamma_{20}, \gamma_{21}, \gamma_{22}, \gamma_{23}).$$

However, the first category comes next to the last category via the option `/ref=first` and thus, first reverse the order of k as follows

$$(\gamma_{20}, \gamma_{21}, \gamma_{22}, \gamma_{23}, \gamma_{10}, \gamma_{11}, \gamma_{12}, \gamma_{13})$$

and then move the first category of j (=0) next to the last category (=3), i.e., the final revised order is

$$(\gamma_{21}, \gamma_{22}, \gamma_{23}, \gamma_{20}, \gamma_{11}, \gamma_{12}, \gamma_{13}, \gamma_{10})$$

(see the order of the interaction effect `group*week` in the table labeled "Solution for Fixed Effects" of the SAS output). Then, the coefficients of the linear contrast for the average treatment effect, τ_{21} needs the following change

$$(3, -1, -1, -1, -3, 1, 1, 1) \to (1, 1, 1, -3, -1, -1, -1, 3).$$

Furthermore, it should be noted that the statistical inferential results about the fixed effects depend on the covariance structure $\mathbf{\Sigma}_k$ used in the analysis. So, it is important to select an appropriate model for the covariance structure. To illustrate this point, we shall fit four different covariance structures to the *Rat Data*, i.e., compound symmetry, first-order autoregressive, general autoregressive, and unstructured described above. The SAS programs used are shown in Program 3.1.

Program 3.1. SAS procedure `PROC MIXED` for the *Rat Data*

```
data d1;
infile 'c:\book\RepeatedMeasure\experimentRat.dat' missover;
input id group week y;

proc mixed data = d1 method=reml covtest;
   class id group week/ ref=first ;
   model y = group week group*week / s cl ddfm=sat ;
   repeated / type = cs     subject = id r  rcorr ;
 ( repeated / type = ar(1) subject = id r  rcorr ; )
 ( repeated / type = toep subject = id r  rcorr ; )
 ( repeated / type = un     subject = id r  rcorr ; )
   estimate 'mean CFB ' group*week  1 1 1 -3  -1 -1 -1 3
                        / divisor=3 cl alpha=0.05;
 run ;
```

Simple Notes on the SAS procedure shown in Program 3.1.

- The option "`method=reml`" specifies the REML estimation. In this book we always specify REML.
- The variables `group` and `week` are considered as numeric factors by the `CLASS` statement.

- The option "`ddfm=sat`" specifies the Satterthwaite method (see (B.42) for details) for estimating the degrees of freedom in the t-test and F-test for the fixed-effects estimates.

- The `REPEATED` statement is used to specify the repeated effects (here, "`week`"), which defines the ordering of the repeated measurements within each subject. However, if the data are ordered similarly for each subject as in the case of the *Rat Data*, then specifying a repeated effect can be omitted. The option `type=` specifies the model for covariance structure $\boldsymbol{\Sigma}_k$: `type = cs` (compound symmetry), `type = ar(1)` (first-order autoregressive), `type = toep` (general autoregressive), and `type = un` (unstructured). In Program 3.1, all the treatment groups are assumed to have homogeneous covariance structure, i.e., $\boldsymbol{\Sigma}_k = \boldsymbol{\Sigma}$.

- The `ESTIMATE` statement allows estimation and testing of the linear contrast specified.

- See the SAS/STAT User's Guide for other details.

The results are shown in Output 3.1a for the CS model with `type=cs` and Output 3.1b for the UN model with `type=un`.

Output 3.1a The CS model for the *Rat Data*

```
Fit statistics
-2 Res Log Likelihood 140.8
AIC (smaller is better) 144.8
BIC (smaller is better) 145.8

Covariance Parameter Estimates
Cov Parm Subject      Estimate S.E.  Z value Pr > Z
CS           id       4.0382 1.8736 2.16 0.0311
Residual              0.6017 0.1553 3.87 <.0001

Solution for Fixed Effects
Effect group week Estimate S.E. DF t Value Pr>|t| Alpha Lower Upper
Intercept      10.9333 0.8794 12.2 12.43 <.0001 0.05  9.021 12.846
group      2   -1.0167 1.2436 12.2 -0.82 0.4293 0.05 -3.721 1.6875
group      1     0 . . . . . . .
week          1  0.2000 0.4478 30  0.45 0.6584 0.05 -0.7146  1.1146
week          2 -0.6500 0.4478 30 -1.45 0.1570 0.05 -1.5646  0.2646
week          3 -2.8500 0.4478 30 -6.36 <.0001 0.05 -3.7646 -1.9354
week          0  0 . . . . . . .
group*week 2 1  0.7000 0.6333 30  1.11 0.2778 0.05 -0.5934  1.9934
group*week 2 2 -0.4000 0.6333 30 -0.63 0.5324 0.05 -1.6934  0.8934
group*week 2 3 -3.7667 0.6333 30 -5.95 <.0001 0.05 -5.0601 -2.4732
group*week 2 0  0 . . . . . . .
group*week 1 1  0 . . . . . . .
group*week 1 2  0 . . . . . . .
group*week 1 3  0 . . . . . . .
group*week 1 0  0 . . . . . . .

Type 3 Tests of Fixed Effects
Effect      Num DF  Dem DF  F Value Pr > F
group         1 10     2.54  0.1420
week          3 30  113.66    <.0001
group*week    3 30   19.67    <.0001

Estimates
Label         Estimate S.E.  DF  t Value Pr>|t| Alpha Lower Upper
mean CFB       -1.1556 0.5171 30 -2.23 0.0330 0.05 -2.2116 -0.09947
```

Output 3.1b The UN model for the *Rat Data*

```
Fit Statistics
-2 Res Log Likelihood 88.3
AIC (smaller is better) 108.3
BIC (smaller is better) 113.1

Estimated R Matrix for id 2 (Common Covariance)
Row  Col1    Col2    Col3    Col4
1  3.5122 3.4202 3.4787 4.4183
2  3.4202 3.3682 3.3967 4.3453
3  3.4787 3.3967 3.7782 5.1698
4  4.4183 4.3453 5.1698 7.9008

Estimated R Correlation Matrix for id2
Row Col1 Col2 Col3 Col4
1 1.0000 0.9944 0.9550 0.8388
2 0.9944 1.0000 0.9522 0.8423
3 0.9550 0.9522 1.0000 0.9462
4 0.8388 0.8423 0.9462 1.0000

Solution for Fixed Effects
Effect group week Estimate S.E. DF t Value Pr>|t| Alpha Lower Upper
group      2      -1.0167 1.0820 10 -0.94 0.3696 0.05 -3.4275 1.3942
group*week 2 1     0.7000 0.1155 10  6.06 0.0001 0.05  0.4427  0.9573
group*week 2 2    -0.4000 0.3332 10 -1.20 0.2576 0.05 -1.1423  0.3423
group*week 2 3    -3.7667 0.9267 10 -4.06 0.0023 0.05 -5.8315 -1.7018

Type 3 Tests of Fixed Effects
Effect      Num DF  Dem DF   F Value Pr > F
group          1            10       2.54  0.1420
week           3            10      81.17  <.0001
group*week     3            10      23.61  <.0001

Estimates
Label        Estimate S.E.   DF   t Value Pr>|t| Alpha Lower   Upper
mean CFB      -1.1556 0.4117 10 -2.81   0.0186  0.05 -2.0730 -0.2381
```

In the CS (compound symmetry) model, two variance estimates, $\hat{\sigma}_B^2$, $\hat{\sigma}_E^2$ of the analysis of variance model (3.18) are shown in the table labeled "Covariance Parameter Estimates"

$$\hat{\sigma}_B^2 = 4.0382(\texttt{CS}),\ \hat{\sigma}_E^2 = 0.6017(\texttt{Residual}).$$

Correlation matrices are omitted here since we can easily compute $\rho = 0.8703$ from equation (3.21). Estimates of treatment effect at each time and of average treatment effect are shown in the table labeled "Solution for Fixed Effects" and the table labeled "Estimates," respectively.

1. `group*week 2 1` : $\hat{\tau}_{21}^{(1)} = 0.7000 \pm 0.6333, p = 0.28$
2. `group*week 2 2` : $\hat{\tau}_{21}^{(2)} = -0.4000 \pm 0.6333, p = 0.53$

3. `group*week 2 3` : $\hat{\tau}_{21}^{(3)} = -3.7667 \pm 0.6333, p < .0001$

4. `mean CFB` : $\hat{\tau}_{21} = -1.1556 \pm 0.5171, p = 0.033$

In the unstructured model, the estimated covariance matrix is shown in the table labeled "Estimated R Matrix for id 2" (R means residual covariance) and also in the table "Covariance Parameter Estimates." The latter table is omitted here but includes more detailed information such as standard errors, Z-value and p value (see Output 3.2b in the next section). The estimated correlation matrix is shown in the table labeled "Estimated R Correlation Matrix for id 2." It should be noted that the parameter α_2 is estimated as -1.0167 ± 1.0820 ($p = 0.37$) in the unstructured model (see `group 2` in the table "Solution for Fixed Effects"), which is identical to the *difference in means at baseline between two groups* shown in Table 2.2. Furthermore, the test result for the null hypothesis of no differences between treatment groups (3.22), which is not related to the treatment effect at all, is shown in the row `group` of the table labeled "Type 3 Tests of Fixed Effects" and the result $F = 2.54$, $p = 0.142$ is identical to that in the split-plot ANOVA (Table 3.4) **without reference to the type of covariance structure** as explained in Section 3.4.

A summary of the results of application of the four kinds of analysis of variance models based on REML to the *Rat Data* are shown in Table 3.6. According to the value of AIC, the best fit model was the unstructured model (AIC = 108.3). The BIC value also chose the same model as the best fit model. Although the average treatment effect was estimated as $\hat{\tau}_{21} = -1.16$ without reference to the type of covariance structure, the estimate of standard errors changed depending on the type of covariance structure.

- In the unstructured model, the estimate of standard errors is $S.E. = 0.41 (p = 0.019)$, which is identical to the result of Student's two-sample t-test (3.16) shown in Table 3.1.

- Furthermore, the treatment effect at week 1 ($\hat{\tau}_{21}^{(1)} \Rightarrow$ `group*week 2 1`) and 3 ($\hat{\tau}_{21}^{(3)} \Rightarrow$ `group*week 2 3`) is also identical to the corresponding result of Student's two-sample t-test based on CFB as shown in Table 2.3, respectively.

These results indicate that, **when the unstructured covariance is the best fitted model, the result of the analysis of variance model is identical to the result of Student's two-sample t-test for the difference in means of CFB between groups using only the data necessary for the comparison.**

TABLE 3.6
Results of analysis of variance model (3.3) based on REML, applied to the *Rat Data* (Table 2.1). The results of the best fit model are indicated in boldface.

	Covariance structure			
		Autoregressive model		
	CS	First-order	General	Unstructured
(1) AIC				
	144.80	131.8	133.1	**108.3**
(2) Interaction: time × treatment				
F(df)	19.7 (3, 30)	22.53 (3, 30)	20.05 (3, 30)	**23.61 (3, 10)**
p	$< .0001$	$< .0001$	$< .0001$	**<. 0001**
(3) CFB over time: $\hat{\tau}_{21}$= -1.16				
SE	0.52	0.54	0.63	**0.41**
t(df)	-2.23(30)	-2.15(30)	-1.84(30)	**-2.81(10)**
p	0.033	0.040	0.075	**0.019**
(4) CFB at week 3: $\hat{\tau}_{21}^{(3)} = -3.77$				
SE	0.63	0.74	0.88	**0.93**
t(df)	-5.95(30)	-5.07(30)	-4.27(30)	**-4.06(10)**
p	<0.001	<0.001	0.002	**0.002**
(5) CFB at week 1: $\hat{\tau}_{21}^{(1)} = 0.7$				
SE	0.63	0.44	0.44	**0.12**
t(df)	1.11(30)	1.59(30)	1.59(30)	**6.06(10)**
p	0.278	0.122	0.119	**<0.001**

3.6 Heterogeneous covariance

So far, homogeneous covariance structure is assumed for all the treatment groups, i.e., $\mathbf{\Sigma}_k = \mathbf{\Sigma}$. In this section, to check the homogeneity assumption, we shall consider the analysis of variance model with heterogeneous covariance. To do this in `PROC MIXED`, we have only to add the option `group = group` to the `REPEATED` statement, where the former `group` is the SAS statement and the latter `group` is a numeric factor denoting the treatment group. Then the modified REPEATED statement will be

```
repeated / type = cs subject = id r rcorr group = group;
```

In this case, the variable `group` must be declared as a numeric factor in the `CLASS` statement. Now we shall fit the two models, CS and UN, to the *Rat Data*. The respective sets of SAS programs appear in Program 3.2.

Program 3.2 SAS procedure PROC MIXED for the *Rat Data* - Unequal Covariance between treatment groups

```
data d1;
infile 'c:\book\RepeatedMeasure\experimentRat.dat' missover;
input id group week y;

proc mixed data = d1 method=reml covtest;
   class id group week/ ref=first ;
   model y = group week group*week / s cl ddfm=sat ;
   repeated / type = cs subject = id r  rcorr group = group;
 ( repeated / type = un subject = id r  rcorr group = group; )
   estimate 'mean CFB ' group*week  1 1 1 -3  -1 -1 -1 3
                         / divisor=3 cl alpha=0.05;
run ;
```

Here also, we shall show the results of two models, the CS model and the UN model. The results are shown in Output 3.2a for the CS model with `type=cs` and Output 3.2b for the UN model with `type=un`.

Output 3.2a CS model for the *Rat Data* - Unequal Covariance between treatment groups

```
Fit Statistics
-2 Res Log Likelihood 140.4
AIC (smaller is better) 148.4

Covariance Parameter Estimates
Cov Parm Subject Estimate S.E.  Z value Pr > Z
Variance id group 2  0.6950 0.2538 2.74 0.0031
CS       id group 2  3.9975 2.6389 1.51 0.1298
Variance id group 1  0.5083 0.1856 2.74 0.0031
CS       id group 1  4.0788 2.6605 1.53 0.1252

Solution for Fixed Effects
Effect group week Estimate S.E. DF t Value Pr>|t|  Alpha Lower Upper
group*week 2  1     0.7000 0.6333 29.3  1.11 0.2780 0.05 -0.5947 1.9947
group*week 2  2    -0.4000 0.6333 29.3 -0.63 0.5326 0.05 -1.6947 0.8947
group*week 2  3    -3.7667 0.6333 29.3 -5.95 <.0001 0.05 -5.0614 -2.4719

Type 3 Tests of Fixed Effects
Effect      Num DF  Dem DF   F Value  Pr > F
group       1         10       2.54   0.1420
week        3         29.3  113.66   <.0001
group*week  3         29.3   19.67   <.0001

Estimates
Label        Estimate   S.E. DF  t Value Pr>|t|  Aalpha Lower  Upper
mean CFB     -1.1556  0.5171 29.3 -2.23 0.0332  0.05 -2.2127 -0.09840
```

Output 3.2b UN model for the *Rat Data* - Unequal Covariance between treatment groups

```
Fit Statistics
-2 Res Log Likelihood 71.2
AIC (smaller is better) 111.2

Covariance Parameter Estimates (by group)
Cov Parm Subject Group Estimate S.E. Z Pr > |Z|
UN(1,1) id group 2 3.6217 2.2905 1.58 0.0569
UN(2,1) id group 2 3.5637 2.2633 1.57 0.1154
UN(2,2) id group 2 3.5657 2.2551 1.58 0.0569
UN(3,1) id group 2 3.4147 2.2145 1.54 0.1231
UN(3,2) id group 2 3.4187 2.2067 1.55 0.1213
UN(3,3) id group 2 3.5507 2.2456 1.58 0.0569
UN(4,1) id group 2 4.2820 3.0798 1.39 0.1644
UN(4,2) id group 2 4.3120 3.0735 1.40 0.1606
UN(4,3) id group 2 4.9940 3.2698 1.53 0.1267
UN(4,4) id group 2 8.0320 5.0799 1.58 0.0569

UN(1,1) id group 1 3.4027 2.1520 1.58 0.0569
UN(2,1) id group 1 3.2767 2.0749 1.58 0.1143
UN(2,2) id group 1 3.1707 2.0053 1.58 0.0569
UN(3,1) id group 1 3.5427 2.2882 1.55 0.1216
UN(3,2) id group 1 3.3747 2.1949 1.54 0.1242
UN(3,3) id group 1 4.0057 2.5334 1.58 0.0569
UN(4,1) id group 1 4.5547 3.0719 1.48 0.1382
UN(4,2) id group 1 4.3787 2.9600 1.48 0.1391
UN(4,3) id group 1 5.3457 3.4554 1.55 0.1219
UN(4,4) id group 1 7.7697 4.9140 1.58 0.0569

Solution for Fixed Effects
Effect group week Estimate S.E. DF t Value Pr>|t|  Alpha Lower Upper
group*week 2 1     0.7000 0.1155 8      6.06 0.0003 0.05 0.4337 0.9663
group*week 2 2    -0.4000 0.3332 9.99 -1.20 0.2576 0.05 -1.1424 0.3424
group*week 2 3    -3.7667 0.9267 9.62 -4.06 0.0025 0.05 -5.8427 -1.6907

Estimates
Label      Estimate S.E.  DF  t Value Pr>|t|  Alpha Lower Upper
mean CFB    -1.1556 0.4117 9.5 -2.81 0.0195   0.05 -2.0796 -0.2315
```

In the CS model, two variance estimates, $\hat{\sigma}_B^2$ and $\hat{\sigma}_E^2$, are shown in the table labeled "Covariance Parameter Estimates" by treatment group. You can see that the difference between groups is small for both variances. In the unstructured model, the covariance matrix is shown by treatment group in the table labeled "Covariance Parameter Estimates" in the form of UN(j_1, j_2). Here also, we can observe small differences between groups. When we observe the change of AICs from the homogeneous model to the heterogeneous model, we have 144.8 $\rightarrow$ 148.4 for the CS model and 108.3 $\rightarrow$ 111.2 for the UN model, indicating that the homogeneous models are preferred to the heterogeneous ones.

3.7 ANCOVA-type models

So far, the baseline data y_{ij0} was used as one value of the response variable. In this section, we shall introduce some ANCOVA-type models adjusting for the baseline data y_{ij0}. To compare the ANOVA model, we shall consider the following two ANCOVA-type models:

$$
\begin{aligned}
\text{Model A: } y_{kij} &= \mu + \alpha_k + \beta_j + \gamma_{kj} + \epsilon_{kij} \ (k = 0, 1, ..., T) && (3.33)\\
\text{Model B: } y_{kij} &= \mu + \theta y_{ki0} + \alpha_k^{'} + \beta_j^{'} + \gamma_{kj}^{'} + \epsilon_{kij}^{'} \ (k = 1, 2, ..., T) && (3.34)\\
\text{Model C: } y_{kij} &= \mu + \theta y_{ki0} + \alpha_i^{'} + \beta_j^{'} + \phi_j(y_{ki0} \times \texttt{Time}_j) + \gamma_{kj}^{'} + \epsilon_{kij}^{'} \\
& \qquad (k = 1, 2, ..., T) && (3.35)\\
\boldsymbol{\epsilon}_{ki}^{'} &= (\epsilon_{ki1}^{'}, ..., \epsilon_{kiT}^{'})^t \sim N(\mathbf{0}, \boldsymbol{\Sigma})
\end{aligned}
$$

where

$\alpha_k^{'}$:	the fixed effects of the kth treatment group
$\beta_j^{'}$:	the fixed effects of the jth measurement time
$\gamma_{kj}^{'}$:	the fixed effects of the interaction between the kth group and the jth time
$\texttt{Time}_j$:	a dummy variable indicating the jth time
θ :	coefficient for baseline data
ϕ_j :	coefficients for the interaction term $(y_{ki0} \times \texttt{Time}_j)$

Model A denotes the ANOVA model, Model B denotes an ANCOVA-type model with the *baseline effects* θ constant over time, and Model C denotes an ANCOVA-type model with the *baseline effects* $\theta + \phi_j$ which varies over time. Furthermore, let us consider the following three models which replace y_{kij} with CFB, $d_{kij} = y_{kij} - y_{ki0}$:

$$
\begin{aligned}
\text{Model A}_d\text{: } d_{kij} &= \mu + \alpha_k^{'} + \beta_j^{'} + \gamma_{kj}^{'} + \epsilon_{kij}^{'} && (3.36)\\
\text{Model B}_d\text{: } d_{kij} &= \mu + \theta y_{ki0} + \alpha_k^{'} + \beta_j^{'} + \gamma_{kj}^{'} + \epsilon_{kij}^{'} && (3.37)\\
\text{Model C}_d\text{: } d_{kij} &= \mu + \theta y_{ki0} + \alpha_i^{'} + \beta_j^{'} + \phi_j(y_{ki0} \times \texttt{Time}_j) + \gamma_{kj}^{'} + \epsilon_{kij}^{'} \\
k &= 1, 2, ..., T && (3.38)\\
\boldsymbol{\epsilon}_{ki}^{'} &= (\epsilon_{ki1}^{'}, ..., \epsilon_{kiT}^{'})^t \sim N(\mathbf{0}, \boldsymbol{\Sigma})
\end{aligned}
$$

Theoretically, it can be shown that the treatment effect estimated from Model

A is identical to that from Model A$_d$ (see Chapter 4). Similarly, the estimated treatment effect from Model B and Model C are identical to those of Model B$_d$ and Model C$_d$, respectively. Therefore, when we want to compare the three models A, B and C, we have only to compare the models A$_d$, B$_d$ and C$_d$ using AIC or BIC. It should be noted, however, that the treatment effect for Models A$_d$, B$_d$ and C$_d$ should be changed to

$$\tau_{21}^{(j)} = (\alpha_2^{'} - \alpha_1^{'}) + (\gamma_{2j}^{'} - \gamma_{1j}^{'}) \quad (3.39)$$

$$\tau_{21}(j_s, j_e) = (\alpha_2^{'} - \alpha_1^{'}) + \frac{1}{j_e - j_s + 1}\sum_{j=j_s}^{j_e}(\gamma_{2j}^{'} - \gamma_{1j}^{'}). \quad (3.40)$$

For example, when you are interested in the difference in mean changes from baseline at time $j = 3$, you can set

$$\tau_{21}^{(3)} = (-1, 1)(\alpha_1^{'}, \alpha_2^{'})^t + (0, 0, -1, 0, 0, 1)(\gamma_{11}^{'}, \gamma_{12}^{'}, \gamma_{13}^{'}, \gamma_{21}^{'}, \gamma_{22}^{'}, \gamma_{23}^{'})^t.$$

When you are interested in the average difference in mean changes from baseline over the evaluation period $[1, 3]$, then you can set the following linear contrasts

$$\begin{aligned}\tau_{21}(1, 3) &= (-1, 1)(\alpha_1^{'}, \alpha_2^{'})^t \\ &\quad + \frac{1}{3}(-1, -1, -1, 1, 1, 1)(\gamma_{11}^{'}, \gamma_{12}^{'}, \gamma_{13}^{'}, \gamma_{21}^{'}, \gamma_{22}^{'}, \gamma_{23}^{'})^t \\ &= \frac{1}{3}\{(-3, 3)(\alpha_2^{'}, \alpha_1^{'})^t \\ &\quad + (-1, -1, -1, 1, 1, 1)(\gamma_{11}^{'}, \gamma_{12}^{'}, \gamma_{13}^{'}, \gamma_{21}^{'}, \gamma_{22}^{'}, \gamma_{23}^{'})^t\}.\end{aligned}$$

In the application of the ANOVA model to the *Rat Data* (Table 3.5) using SAS `PROC MIXED` in Section 3.5, we used the option `/ref=first` in the CLASS statement and changed the order of the coefficients for the linear contrast to output the treatment effect by time, $\gamma_{21}, \gamma_{22}, \gamma_{23}$ directly. However, here, we use the above linear contrasts (3.39), (3.40) and thus we need no special arrangements.

Now, we shall fit the above three models A$_d$, B$_d$ and C$_d$ with the changes from baseline as outcome variables to the *Rat Data*. Here also, the first step for the analysis is to rearrange the data structure from the long format shown in Table 3.5 into another long format shown in Table 3.7 where the baseline records were deleted and the new variable `ybase` indicating baseline data was created. In other words, when we have p variables, N cases, and the number of repeated measures is $T + 1$ including one baseline time point, the data

TABLE 3.7
The *Rat Data* for the ANCOVA-type model: the baseline data of response variable y in Table 3.5 was deleted and added as a new variable `ybase` (only the data for the first three rats are shown).

	Rat id	Treatment	Time	Response	Baseline data
Variable in SAS	`id`	`group`	`week`	`y`	`ybase`
	1	2	1	8.60	7.50
	1	2	2	6.90	7.50
	1	2	3	0.80	7.50
	2	2	1	11.70	10.60
	2	2	2	8.80	10.60
	2	2	3	1.60	10.60
	3	2	1	13.00	12.40
	3	2	2	11.00	12.40
	3	2	3	5.60	12.40

structure for the ANOVA model is a long format with $(T+1)N \times p$ but the one for the ANCOVA-type model including one baseline data needs a long format with $TN \times (p+1)$. We shall use the SAS program shown in Program 3.3 to fit each of the above three models.

Program 3.3 SAS `PROC MIXED` (Unstructured Σ) for the *Rat Data* for fitting three models: Model $\mathbf{A}_d$, $\mathbf{B}_d$ and $\mathbf{C}_d$. For comparing these models based on AIC and BIC, we have to replace the option `method=reml` with `method=ml`.

```
<data input>
data d3;
  infile 'c:\book\RepeatedMeasure\experimentRatPre.dat' missover;
  input id group week y ybase;
  cfb=y-ybase;

proc mixed data = d3 method=reml covtest;
class id group week ;
  model cfb =          group week group*week / s ddfm=sat;
 ( model cfb = ybase group week group*week / s ddfm=sat; )
 ( model cfb = ybase ybase*week group week group*week / s ddfm=sat; )
repeated / type = un subject = id r  rcorr ;
estimate 'CFB at week 1'
 group -1 1 group*week -1  0  0  1 0 0 / divisor=1 cl alpha=0.05;
estimate 'CFB at week 2'
 group -1 1 group*week  0 -1  0  0 1 0 / divisor=1 cl alpha=0.05;
estimate 'CFB at week 3'
 group -1 1 group*week  0  0 -1  0 0 1 / divisor=1 cl alpha=0.05;
estimate 'mean CFB '
 group -3 3 group*week -1 -1 -1  1 1 1 / divisor=3 cl alpha=0.05;
run ;
```

When we fitted the ANOVA model (3.3) to the *Rat Data*, the best-fit model for covariance structure is unstructured (`type=un`). Thus here also we shall assume the same *unstructured covariance*. As these three models have different sets of fixed-effects parameters, as explained in Section 3.5, for comparing these models, one should consider AIC and BIC based on the maximum likelihood (ML) estimation. To do so, we have only to replace the option `method=reml` with `method=ml`. The partial results are shown in Output 3.3 where the values of AIC and BIC are only based on the maximum likelihood estimation.

Output 3.3 SAS PROC MIXED for the *Rat Data* (Unstructured Σ) Only the values of AIC and BIC are based on the maximum likelihood estimation

```
<Model Ad>
Fit statistics
AIC (smaller is better) 63.8
BIC (smaller is better) 69.7

Solution for Fixed Effects
Effect group week Estimate S.E. DF t Value Pr>|t| Alpha Lower Upper
CFB at week 1  0.7000 0.1155 10 6.06 0.0001 0.05 0.4427 0.9573
CFB at week 2 -0.4000 0.3332 10 -1.20 0.2576 0.05 -1.1423 0.3423
CFB at week 3 -3.7667 0.9267 10 -4.06 0.0023 0.05 -5.8315 -1.7018
mean CFB      -1.1556 0.4117 10 -2.81 0.0186 0.05 -2.0730 -0.2381

<Model Bd>
Fit statistics
AIC (smaller is better) 62.9
BIC (smaller is better) 69.2

Solution for Fixed Effects
Effect group week Estimate S.E. DF t Value Pr>|t| Alpha Lower Upper
ybase         -0.0545 0.02929 9  -1.86  0.0959 0.05 -0.1207 0.01179
CFB at week 1  0.6446 0.1239 8.83 5.20  0.0006 0.05  0.3634 0.9258
CFB at week 2 -0.4554 0.3393 10.1 -1.34 0.2090 0.05 -1.2106 0.2999
CFB at week 3 -3.8220 0.9471 9.98 -4.04 0.0024 0.05 -5.9330 -1.7111
mean CFB      -1.2109 0.4294 9.93 -2.82 0.0183 0.05 -2.1685 -0.2533

<Model Cd>
Fit statistics
AIC (smaller is better) 63.0
BIC (smaller is better) 70.3

Solution for Fixed Effects
Effect group week Estimate S.E. DF t Value Pr>|t| Alpha Lower Upper
CFB at week 1  0.6734 0.1231 9 5.47 0.0004 0.05 0.3949 0.9518
CFB at week 2 -0.4097 0.3662 9 -1.12 0.2922 0.05 -1.2381 0.4187
CFB at week 3 -3.5044 0.9717 9 -3.61 0.0057 0.05 -5.7025 -1.3062
mean CFB      -1.0802 0.4441 9 -2.43 0.0378 0.05 -2.0849 -0.07560
```

From the results of the three models assuming unstructured covariance $\mathbf{\Sigma}$ common to both treatment groups, we have the following findings:

- All the treatment effects estimated from Model A_d without adjusting for baseline data are the same for those from the ANOVA model (OUTPUT 3.1b). Furthermore, these estimated treatment effects are the same as the results of the repeated application of Student's t test for the difference in means of CFB at each time (Table 2.3).

- Model C_d, in which the *baseline effects* varies over time, gives the same estimate at time 3 as the result of analysis of covariance based on a pair of data (y_{ki0}, y_{ki3}) (Figure 2.5). This indicates that the treatment effect by time from the ANCOVA-type model including the interaction term between baseline data and time is identical to the results from the analysis of variance for adjusting for baseline at each time point.

- Judging from AIC (Model A_d = 63.8, Model B_d = 62.9, Model C_d = 63.0) and BIC (Model A_d = 69.7, Model B_d = 69.2, Model C_d = 70.3), the best-fit model is shown to be Model B model adjusting for baseline data with the baseline effect constant over time. However, the differences in values of AIC and BIC are very small among three models. For example, the treatment effects at time 3 are estimated as follows:

  Model A_d: $\hat{\tau}_{21}^{(3)} = -3.7667$ (s.e. $= 0.9267$), $p = 0.0023$
  Model B_d: $\hat{\tau}_{21}^{(3)} = -3.8220$ (s.e. $= 0.9471$), $p = 0.0024$
  Model C_d: $\hat{\tau}_{21}^{(3)} = -3.5044$ (s.e. $= 0.9717$), $p = 0.0057$

The overall message from the above result will be that (1) **a usual analysis of covariance (ANCOVA) based on a pair of data (y_{ki0}, y_{kij}) does not tell us whether or not to adjust for baseline** and (2) **although it is a general practice of randomized controlled trials to use ANCOVA alone to adjust for the baseline measurement, adding "mean change from baseline" (Model A_d) could be a good method to get a good estimate of the treatment effect.**

4

From ANOVA models to mixed-effects repeated measures models

4.1 Introduction

In Section 2.4, we conducted an analysis of covariance adjusting for the baseline data to estimate the treatment effect where we observed a high positive correlation coefficient $\rho = 0.782$ between the baseline measurement and the measurement at week 3 (Figure 2.4). Similar positive correlation coefficients were also observed for the log-transformed serum levels of glutamate pyruvate transaminase (GPT) for each of treatment groups between the baseline measurement and the measurement at week 4 (Figure 4.1) in a randomized controlled trial with a *1:4* repeated measures design for chronic hepatitis patients to investigate whether the anti-hepatitis drug Gritiron tablets improve liver function abnormality[1] (Yano et al., 1989). In the previous chapter, the *Rat Data* was analyzed using the SAS procedure PROC MIXED, which allowed you to choose the good-fit covariance model from many candidate covariance models. However, this type of ad hoc analysis based on *the best-fit covariance* without rhyme or reason will not tell us why and how these positive correlation coefficients arise while repeated measures were usually taken *independently* for each patient. Furthermore, to estimate the treatment effect in the *1:1* pre-post design, an analysis of covariance is usually carried out to adjust for baseline data. *But why?*

To understand these problems, which are not always trivial, we need to change the model framework from the *ANOVA* model to the *mixed-effects* repeated measures model.

[1]This data set called *Gritiron Data* will be analyzed to illustrate the latent profile models in addition to the linear mixed-effects models in Chapter 11.

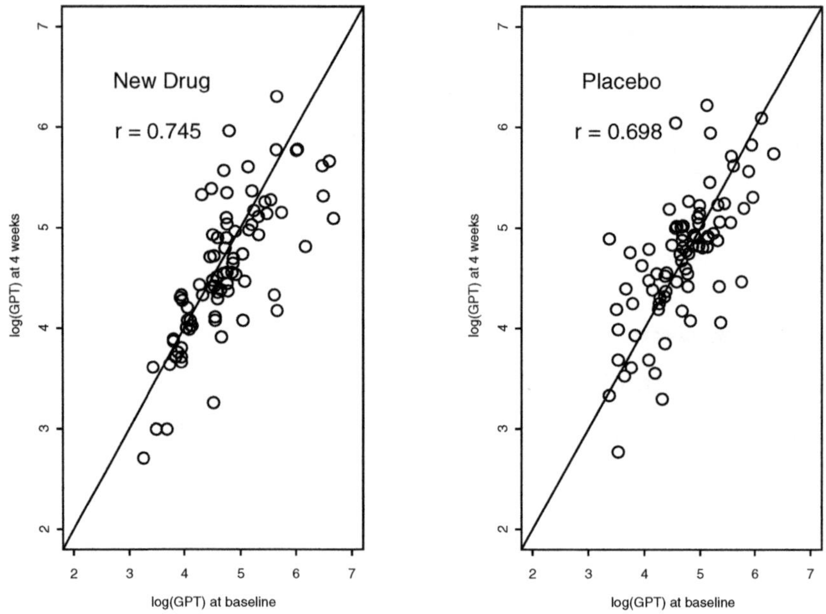

FIGURE 4.1
Gritiron Data: Scatter plots, correlation coefficients, and regression line for the log-transformed serum levels of glutamate pyruvate transaminase (GPT) between the baseline measurement and the measurements at week 4 by treatment group in a randomized controlled trial for chronic hepatitis patients (Yano et al., 1989).

4.2 Shift to mixed-effects repeated measures models

To understand the situation, let us consider the relationship between a pair of data points, the baseline data y_{ki0} and the data y_{kij} measured at time $j(> 0)$ for the same subject i of the treatment group k in the ANOVA model (3.3). For simplicity, consider here the comparison of two treatment groups ($G = 2$) where $k = 1$ denotes the control group and $k = 2$ denotes the new treatment group.

In the ANOVA model, as was illustrated with the *Rat Data* in Section 3.5, you can choose the best model for the covariance structure $\mathbf{\Sigma}_k$ (3.4) from many candidates. However, with this approach, you may not be able to understand the reason why the selected covariance model has arisen. So, to understand the covariance structure, let us decompose the error term ϵ_{kij} into

two independent components, one relating to the *inter-subject variability* and the other relating to the *residual* error term ϵ_{kij}. For example, we can consider the following decompositions:

$$\begin{aligned} y_{ki0} &= \mu + \alpha_k + \beta_0 + \gamma_{k0} + \epsilon_{ki0} \\ &= \mu + \alpha_k + 0 + 0 + (b_{0ki} + \epsilon_{ki0}) \\ y_{kij} &= \mu + \alpha_k + \beta_j + \gamma_{kj} + \epsilon_{kij} \\ &= \mu + \alpha_k + \beta_j + \gamma_{kj} + (b_{0ki} + b_{1ki} + \epsilon_{kij}), \end{aligned}$$

where b_{0ki} denotes the *random intercept*, which may reflect inter-subject variability due to possibly many unobserved prognostic factors in the baseline period, and b_{1ki} denotes the *random slope*, which may reflect inter-subject variability of the response to the treatment and assumed to be constant here regardless of the measurement time j. It should be noted that the *random slope* introduced here does not mean the *slope* on the time or a linear time trend. Furthermore, these two random variables are assumed to have the bivariate normal distribution:

$$\boldsymbol{b}_{ki} = (b_{0ki}, b_{1ki})^t \sim N(0, \Phi), \tag{4.1}$$

where

$$\boldsymbol{\Phi} = \begin{pmatrix} \sigma^2_{B0} & \rho_B\sigma_{B0}\sigma_{B1} \\ \rho_B\sigma_{B0}\sigma_{B1} & \sigma^2_{B1} \end{pmatrix}. \tag{4.2}$$

In other words, the decomposed model mixes up two types of variables, the random-effects variables (b_{0ki}, b_{1ki}) and the fixed-effects parameters $(\mu, \alpha_i, \beta_0, \beta_j, \gamma_{ij})$, leading to a mixed-effects model or mixed model.

Here, let us get back to the notation of *repeated measures design* defined in Chapter 1, i.e., using the following notational change

$$ki \to i, \quad j \text{ (as it is)}. \tag{4.3}$$

Then we have

$$\boldsymbol{y}_i = (y_{i0}, y_{i1}, ..., y_{iT}), \; i = 1, ..., (n_1 + n_2),$$

and let us introduce the variable x_{1i}

$$x_{1i} = \begin{cases} 1, & \text{if the } i\text{th subject is assigned to the new treatment} \\ 0, & \text{if the } i\text{th patient is assigned to the control.} \end{cases} \tag{4.4}$$

Then, the above ANOVA model can be replaced by the following mixed-effects repeated measures model:

A mixed-effects repeated measures model

$$y_{ij} \mid \boldsymbol{b}_i = \begin{cases} \beta_0 + \beta_1 x_{1i} + b_{0i} + \epsilon_{i0} & \text{for } j = 0 \\ \beta_0 + \beta_1 x_{1i} + \beta_{2j} + \beta_{3j} x_{1i} + b_{0i} + b_{1i} + \epsilon_{ij} & \text{for } j \geq 1 \end{cases} \tag{4.5}$$

where the same symbol β's as the ANOVA model are used here but their meanings are different as follows:

1. β_1 ($= \alpha_2$ in the ANOVA model) denotes the difference in means at baseline $j = 0$.

2. β_{2j} denotes the mean change from baseline at time j in the control group.

3. The change from baseline (CFB) at time j defined in (3.7) is changed to

$$d_{ij} = y_{ij} - y_{i0}, \quad (j = 1, ..., T). \tag{4.6}$$

4. β_{3j} denotes the treatment effect at time j (corresponding to $\tau_{21}^{(j)} = \gamma_{2j}$ (3.10) in the ANOVA model).

5. ϵ_{ij} denote mutually independent random errors distributed with normal distribution with mean 0 and variance σ_E^2.

6. $\boldsymbol{b}_i = (b_{0i}, b_{1i})^t$ and error terms $\{\epsilon_{ij}, j = 0, ..., T\}$ are independent.

The repeated measures model (4.5) can be expressed in the matrix form

$$\boldsymbol{y}_i \mid \boldsymbol{b}_i = \boldsymbol{X}_i\boldsymbol{\beta} + \boldsymbol{Z}\boldsymbol{b}_i + \boldsymbol{\epsilon}_i = \boldsymbol{X}_i\boldsymbol{\beta} + \boldsymbol{\epsilon}_i^*$$

where

$$\boldsymbol{b}_i \sim N(\boldsymbol{0}, \boldsymbol{\Phi}), \ \boldsymbol{\epsilon}_i \sim N(\boldsymbol{0}, \sigma_E^2 \boldsymbol{I}), \ \boldsymbol{\epsilon}_i^* \sim N(\boldsymbol{0}, \boldsymbol{\Sigma})$$

and

$$\boldsymbol{\Sigma} = \sigma_E^2 \boldsymbol{I} + \boldsymbol{Z\Phi Z}^t. \tag{4.7}$$

Then, we have

$$\begin{aligned}
E(y_{i0}) &= \beta_0 + \beta_1 x_{1i} \\
E(y_{ij}) &= \beta_0 + \beta_1 x_{1i} + \beta_{2j} + \beta_{3j} x_{1i} \\
E(d_{ij}) &= \beta_{2j} + \beta_{3j} x_{1i} \\
Var(d_{ij}) &= \sigma_{B1}^2 + 2\sigma_E^2 \\
Var(y_{i0}) &= (\boldsymbol{\Sigma})_{11} = \sigma_{B0}^2 + \sigma_E^2 \\
Var(y_{ij}) &= (\boldsymbol{\Sigma})_{(j+1)(j+1)} = \sigma_{B0}^2 + \sigma_{B1}^2 + 2\rho_B \sigma_{B0} \sigma_{B1} + \sigma_E^2 \\
Cov(y_{i0}, y_{ij}) &= (\boldsymbol{\Sigma})_{1(j+1)} = \sigma_{B0}^2 + \rho_B \sigma_{B0} \sigma_{B1} \\
Cov(y_{ij_1}, y_{ij_2}) &= (\boldsymbol{\Sigma})_{(j_1+1)(j_2+1)} = \sigma_{B0}^2 + \sigma_{B1}^2 + 2\rho_B \sigma_{B0} \sigma_{B1} \\
&\qquad (\text{for } j_1, j_2 > 0),
\end{aligned}$$

where (y_{i0}, y_{ij}) has the bivariate normal distribution with correlation coefficient ρ_{0j}

$$\rho_{0j} = \frac{\sigma_{B0}^2 + \rho_B \sigma_{B0} \sigma_{B1}}{\sqrt{\sigma_{B0}^2 + \sigma_E^2}\sqrt{\sigma_{B0}^2 + \sigma_{B1}^2 + 2\rho_B \sigma_{B0} \sigma_{B1} + \sigma_E^2}}. \tag{4.8}$$

Furthermore, (y_{ij_1}, y_{ij_2}) also has the bivariate normal distribution with correlation coefficient $\rho_{j_1 j_2}$:

$$\rho_{j_1 j_2} = \frac{\sigma_{B0}^2 + \sigma_{B1}^2 + 2\rho_B \sigma_{B0} \sigma_{B1}}{\sigma_{B0}^2 + \sigma_{B1}^2 + 2\rho_B \sigma_{B0} \sigma_{B1} + \sigma_E^2}. \tag{4.9}$$

Especially when we can ignore the inter-subject variability of the response to the treatment, i.e.,$\sigma_{B1}^2 = 0$ we have

$$\rho_{0j} = \rho_{j_1 j_2} = \frac{\sigma_{B0}^2}{\sigma_{B0}^2 + \sigma_E^2}. \tag{4.10}$$

In this case, the structure of covariance matrix $\boldsymbol{\Sigma}$ becomes *compound symmetry* (3.29). Namely, the existence of inter-subject variability in the baseline data produces a positive correlation coefficient between points in time, and the larger the inter-subject variability σ^2_{B0}, the larger the correlation. Next, consider the following mixed-effects repeated measures model:

Another mixed-effects repeated measures model

$$y_{ij} \mid \boldsymbol{b}_i = \begin{cases} \beta_0 + \beta_1 x_{1i} + b_{0i} + \epsilon_{i0} & \text{for } j = 0 \\ \beta_0 + \beta_1 x_{1i} + \beta_{2j} + \beta_{3j} x_{1i} + b_{0i} + b_{1ij} + \epsilon_{ij} & \text{for } j \geq 1 \end{cases} \tag{4.11}$$

where $(b_{0i}, b_{1i1}, ..., b_{1iT})$ and error terms $\{\epsilon_{ij}, j = 0, ..., T\}$ are independent and b_{1ij} denote the *random slope*, which may change over time. In other words,

$$\boldsymbol{b}_i = (b_{0i}, b_{1i1}, ..., b_{1iT})^t \sim N(0, \boldsymbol{\Phi}) \tag{4.12}$$

where the (l, m)th element of $\boldsymbol{\Phi}$ is

$$(\boldsymbol{\Phi})_{lm} = \rho_{B(l-1)(m-1)} \sigma_{B(l-1)} \sigma_{B(m-1)}, \quad (l, m = 1, ..., T+1). \tag{4.13}$$

In this model, we have

$$\begin{aligned} Var(d_{ij}) &= \sigma^2_{Bj} + 2\sigma^2_E \\ Var(y_{i0}) &= (\boldsymbol{\Sigma})_{11} = \sigma^2_{B0} + \sigma^2_E \\ Var(y_{ij}) &= (\boldsymbol{\Sigma})_{(j+1)(j+1)} = \sigma^2_{B0} + \sigma^2_{Bj} + 2\rho_{B0j}\sigma_{B0}\sigma_{Bj} + \sigma^2_E \\ Cov(y_{i0}, y_{ij}) &= (\boldsymbol{\Sigma})_{1(j+1)} = \sigma^2_{B0} + \rho_{B0j}\sigma_{B0}\sigma_{Bj} \\ Cov(y_{ij_1}, y_{ij_2}) &= (\boldsymbol{\Sigma})_{(j_1+1)(j_2+1)} \\ &= \sigma^2_{B0} + \rho_{B0j_1}\sigma_{B0}\sigma_{Bj_1} + \rho_{B0j_2}\sigma_{B0}\sigma_{Bj_2} + \rho_{Bj_1j_2}\sigma_{Bj_1}\sigma_{Bj_2} \\ &\qquad (\text{for } j_1, j_2 > 0), \end{aligned}$$

where (y_{i0}, y_{ij}) has the bivariate normal distribution with correlation coefficient ρ_{0j}

$$\begin{aligned} \rho_{0j} &= \frac{\sigma^2_{B0} + \rho_{B0j}\sigma_{B0}\sigma_{Bj}}{\sqrt{\sigma^2_{B0} + \sigma^2_E}\sqrt{\sigma^2_{B0} + \sigma^2_{Bj} + 2\rho_{B0j}\sigma_{B0}\sigma_{Bj} + \sigma^2_E}} \\ &= \frac{\sigma^2_{B0} + \rho_{B0j}\sigma_{B0}\sigma_{Bj}}{\sqrt{\sigma^2_{B0} + \sigma^2_E}\sqrt{V_j}}. \end{aligned} \tag{4.14}$$

Furthermore, (y_{ij_1}, y_{ij_2}) also has the bivariate normal distribution with correlation coefficient $\rho_{j_1 j_2}$:

$$\rho_{j_1 j_2} = \frac{\sigma_{B0}^2 + \rho_{B0j_1}\sigma_{B0}\sigma_{Bj_1} + \rho_{B0j_2}\sigma_{B0}\sigma_{Bj_2} + \rho_{Bj_1j_2}\sigma_{Bj_1}\sigma_{Bj_2}}{\sqrt{V_{j_1}V_{j_2}}} \tag{4.15}$$

Namely, in this model, the structure of covariance matrix $\mathbf{\Sigma}$ becomes quite close to *unstructured* (3.32) which is illustrated in Section 7.4.4.

It should be noted here that

1. the *repeated measures data* is also called *hierarchically structured two-level clustered data* where the same subject is called a *cluster* and that the subject is at the level two and the measurements are at the level one, and

2. these correlations (4.8, 4.9, 4.10, 4.14, 4.15) are called *intra-cluster correlations* or ICC.

4.3 ANCOVA-type mixed-effects models

In contrast with the repeated measures model (4.5), we can consider a model to adjust for baseline measurement as a covariate only for *1:T* repeated measures design as is already described in Section (3.7). We shall call this model the *ANCOVA-type mixed-effects model*:

An ANCOVA-type mixed-effects model

$$y_{ij} \mid b_{i(Ancova)} = \begin{cases} \beta_0' + b_{i(Ancova)} + \beta_{2j}' + \theta y_{i0}, + \epsilon_{ij} \text{ (control group)} \\ \beta_0' + b_{i(Ancova)} + \beta_{2j}' + \theta y_{i0} + \beta_1' + \beta_{3j}' + \epsilon_{ij}, \\ \qquad \text{(new treatment group)} \end{cases}$$

$$j = 1, ..., T, \tag{4.16}$$

where $b_{i(Ancova)}$ denotes the *random intercept*, which may reflect the inter-subject variability assumed to be constant during the treatment period, θ is a coefficient for the baseline measurement y_{i0}, and $\beta_1' + \beta_{3j}'$ denotes the treatment effect at the jth time point. For more details and illustrations, see Section (7.7).

4.4 Unbiased estimator for treatment effects

This section involves methodological elements to a certain extent. So, readers who are not interested in methodological details can skip this section and go straight to the next chapter.

Let us consider here several kinds of estimators of treatment effect β_{3j} at time j of the mixed-effects repeated measures model (4.5).

4.4.1 Difference in mean changes from baseline

First, given the variance covariance parameters $(\sigma_E^2, \mathbf{\Phi})$, the maximum likelihood estimator (MLE) of β_{3j} is equal to the difference in mean changes from baseline

$$\hat{\beta}_{3j} = \frac{1}{n_2}\sum_{i=1}^{N} d_{ij}x_{1i} - \frac{1}{n_1}\sum_{i=1}^{N} d_{ij}(1-x_{1i}) \quad (= \hat{\tau}_{21}^{(j)} = \hat{\gamma}_{2j}), \qquad (4.17)$$

which is unbiased estimator of β_{3j}, i.e.,

$$E(\hat{\beta}_{3j}) = \beta_{3j}. \qquad (4.18)$$

Its variance is given by

$$\text{Var}(\hat{\beta}_{3j}) = \frac{n_1+n_2}{n_1 n_2}(\sigma_{B1}^2 + 2\sigma_E^2). \qquad (4.19)$$

where σ_{B1}^2 can be replaced by σ_{Bj}^2 in the model (4.11). For the analysis of the *Rat Data*, the results are shown in Table 2.3 in which Student's t-test for the difference in means of CFB between two groups were repeated at each time point.

4.4.2 Difference in means

On the other hand, as is shown in Table 2.2, the difference in means at the specified time point j, $\hat{\beta}_{3j,Mean}$, is often used as the primary statistical analysis for repeated measures data. The expected value of the difference in means at time j is

$$E(\hat{\beta}_{3j,Mean}) = E\left(\frac{1}{n_2}\sum_{i=1}^{N} y_{ij}x_{1i} - \frac{1}{n_1}\sum_{i=1}^{N} y_{ij}(1-x_{1i})\right) = \beta_{3j} + \beta_1, \tag{4.20}$$

except when $\beta_1 = 0$, $\hat{\beta}_{3j,Mean}$ is a biased estimator of β_{3j}. However, in a well-controlled randomized trial, one would expect that the baseline measurements y_{i0} would be comparable between treatment groups and β_1 would be expected to be zero. Its variance is

$$\text{Var}(\hat{\beta}_{3j,Mean}) = \frac{n_1+n_2}{n_1 n_2}(\sigma_{B0}^2 + \sigma_{B1}^2 + 2\rho_B\sigma_{B0}\sigma_{B1} + \sigma_E^2). \tag{4.21}$$

By comparing the variances of these two estimators, we can say that $\hat{\beta}_{3j}$ could be better than $\hat{\beta}_{3j,Mean}$ if

$$\begin{aligned} & \sigma_{B0}^2 + \sigma_{B1}^2 + 2\rho_B\sigma_{B0}\sigma_{B1} + \sigma_E^2 > \sigma_{B1}^2 + 2\sigma_E^2 \\ \rightarrow\ & \sigma_{B0}^2 + 2\rho_B\sigma_{B0}\sigma_{B1} > \sigma_E^2. \end{aligned} \tag{4.22}$$

Especially when $\sigma_{B1}^2 = 0$, the condition will be

$$Cor(y_{i0}, y_{ij}) = \rho_{0j} > \frac{1}{2}. \tag{4.23}$$

4.4.3 Adjustment due to regression to the mean

First, assume that $\beta_1 = 0$. Then, the expectation of $d_{ij} = y_{ij} - y_{i0}$ conditional on y_{i0} is

$$\begin{aligned} E(d_{ij} \mid y_{i0}) &= E(d_{ij}) + \rho_{d,y0}\sqrt{\frac{\text{Var}(d_{ij})}{\text{Var}(y_{i0})}}(y_{i0} - E(y_{i0})) \\ &= \beta_{2j} + \beta_{3j}x_{1i} - (1-\phi)(y_{i0} - \beta_0) \end{aligned} \tag{4.24}$$

where

$$\phi = \frac{\sigma_{B0}^2 + \rho_B \sigma_{B0}\sigma_{B1}}{\sigma_{B0}^2 + \sigma_E^2} (= \rho_{0j}, \text{ for } \sigma_{B1}^2 = 0). \tag{4.25}$$

and the quantity $-(1-\phi)(y_{i0} - \beta_0)$ is due to so-called *regression to the mean* when $\phi < 1$ (which is usually satisfied). If y_{i0} is greater than the baseline mean β_0, then the term is negative, and if y_{i0} is less than β_0, then the term is positive. In this case, given the variance covariance parameters $(\sigma_E^2, \mathbf{\Phi})$, the unbiased estimator of the treatment effect β_{3j} is given by

$$\tilde{\beta}_{3j} = \hat{\beta}_{3j} + (1-\phi)\left\{\frac{1}{n_2}\sum_{i=1}^{N} y_{i0}x_{1i} - \frac{1}{n_1}\sum_{i=1}^{N} y_{i0}(1-x_{1i})\right\} \tag{4.26}$$

which is equivalent to the estimator $\hat{\beta}_{3j,Ancova}$ based on the ANCOVA approach adjusting for the baseline measurement y_{i0}. In other words, under the mixed-effects repeated measures model (4.5) with $\beta_1 \neq 0$, the ANCOVA estimator has a bias $(1-\phi)\beta_1$ introduced by misspecifying the model (Stanek, 1988; Liang and Zeger, 2000), i.e.,

$$\beta_{3j,Ancova} = \beta_{3j} + (1-\phi)\beta_1. \tag{4.27}$$

However, this bias is also expected to be zero in a well-controlled randomized trial. Furthermore, the variance of $\hat{\beta}_{3j,Ancova}$ is

$$\begin{aligned}\text{Var}(\hat{\beta}_{3j,Ancova}) &= \frac{n_1+n_2}{n_1 n_2}(\sigma_{B1}^2 + 2\sigma_E^2)\left\{1 - \frac{(\sigma_E^2 - \rho_B\sigma_{B0}\sigma_{B1})^2}{(\sigma_{B1}^2 + 2\sigma_E^2)(\sigma_{B0}^2 + \sigma_E^2)}\right\} \\ &= \text{Var}(\hat{\beta}_{3j})\left\{1 - \frac{(\sigma_E^2 - \rho_B\sigma_{B0}\sigma_{B1})^2}{(\sigma_{B1}^2 + 2\sigma_E^2)(\sigma_{B0}^2 + \sigma_E^2)}\right\}. \end{aligned} \tag{4.28}$$

Namely, $\hat{\beta}_{3j,Ancova}$ is more precise than $\hat{\beta}_{3j}$, however, the gain in efficiency by using $\hat{\beta}_{3j,Ancova}$ seems to be small in many cases.

Second, assume that $\beta_1 \neq 0$. Then, the expectation of $d_{ij} = y_{ij} - y_{i0}$ conditional on y_{i0} is

$$E(d_{ij} \mid y_{i0}) = \beta_{2j} + \beta_{3j}x_{1i} - (1-\phi)(y_{i0} - \beta_0 - \beta_1 x_{1i}) \tag{4.29}$$

In this case, given the variance covariance parameters $(\sigma_E^2, \mathbf{\Phi})$, the unbiased estimator of the treatment effect β_{3j} is equivalent to the maximum likelihood estimator $\hat{\beta}_{3j}$.

Example. The *Rat Data*

For illustrating the characteristics of these three estimators, consider the treatment effect at week 3 ($j = 3$). In this experiment, we have the following estimates (s.e.) and p values:

1. $\hat{\beta}_{33} = -3.77\ (\pm 0.093),\ p = 0.0023$ (see Table 2.3, Output 3.1b, Output 3.3)

2. $\hat{\beta}_{33,Mean} = -4.78\ (\pm 0.162),\ p = 0.0146$ (see Table 2.2)

3. $\hat{\beta}_{33,Ancova} = -3.50\ (\pm 0.097),\ p = 0.0057$ (see Program and Output 2.2, Output 3.3)

From these estimates, we have the following:

1. The difference in means $\hat{\beta}_{33,Mean}$ is larger than $\hat{\beta}_{33}$ by $-4.78 - (-3.77) = -1.01$, leading to $\hat{\beta}_1 = -1.01$.

2. The ANCOVA's estimate is larger than $\hat{\beta}_{33}$ by $-3.50 - (-3.77) = 0.027$, leading to $(1 - \phi)\beta_1 = 0.027$. So we have $\hat{\phi} = 1.27$.

Regarding the standard error estimates, the difference in mean CFBs, $\hat{\beta}_{33}$, has the lowest. As shown in Output 3.3, the ANOVA model, without adjusting for baseline data, was shown to fit better than the ANCOVA-type model.

In this section, we compared the three estimators for treatment effect in the ordinary *1:T* repeated measures design. However, when we consider an *S:T* repeated measures design, the ANCOVA-type model adjusting for plural baseline measurements will be unnatural and the mixed-effects repeated measures model (4.5) will be much more natural.

5

Illustration of the mixed-effects models

5.1 Introduction

In this chapter, we shall illustrate the linear mixed-effects models with real data in more detail, especially for readers who have skipped Chapter 4 and are not interested in or not familiar with the technical details described in Chapter 4. To understand mixed-effects models intuitively and visually, the growth curve model to be introduced in the next section would probably be the best example. Then we are going to move on to the *Rat Data* again where the linear mixed-effects models discussed in Chapter 4 are illustrated.

5.2 The Growth Data

First, let us consider here a linear regression model for growth curves arising from an animal experiment with *0:5* repeated measures designs to understand what the mixed-effects models mean. Table 5.1 shows repeated measures on weights for each of 30 rats, measured weekly for five weeks (Gelfand *et al.*, 1990). Figure 5.1 presents subject-specific growth profiles of weight.

5.2.1 Linear regression model

Let y_{ij} denote the weight of the ith rat measured at age t_j. Then, a possible naive model for the repeated measures might be the following linear regression model

$$\begin{aligned} y_{ij} &= \beta_0 + \beta_1 t_j + \epsilon_{ij}, \quad \epsilon_{ij} \sim N(0, \sigma_E^2), \\ & \quad i = 1, ..., 30; \; j = 1, ..., 5 \end{aligned} \tag{5.1}$$

where both the intercept β_0 (weight at birth) and the slope β_1 (growth rate) are assumed to be the same (i.e., *fixed*) for all the rats. In this sense, these two parameters (β_0, β_1) are called *fixed-effects*. Furthermore, the residuals ϵ_{ij}

TABLE 5.1
Growth Data: weight for each of 30 rats, measured weekly for five weeks (Gelfand *et al.*, 1990).

	Days				
Rat No.	8	15	22	29	36
1	151.0	199.0	246.0	283.0	320.0
2	145.0	199.0	249.0	293.0	354.0
3	147.0	214.0	263.0	312.0	328.0
4	155.0	200.0	237.0	272.0	297.0
5	135.0	188.0	230.0	280.0	323.0
6	159.0	210.0	252.0	298.0	331.0
7	141.0	189.0	231.0	275.0	305.0
8	159.0	201.0	248.0	297.0	338.0
9	177.0	236.0	285.0	350.0	376.0
10	134.0	182.0	220.0	260.0	296.0
11	160.0	208.0	261.0	313.0	352.0
12	143.0	188.0	220.0	273.0	314.0
13	154.0	200.0	244.0	289.0	325.0
14	171.0	221.0	270.0	326.0	358.0
15	163.0	216.0	242.0	281.0	312.0
16	160.0	207.0	248.0	288.0	324.0
17	142.0	187.0	234.0	280.0	316.0
18	156.0	203.0	243.0	283.0	317.0
19	157.0	212.0	259.0	307.0	336.0
20	152.0	203.0	246.0	286.0	321.0
21	154.0	205.0	253.0	298.0	334.0
22	139.0	190.0	225.0	267.0	302.0
23	146.0	191.0	229.0	272.0	302.0
24	157.0	211.0	250.0	285.0	323.0
25	132.0	185.0	237.0	286.0	331.0
26	160.0	207.0	257.0	303.0	345.0
27	169.0	216.0	261.0	295.0	333.0
28	157.0	205.0	248.0	289.0	316.0
29	137.0	180.0	219.0	258.0	291.0
30	153.0	200.0	244.0	286.0	324.0

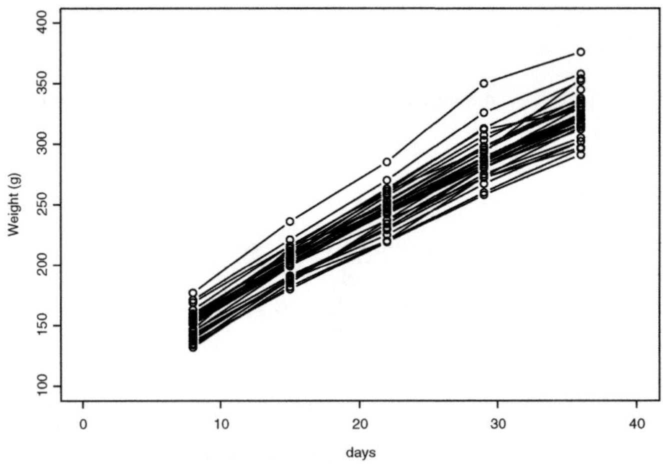

FIGURE 5.1
Growth Data: Growth profiles of weight for each of 30 rats, measured weekly for five weeks.

are assumed to be normally distributed with zero mean and variance σ_E^2 and *any pair of residuals* ϵ_{ij} *and* ϵ_{ik} *are assumed to be independent.* The independence assumption, however, does not fit well to the repeated measures because there usually occur correlations among the repeated measures as described in Chapter 4. For example, Figure 5.2 shows a scatter plot of weight at age 15 days and weight at age 29 days in which a large correlation coefficient 0.844 is observed. These correlations are theoretically shown to be induced by the inter-subject variability or heterogeneity in the baseline data (see (4.8), (4.9), (4.14) and (4.15)). In the growth curve experiment data, the baseline data will correspond to weight at age 8 days.

5.2.2 Random intercept model

Figure 5.1 suggests the existence of inter-subject variability of weight at age 8 days (baseline). Such inter-subject variability may reflect many unobserved characteristics of subjects. To take the inter-subject variability into account, consider the following model, called the *random intercept model*:

$$y_{ij} \mid b_{0i} = (\beta_0 + b_{0i}) + \beta_1 t_j + \epsilon_{ij}, \; \epsilon_{ij} \sim N(0, \sigma_E^2) \quad (5.2)$$

$$b_{0i} \sim N(0, \sigma_{B0}^2) \quad (5.3)$$

where b_{0i} denotes the unobserved random effects, called *random intercept*, which may reflect inter-subject variability due to unobserved characteristics of that subject and is assumed to be independently normally distributed with

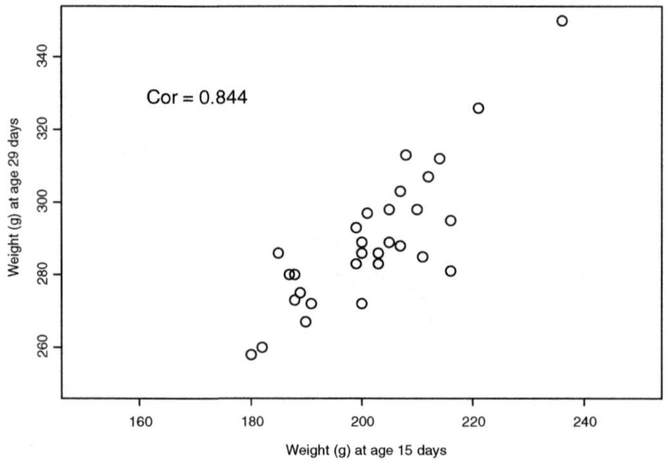

FIGURE 5.2
Growth Data: Scatter plot of weight at age 15 days and weight at age 29 days in which the correlation coefficient is 0.844.

mean 0 and variance σ_{B0}^2 and $(\beta_0 + b_{0i})$ denotes the subject-specific intercept. This model is also called the *mixed-effects* model in that it includes both fixed effects and random effects. *In the mixed-effects model, conditional on the values of the random effects b_{0i}, the repeated measurements are assumed to be independent and follow the linear model $\beta_0 + \beta_1 t_j + (b_{0i} + \epsilon_{ij})$, and any pair of residuals ϵ_{ij} and ϵ_{ik}, i.e., the repeated measurements, are assumed to be independent.* Then, the residual that would be present in the naive model (5.1) has been decomposed into two parts: random effects b_{0i}, which is constant over time, and a residual ϵ_{ij}, which varies randomly over time. The b_{0i} and ϵ_{ij} are assumed to be independent of each other. Then, the variance of each repeated measurement is

$$\text{Var}(y_{ij}) = \sigma_{B0}^2 + \sigma_E^2 \tag{5.4}$$

and the covariances between any two repeated measurements, y_{ij} at age j and y_{ik} at age k, are all the same as

$$\text{Cov}(y_{ij}, y_{ik}) = \sigma_{B0}^2. \tag{5.5}$$

Namely, it follows from the two relations (5.4) and (5.5) that the correlation between y_{ij} and y_{ik} is given by

$$\text{Cor}(y_{ij}, y_{ik}) = \frac{\sigma_{B0}^2}{\sigma_{B0}^2 + \sigma_E^2}, \tag{5.6}$$

which is the *intra-class correlation* or *intra-cluster correlation* where the *subject* is called *class* or *cluster*. This correlation also indicates the proportion of the total variance that is due to inter-subject variability. This is also called the *compound symmetry* structure or the *exchangeable* structure because of equal variance and equal covariance regardless of measurement times (see (3.29)).

5.2.3 Random intercept plus slope model

In a similar manner, we can introduce the following *random intercept plus slope* model that takes account of a possible inter-subject variability of the *growth rate* in addition to the intercept:

$$y_{ij} \mid \boldsymbol{b}_i = (\beta_0 + b_{0i}) + (\beta_1 + b_{1i})t_j + \epsilon_{ij}, \ \epsilon_{ij} \sim N(0, \sigma_E^2) \tag{5.7}$$

$$\boldsymbol{b}_i = (b_{0i}, b_{1i})^t \sim N(0, \boldsymbol{\Phi}) \tag{5.8}$$

$$\boldsymbol{\Phi} = \begin{pmatrix} \sigma_{B0}^2 & \rho_B \sigma_{B0} \sigma_{B1} \\ \rho_B \sigma_{B0} \sigma_{B1} & \sigma_{B1}^2 \end{pmatrix}, \tag{5.9}$$

where b_{1i} denotes the *random slope*, $(\beta_1 + b_{1i})$ denotes the subject-specific slope reflecting inter-subject variability of growth rate, and the two random effects are assumed to have a bivariate normal distribution with zero mean and covariance matrix Φ. Here also, the (b_{0i}, b_{1i}) and ϵ_{ij} are assumed to be independent of each other. With this model, we have

$$\text{Var}(y_{ij}) = \sigma_{B0}^2 + 2\rho_B \sigma_{B0} \sigma_{B1} + \sigma_{B1}^2 t_j^2 + \sigma_E^2 \tag{5.10}$$

$$\text{Cov}(y_{ij}, y_{ik}) = \sigma_{B0}^2 + \rho_B \sigma_{B0} \sigma_{B1}(t_j + t_k) + \sigma_{B1}^2 t_j t_k, \tag{5.11}$$

which shows that the correlation is no longer the same for all pairs of measurement times. The above story tells us that some correlation structure among the repeated measures data can naturally arise from an introduction of random effects. This is an interesting and important feature of the mixed-effects model.

5.2.4 Analysis using SAS

First, we shall fit the ordinary regression model (5.1) to the *Growth Data* shown in Table 5.1 using the SAS procedure `PROC GLM`. The data structure

TABLE 5.2
Growth Data (Table 5.1): Data structure for SAS `PROC GLM` (Data for the first two rats are shown).

no	Weight y	id	day
1	151	1	8
2	199	1	15
3	246	1	22
4	283	1	29
5	320	1	36
6	145	2	8
7	199	2	15
8	249	2	22
9	293	2	29
10	354	2	36

for SAS appears in Table 5.2. A list of variables used in the analysis is as follows:

1. `y` weight
2. `day` age
3. `id` the subject id $(= 1, 2, ..., 30)$

The SAS program used to fit the model and a part of the results is shown in Program and Output 5.1.

Program and Output 5.1. SAS `PROC GLM` for the model (5.1)

```
<program>
data d3;
  infile 'c:\book\RepeatedMeasure\ratlong.dat' missover;
  input no y id day;
proc glm data=d3;  class group;
model y  =  day  /solution clparm;
run;

<output>
R-Square Coeff Var Root MSE   y Mean
0.935910 6.648275  16.13226   242.6533

Parameter Estimate Standard Error t Value Pr > |t|  Lower Upper
Intercept 106.5676          3.20994 33.20  <.0001  100.2243 112.9108
day         6.1857          0.13305 46.49  <.0001    5.9227   6.4486
```

The estimated regression line is $y = 106.6 + 6.19x$ and the estimates of the standard error of the intercept and the slope are 3.21, 0.133, respectively.

From the value of "Root MSE", we have $\hat{\sigma}_E^2 = 16.13^2 = 260.2$. The test result for the slope: $H_0 : \beta_1 = 0$ is highly significant ($p < .0001$).

Second, we shall fit the *random intercept model* (5.2) to the *Growth Data*. The SAS program and a part of the output are shown in Program and Output 5.2. To indicate the *random intercept* in `PROC MIXED`, we can use the following `RANDOM` statement

```
random intercept / subject = id, g gcorr;
```

In this case, to indicate *error terms* ϵ_{ij} distributed with a normal distribution with mean 0 and variance σ_E^2, we use the option `type = simple` in the `REPEATED` statement like this

```
repeated day / type = simple subject = id, r rcorr;
```

Program and Output 5.2. SAS `PROC MIXED` for the model (5.2)

```
<program>
proc mixed data = d3 method=reml covtest;
   class id ;
   model y =  day / s cl ddfm=sat;
   random  intercept /  subject=id g gcorr ;
   repeated  / type=simple subject=id r rcorr;
   run ;

<output>
Covariance Parameter Estimates
Cov Parm Subject     Estimate S.E.   Z value Pr > Z
Intercept  id         196.94   55.2812 3.56 0.0002
Residual   id          67.3025  8.7251 7.71 <.0001

Fit Statistics
-2 Res Log Likelihood 1137.3
AIC (smaller is better) 1141.3

Solution for Fixed Effects
Effect    Estimate     S.E. DF t Value Pr>|t| Alpha Lower Upper
Intercept 106.57  3.0380   49 35.08 <.0001 0.05 100.46  112.67
day        6.1857 0.06766 119 91.42 <.0001 0.05   6.0517  6.3197
```

Although the estimated linear regression line was the same $y = 106.6 + 6.19x$ as the model (5.1), we have here $\hat{\sigma}_{B0}^2 = 196.9$ and $\hat{\sigma}_E^2 = 67.3$. Namely, the error variance σ_E^2 of the model (5.1) is decomposed into the two variance components, σ_{B0}^2 and σ_E^2, of the random intercept model. As a result, the standard errors of the intercept and the slope $(3.04, 0.068)$ were smaller than $(3.21, 0.13)$ of the model (5.1) and the corresponding t-values were bigger, indicating the increase of the precision of estimates of the fixed-effects parameters.

Finally, let us fit the *random intercept plus slope model* (5.7). The SAS program and outputs are shown in Program and Output 5.3. It should be noted that to specify the *random intercept and slope model* in `PROC MIXED`, we need the following RANDOM statement: When you would like to fit the model with $\rho_B \neq 0$, you have to use the following

```
random  intercept day / type=un subject=id g gcorr ;
```

When you would like to fit the model with $\rho_B = 0$, then

```
random  intercept day / type=simple subject=id g gcorr ;
```

To compare these two models, you can use AIC and BIC.

Program and Output 5.3. SAS PROC MIXED **for the model (5.7)**

```
<program>
 proc mixed data = d3 method=reml covtest;
   class id ;
   model y =  day / s cl ddfm=sat cl ;
   random  intercept day / type=un subject=id g gcorr ;
  ( random  intercept day / type=simple subject=id g gcorr ; )
   repeated / type=simple subject=id r rcorr;
run ;

<A part of output: type=un >
Covariance Parameter Estimates
Cov Parm Subject  Estimate S.E.    Z value Pr > Z
UN(1,1)     id    115.42   42.0847  2.74 0.0030
UN(2,1)     id     -0.8731  1.4493 -0.60 0.5469
UN(2,2)     id      0.2607  0.08853 2.94 0.0016
Residual    id     36.1756  5.3927  6.71 <.0001

Fit Statistics
-2 Res Log Likelihood 1095.4
AIC (smaller is better) 1103.4

Solution for Fixed Effects
Effect    Estimate S.E. DF t Value Pr>|t| Alpha Lower Upper
Intercept 106.57   2.2977 29 46.38 <.0001 0.05 101.87 111.27
day         6.1857 0.1056 29 58.58 <.0001 0.05 5.9698 6.4017

<A part of output : type=simple>
Covariance Parameter Estimates
Cov Parm Subject      Estimate S.E.  Z value Pr > Z
Intercept id 106.31   37.4931  2.84 0.0023
day       id   0.2417  0.07887 3.06 0.0011
Residual  id  36.8340  5.4817  6.72 <.0001

Fit Statistics
-2 Res Log Likelihood 1095.8
AIC (smaller is better) 1101.8

Solution for Fixed Effects
Effect group week Estimate S.E. DF t Value Pr>|t| Alpha Lower Upper
Intercept 106.57   2.2365 32.6 47.65 <.0001 0.05 102.02 111.12
day         6.1857 0.1028 32.6 60.18 <.0001 0.05 5.9765 6.3949
```

AIC chose the independence model ($\rho_B = 0$). In this model also, we have the same regression line with variance estimates: $\hat{\sigma}^2_{B0} = 106.31$, $\hat{\sigma}^2_{B1} = 0.2417$, and $\hat{\sigma}^2_E = 36.83$. The error variance 36.83 was smaller than 67.3 of the random-intercept model and the resultant standard errors $(2.24, 0.103)$ for the intercept and the slope were smaller than $(3.21, 0.133)$ of the random intercept model. Judging from AIC, the *random intercept plus slope model* with $\rho_B = 0$ was the best fit to the *Growth Data.* One purpose of this experiment is to estimate the mean weight at birth β_0, which was estimated to be 106.6 $(95\%CI : 102.0 - 111.1)$ in the *random intercept plus slope model.*

5.3 The Rat Data

In Section 3.5, we applied an analysis of variance model (3.3) to the *Rat Data* shown in Table 3.5 using `PROC MIXED`. In this section, let us apply a *random intercept model* and a *random intercept plus slope model* to the data via the expression of mixed-effects repeated measures model (4.5), introduced in Chapter 4.

5.3.1 Random intercept model

First, a *random intercept model* expressing the inter-subject variability at week 0 (baseline) can be given as

$$y_{ij} \mid b_{0i} = \begin{cases} \beta_0 + \beta_1 x_{1i} + b_{0i} + \epsilon_{i0} & \text{for } j = 0 \\ \beta_0 + \beta_1 x_{1i} + \beta_{2j} + \beta_{3j} x_{1i} + b_{0i} + \epsilon_{ij} & \text{for } j \geq 1, \end{cases} \tag{5.12}$$

where b_{0i} denotes the unobserved random effects, called *random intercept,* which may reflect inter-subject variability due to possibly many unobserved prognostic factors at baseline and is assumed to be independently normally distributed with mean 0 and variance σ^2_{B0}, and $(\beta_0 + b_{0i})$ denotes the subject-specific intercept. The residuals ϵ_{ij} are assumed to be normally distributed with zero mean and variance σ^2_E and the b_{0i} and ϵ_{ij} are assumed to be independent of each other and

$$x_{1i} = \begin{cases} 1, & \text{if the } i\text{th subject is assigned to the new treatment} \\ 0, & \text{if the } i\text{th subject is assigned to the control.} \end{cases} \tag{5.13}$$

Interpretations of the fixed effects β's are as follows:

1. β_1 denotes the difference in means at time 0.

2. β_{2j} denotes the mean change from baseline at time j in the control group.

3. $\beta_{2j} + \beta_{3j}$ denotes the mean change from baseline at time j in the new treatment group.

4. β_{3j} denotes the difference in mean changes from baseline between two groups, or an effect for the treatment-by-time interaction. In other words, it denotes the effect size of the new treatment compared with the control treatment at time j (corresponding to $\tau_{21}^{(j)}$ defined in (3.10)).

Then, the model (5.12) can be re-expressed as the following model:

$$\begin{aligned} y_{ij} \mid b_{0i} &= \beta_0 + \beta_1 x_{1i} + \beta_{2j} x_{2ij} + \beta_{3j} x_{1i} x_{2ij} + b_{0i} + \epsilon_{ij} \\ & \quad b_{0i} \sim N(0, \sigma_{B0}^2), \quad \epsilon_{ij} \sim N(0, \sigma_E^2) \\ & \quad j = 0, 1, 2, 3; \; \beta_{20} = 0, \; \beta_{30} = 0, \end{aligned} \tag{5.14}$$

where

$$x_{2ij} = \begin{cases} 1, & \text{for } j \geq 1 \text{ (evaluation period)} \\ 0, & \text{for } j \leq 0 \text{ (baseline period).} \end{cases} \tag{5.15}$$

In this mixed-effects model, the treatment effect at time j can be expressed as

$$\beta_{3j} = \beta_{3j} - \beta_{30} = \beta_{3j} \; (j = 1, 2, 3), \tag{5.16}$$

which corresponds to $\tau_{21}^{(j)}$ (3.9) defined in the ANOVA model. For example, the treatment effect at week 3 can be expressed using linear contrast:

$$\beta_{33} - \beta_{30} = (-1, 0, 0, 1)(\beta_{30}, \beta_{31}, \beta_{32}, \beta_{33})^t \; (= \tau_{21}^{(3)}). \tag{5.17}$$

Therefore, the average treatment effect over the measurement period is

$$\frac{1}{3}\sum_{j=1}^{3}(\beta_{3j} - \beta_{30}) = \frac{1}{3}(-3, 1, 1, 1)(\beta_{30}, \beta_{31}, \beta_{32}, \beta_{33})^t. \tag{5.18}$$

which corresponds to τ_{21} (3.11) in the ANOVA model. Now, let us apply the *random intercept model* to the *Rat Data* using `PROC MIXED`. Although the SAS program used here is quite similar to the one used for the analysis of variance model (Section 3.5), the following points are different:

1. In the ANOVA model, the variable `group` indicating the treatment group (1=control, 2=new treatment), is defined as a numeric factor. However, in here, the variable `group` indicating x_{1i} is defined as a continuous binary variable (0=control, 1=new treatment). Therefore, delete the variable `group` from the `CLASS` statement and add `group = group - 1` in the `DATA` step.

2. Add the following `RANDOM` statement

```
random intercept / subject=id, g, gcorr;
```

   where `intercept` denotes the inter-subject variability at baseline b_{0i}. Then use the following modified `REPEATED` statement

```
repeated week / type=simple subject = id r rcorr ;
```

3. The fixed effects β_{2j} can be expressed via the variable `week` (main factor), which must be specified as a numeric factor by the `CLASS` statement.

4. The fixed effects β_{3j} can be expressed via the `group * week` interaction. However, we have to change the order of the elements in the linear contrast corresponding to the average treatment effect (5.18) in the `ESTIMATE` statement as

```
group*week 1 1 1 -3
```

   due to the option `/ref=first` as explained in Program 3.1 for an ANOVA model in Section 3.5. It should be noted that, in the ANOVA model, the variable `group` is defined as a numeric factor and thus the linear contrast has been set as

```
group*week 1 1 1 -3 -1 -1 -1 3
```

The SAS program and a part of the output are shown in Program and Output 5.4.

Program and Output 5.4 SAS `PROC MIXED` for the model (5.14)

```
< SAS program >
data d1;
  infile 'c:\book\RepeatedMeasure\experimentRat.dat' missover;
  input id group week y;
  group=group-1;

proc mixed data=d1 method=reml covtest;
  class id  week / ref=first ;
  model y = group week group*week / s cl ddfm=sat ;
  random intercept /  subject= id g gcorr ;
  repeated week/ type = simple subject = id r  rcorr ;
  estimate 'mean CFB ' group*week 1 1 1 -3
                     / divisor=3 cl alpha=0.05;
run;

<A part of output: type=simple >
Fit statistics
-2 Res Log Likelihood 140.8
AIC (smaller is better) 144.8
BIC (smaller is better) 145.8

Covariance Parameter Estimates
Cov Parm Subject      Estimate S.E.   Z value Pr > Z
Intercept   id        4.0382  1.8736  2.16 0.0156
Residual    id        0.6017  0.1553  3.87 <.0001

Solution for Fixed Effects
Effect     week Estimate S.E. DF t Value Pr>|t| Alpha Lower Upper
Intercept      10.9333 0.8794 12.2 12.43 <.0001 0.05 9.0212 12.8455
group          -1.0167 1.2436 12.2 -0.82 0.4293 0.05 -3.7208 1.6875
week        1  0.2000 0.4478 30    0.45 0.6584 0.05 -0.7146 1.1146
week        2 -0.6500 0.4478 30   -1.45 0.1570 0.05 -1.5646 0.2646
week        3 -2.8500 0.4478 30   -6.36 <.0001 0.05 -3.7646 -1.9354
week        0  0 . . . . . . .
group*week  1  0.7000 0.6333 30    1.11 0.2778 0.05 -0.5934 1.9934
group*week  2 -0.4000 0.6333 30   -0.63 0.5324 0.05 -1.6934 0.8934
group*week  3 -3.7667 0.6333 30   -5.95 <.0001 0.05 -5.0601 -2.4732
group*week  0  0

Estimates
Label      Estimate S.E.  DF  t Value Pr>|t| Alpha Lower Upper
mean CFB  -1.1556 0.5171 30    -2.23 0.0330 0.05 -2.2116 -0.09947
```

As compared with the SAS outputs (Output 3.1a) of the analysis of variance model (3.3), the variance estimate σ^2_{B0} is shown here as the parameter `Intecept` of the column "Covariance Parameter Estimates," not as the parameter `CS` (compound symmetry model). Other outputs are all the same as those of the analysis of variance model.

5.3.2 Random intercept plus slope model

As the second model, consider a *random intercept plus slope model* by simply adding the random slope b_{1i} taking account of the inter-subject variability of the response assumed to be constant during the treatment period (or to the treatment). It should be noted here that the *random slope* introduced in this model does not mean the *slope* on the time or a linear time trend because the model discussed here aims at estimating the treatment effect at each measurement time point. Using an expression similar to (5.12), the model is expressed as

$$y_{ij} \mid (b_{0i}, b_{1i}) = \begin{cases} \beta_0 + \beta_1 x_{1i} + b_{0i} + \epsilon_{i0} & \text{for } j = 0 \\ \beta_0 + \beta_1 x_{1i} + \beta_{2j} + \beta_{3j} x_{1i} + b_{0i} + b_{1i} + \epsilon_{ij} & \text{for } j \geq 1. \end{cases} \tag{5.19}$$

Then the model is re-expressed as the following mixed-effects model:

$$\begin{aligned} y_{ij} \mid \boldsymbol{b}_i &= \beta_0 + b_{0i} + b_{1i} x_{2ij} + \beta_1 x_{1i} + (\beta_{2j} + b_{1i}) x_{2ij} \\ &\quad + \beta_{3j} x_{1i} x_{2ij} + \epsilon_{ij} \\ &\quad \boldsymbol{b}_i = (b_{0i}, b_{1i})^t \sim N(0, \boldsymbol{\Phi}), \quad \epsilon_{ij} \sim N(0, \sigma_E^2) \\ &\quad j = 0, 1, 2, 3; \ \beta_{20} = 0, \ \beta_{30} = 0, \end{aligned} \tag{5.20}$$

where

$$\boldsymbol{\Phi} = \begin{pmatrix} \sigma_{B0}^2 & \rho_B \sigma_{B0} \sigma_{B1} \\ \rho_B \sigma_{B0} \sigma_{B1} & \sigma_{B1}^2 \end{pmatrix}. \tag{5.21}$$

In the SAS procedure `PROC MIXED`, the random slope b_{1i} can be expressed by a new binary variable `post` indicating x_{2ij}. For example, to apply the model with $\rho_B = 0$, we have only to modify the Program 5.4 as follows:

1. First, create the variable `post` in the `DATA` statement as

```
if week=0 then post=0; else post=1;
```

2. Then, include the variable `post` in the `RANDOM` statement as

```
random intercept post / type=simple subject=id g gcorr;
```

A part of the SAS output is shown in Output 5.5.

Output 5.5: A part of SAS outputs for the model (5.20)

```
Covariance Parameter Estimates
Cov Parm Subject  Estimate    S.E.   Z value   Pr > Z
Intercept  id       4.0382   1.8736   2.16     0.0156
post       id       1.11E-16 . . .
week       id       0.6017   0.1553   3.87     <.0001
```

In this example, the estimated inter-subject variance is $\hat{\sigma}^2_{B1} = 0$ (1.11E-16), Namely, the *random intercept plus slope* model was degenerated to the *random intercept* model, i.e., all the parameter estimates are the same as those of the *random intercept* model shown in Output 5.4.

5.3.3 Random intercept plus slope model with slopes varying over time

As the third model, consider a *random intercept plus slope model* by adding the random effects $b_{1ij}, j = 1, 2, 3$ taking account of the inter-subject variability of the response assumed to be varying during the treatment period. Using an expression similar to (5.12), the model is expressed as

$$y_{ij} \mid \boldsymbol{b}_i = \begin{cases} \beta_0 + \beta_1 x_{1i} + b_{0i} + \epsilon_{i0} & \text{for } j = 0 \\ \beta_0 + \beta_1 x_{1i} + \beta_{2j} + \beta_{3j} x_{1i} + b_{0i} + b_{1ij} + \epsilon_{ij} & \text{for } j \geq 1. \end{cases} \tag{5.22}$$

where $\boldsymbol{b}_i = (b_{0i}, b_{1i1}, b_{1i2}, b_{1i3})^t$. Then the model is re-expressed as the following mixed-effects model:

$$\begin{aligned} y_{ij} \mid \boldsymbol{b}_i &= \beta_0 + b_{0i} + b_{1i} x_{2ij} + \beta_1 x_{1i} + (\beta_{2j} + b_{1ij}) x_{2ij} \\ &\qquad + \beta_{3j} x_{1i} x_{2ij} + \epsilon_{ij} \qquad (5.23) \\ &\quad \boldsymbol{b}_i = (b_{0i}, b_{1i1}, b_{1i2}, b_{1i3})^t \sim N(0, \boldsymbol{\Phi}), \quad \epsilon_{ij} \sim N(0, \sigma_E^2) \\ &\quad j = 0, 1, 2, 3; \ \beta_{20} = 0, \ \beta_{30} = 0. \end{aligned}$$

To do this using the SAS procedure `PROC MIXED`, follow these steps:

1. First, create the three binary variables (`w1, w2, w3`) representing the random slopes $(b_{1i1}, b_{1i2}, b_{1i3})$ in the `DATA` statement as

```
if week=1 then w1=1; else w1=0;
if week=2 then w2=1; else w2=0;
if week=3 then w3=1; else w3=0;
```

2. Then, include these three variables in the RANDOM statement as

```
random intercept w1 w2 w3 / type=un subject=id g gcorr;
```

However, the program did not converge for the *Rat Data* due possibly to the situation where the number of parameters to be estimated (11) is almost equal to the number of subjects (12). As already discussed in Section 4.2, the covariance matrix $\boldsymbol{\Sigma}$ of this model can be quite close to an *unstructured* covariance model (3.32) and it will be shown that the treatment effects of this model can be approximated well by the *unstructured* covariance model for the *Beat the Blues Data* in Chapter 7. So here, let us apply the unstructured covariance model instead of this model. To apply this model using the SAS procedure PROC MIXED, we have only to delete the random statement of Program 5.4 and change the repeated statement to

```
repeated week/ type = un subject = id r  rcorr ;
```

Part of the results are shown in Output 5.6, which is the same as those of the corresponding part of Output 3.1b, although the estimates of $\boldsymbol{\Phi}$ are not available in this program. The details of the results have already been described in Section 3.5 and, based on AIC or BIC, the third model (5.23) with the unstructured covariance is the best fitted model among the three models introduced in this section.

Output 5.6: A part of SAS outputs for the model (5.22)

```
Solution for Fixed Effects
Effect     week Estimate S.E. DF t Value Pr>|t| Alpha Lower Upper
group*week 1  0.7000 0.1155 10  6.06 0.0001 0.05  0.4427 0.9573
group*week 2 -0.4000 0.3332 10 -1.20 0.2576 0.05 -1.1423 0.3423
group*week 3 -3.7667 0.9267 10 -4.06 0.0023 0.05 -5.8315 -1.7018
group*week 0 0 . . . . . . .
```

I would like to re-emphasize here that, if there is no missing data, the statistical inference of the treatment effect at each time point via the analysis of variance model with the unstructured covariance or the linear mixed-effects model (5.23) is identical to the result of Student's two-sample t-test for the difference in means of CFB between groups using only the data necessary for the analysis.

6

Likelihood-based ignorable analysis for missing data

6.1 Introduction

In this chapter, we shall illustrate a good property of the mixed-effects model for handing missing data. We can apply the *likelihood-based ignorable analysis* under the relatively weak assumption of MAR (missing at random) without a list-wise deletion or imputation methods. Before going to illustrations, we would like to discuss how to handle missing data in mixed-effects models.

6.2 Handling of missing data

In any type of longitudinal or repeated measures studies, occurrence of missing data is not unnatural or inevitable. In animal experiments, missing data may often arise by some experimental mistake. In this case, we can say that such missing data arose *at random*. However, missing data may arise even when summarizing the data to report the experimental results. To change the results in the investigator's own direction, deleting some data or setting some data as "missing" by a *deliberate fabrication* may produce missing data. In this case, the investigator makes a decision to set the data as missing depending on the actual value of the data. Needless to say, this is obviously "fraud" but it appears to be "missing data." In any case, we cannot say such "missing data" are "missing at random," rather we can say "missing not at random." In the latter situation, *complete case* analysis or the analysis based on the *observed data only* obviously leads to some biased invalid results.

Similar situations often arise in clinical trials and epidemiological studies. In clinical trials, missing data often occur due to subject dropout (attrition) or intermittent non-visits to the hospital. Dropout indicates the missing patterns in which missing data are always only followed by missing data. The problem is the nature of the "dropout." If some dropout happens due to some adverse effect of the treatment or worsening of the health condition, these dropouts may be called "informative dropouts." Missing data caused by such dropout can also be described as "missing not at random," like the above-stated missing data due to deliberate fabrication in animal experiments, in the sense that *complete case* analysis produces some biased invalid results. In clinical trials, a *standard method* for dealing with missing data in repeated measurements or longitudinal data has been based on *last observation carried forward* (LOCF). EMEA (the European drugs regulator, 2001) wrote that LOCF is likely to be acceptable if measurements are expected to be relatively constant over time. However, it seems that no one can verify the assumption from the observed data. LOCF is indeed a practical tool in the sense of respecting the intention-to-treat principle by including all individuals in the analysis, but unfortunately has no statistical validity.

In epidemiological study, non-response to a questionnaire may produce informative missing data. For example, even if an investigator tries to examine the association of the risk of some diseases with annual income, participants with very low incomes or very high incomes are usually less likely to fill in his/her actual income in the questionnaire. Namely, missing data for the variable "income" are more likely informative.

In this book, when referring to the missing data, we will use a classification of *missing data mechanism* introduced by Rubin (1976, 1987). To introduce his approach, let us define the following:

- $\boldsymbol{y}_i = (y_{i(-S+1)}, ..., y_{i0}, y_{i1}, ..., y_{iT})^t, \ i = 1, ..., N,$
- Let $\boldsymbol{\theta}$ denote the vector that contains the fixed-effects parameters $\boldsymbol{\beta}$ and the variance-covariance components such as σ_E^2 and $\boldsymbol{\Phi}$ that we wish to estimate.
- Let $\boldsymbol{y}_{i,obs}$ denote the subset of repeated measures that are observed and $\boldsymbol{y}_{i,mis}$ denote the subset of repeated measures that are missing.
- Let $\boldsymbol{r}_i = (r_{i(-S+1),...,r_{i0},r_{i1},...,r_{iT}})^t$ denote the vector of an indicator having a value of 1 if y_{ij} is observed and 0 if y_{ij} is missing.

Then, to make a sound statistical inference on $\boldsymbol{\theta}$, we need to consider the following joint probability distribution

$$p(\boldsymbol{y}_i, \boldsymbol{r}_i \mid \boldsymbol{\theta}, \boldsymbol{\xi}) \tag{6.1}$$

where $\boldsymbol{\xi}$ denotes the vector of parameters governing the missing data mechanism and is assumed to be different from $\boldsymbol{\theta}$ to be estimated. Then, the joint distribution is factored into two parts (1) the marginal distribution of data and (2) the conditional probability of observing the data, given their values, i.e.,

$$p(\boldsymbol{y}_i, \boldsymbol{r}_i \mid \boldsymbol{\theta}, \boldsymbol{\xi}) = p(\boldsymbol{y}_i \mid \boldsymbol{\theta}) p(\boldsymbol{r}_i \mid \boldsymbol{y}_i, \boldsymbol{\xi}), \tag{6.2}$$

which is called the *selection model.* Rubin (1976) defines the three classes of missing data mechanisms by modeling the second term of equation (6.2), i.e.,

$$p(\boldsymbol{r}_i \mid \boldsymbol{y}_i, \boldsymbol{\xi}) \quad = \quad p(\boldsymbol{r}_i \mid \boldsymbol{y}_{i,obs}, \boldsymbol{y}_{i,mis}, \boldsymbol{\xi}). \tag{6.3}$$

- **MCAR**: We say data are *Missing Completely at Random* if the probability does not depend either on the observed (non-missing) data or on the actual values of the missing data, i.e.,

$$p(\boldsymbol{r}_i \mid \boldsymbol{y}_{i,obs}, \boldsymbol{y}_{i,mis}, \boldsymbol{\xi}) \quad = \quad p(\boldsymbol{r}_i \mid \boldsymbol{\xi}). \tag{6.4}$$

  The above-stated missing data that occurred *by some experimental mistake* is MCAR.

- **MAR**: We say data are *Missing at Random* if, given the observed data, the probability does not depend on the actual values of the missing data, i.e.,

$$p(\boldsymbol{r}_i \mid \boldsymbol{y}_{i,obs}, \boldsymbol{y}_{i,mis}, \boldsymbol{\xi}) \quad = \quad p(\boldsymbol{r}_i \mid \boldsymbol{y}_{i,obs}, \boldsymbol{\xi}). \tag{6.5}$$

  For example, suppose that younger children are more prone to missing spirometry measurements, in other words, the probability of missing depends on the age group but that the probability of missing is unrelated to the actual value of the missing data within the age group. In this situation, if the variable age is observed and included in the analysis, we can say missing spirometry data would be MAR dependent on age.

- **MNAR**: We say data are *Missing Not at Random* if the probability does depend on the actual values of the missing data. In the missing spirometry example, the spirometry data is MNAR if patients with a low spirometry value are more likely to have their spirometry recorded than other patients of the same age.

As these terminologies have already been used in the above explanation in a conversational manner, readers may understand the typology easily. However, the difficulty in dealing with missing data is that we cannot judge from the data at hand whether the missing data are MCAR, MAR or MNAR because the missing data are not observed.

6.3 Likelihood-based ignorable analysis

Regardless, the MAR assumption may be made more likely by collecting more explanatory variables such as age in the spirometry example, which may explain missing data, or by collecting repeated measures. Under the assumption of MAR, a valid inference can be obtained through either a likelihood-based ignorable analysis or multiple imputations. In the context of likelihood-based inference where the parameters describing the observed data are different from the parameters describing the missing data mechanism, the former parameters can be estimated simply by maximizing the likelihood for the observed data as follows:

$$\begin{aligned}
p(\boldsymbol{y}_{i,obs}, \boldsymbol{r}_i \mid \boldsymbol{\theta}, \boldsymbol{\xi}) &= \int \cdots \int_{\boldsymbol{y}_{i,mis}} p(\boldsymbol{y}_i, \boldsymbol{r}_i \mid \boldsymbol{\theta}, \boldsymbol{\xi}) d\boldsymbol{y}_{i,mis} \\
&= \int \cdots \int_{\boldsymbol{y}_{i,mis}} p(\boldsymbol{y}_i \mid \boldsymbol{\theta}) p(\boldsymbol{r}_i \mid \boldsymbol{y}_{i,obs}, \boldsymbol{y}_{i,mis}, \boldsymbol{\xi}) d\boldsymbol{y}_{i,mis} \\
&= \int \cdots \int_{\boldsymbol{y}_{i,mis}} p(\boldsymbol{y}_{i,obs}, \boldsymbol{y}_{i,mis} \mid \boldsymbol{\theta}) p(\boldsymbol{r}_i \mid \boldsymbol{y}_{i,obs}, \boldsymbol{\xi}) d\boldsymbol{y}_{i,mis} \\
&= p(\boldsymbol{y}_{i,obs} \mid \boldsymbol{\theta}) p(\boldsymbol{r}_i \mid \boldsymbol{y}_{i,obs}, \boldsymbol{\xi}) \\
&\propto p(\boldsymbol{y}_{i,obs} \mid \boldsymbol{\theta}). \qquad (6.6)
\end{aligned}$$

For the generalized linear mixed-effects model, we have (see Appendix B, Section B.1)

$$p(\boldsymbol{y}_{i,obs} \mid \boldsymbol{\theta}) = \int \cdots \int_{\boldsymbol{b}_i} p(\boldsymbol{y}_{i,obs} \mid \boldsymbol{\theta}, \boldsymbol{b}_i) f(\boldsymbol{b}_i \mid \boldsymbol{\Phi}) d\boldsymbol{b}_i. \qquad (6.7)$$

Namely, the likelihood is expressed as

$$\prod_{i=1}^{N} p(\boldsymbol{y}_{i,obs}, \boldsymbol{r}_i \mid \boldsymbol{\theta}, \boldsymbol{\xi}) \propto \prod_{i=1}^{N} \int \cdots \int_{\boldsymbol{b}_i} p(\boldsymbol{y}_{i,obs} \mid \boldsymbol{\theta}, \boldsymbol{b}_i) f(\boldsymbol{b}_i \mid \boldsymbol{\Phi}) d\boldsymbol{b}_i = L(\boldsymbol{\theta}). \qquad (6.8)$$

Therefore, the missing data $\boldsymbol{y}_{i,miss}$ can be said to be *ignorable*. This method is called *likelihood-based ignorable analysis* or the *ignorable maximum likelihood method*. In other words, we can apply the generalized linear mixed-effects models by simply ignoring (deleting) only the record that includes missing data in a *long format* data file without a list-wise deletion.

Multiple imputations (for example, see Schafer 1997; White et al., 2011; van Buuren, 2012; Carpenter and Kenward, 2013), on the other hand, need the following three basic steps:

1. Impute missing data from the pre-specified *imputation model* and generate several data sets each with slightly different imputed values.

2. Perform the *analysis model* on each of the data sets.

3. Summarize all the results to obtain the estimates, standard errors and test statistics using Rubin's rule.

Likelihood-based ignorable analysis and multiple imputations have very similar statistical properties, but I think non-professional (in statistics) readers had better consider the former. Regarding the comparison of these two methods, Allison (2012) argued that the former is better than the latter for several reasons, with which I agree. Some of them are listed below:

1. Multiple imputations are less efficient than the likelihood-based ignorable analysis.

2. Likelihood-based ignorable analysis always produces the same results but multiple imputations produce a different result every time you use it.

3. Use of multiple imputations requires many different decisions, each of which involves uncertainty. Most statistical softwares for multiple imputations have defaults and several options. These choices are not trivial for users unfamilar with multiple imputations.

4. Furthermore, users have to choose an *imputation model* in addition to the analysis model. This selection causes an additional uncertainty for the results. As nobody knows the correct model for imputation, users must be careful in choosing the imputation model.

Furthermore, the traditional *1:1* design is easily influenced by missing data after randomization and some kind of imputation methods such as LOCF and multiple imputations are inevitably needed for ITT (intention-to-treat) analysis. However, if we adopt an *S:T* design, the necessity for multiple imputations would be quite low. So, in this book, I would like to focus on the likelihood-based ignorable analysis, which is easily applicable via the SAS procedures `PROC MIXED` or `PROC GLIMMIX`.

6.4 Sensitivity analysis

However, in practice, sensitivity analyses are recommended to consider a range of plausible alternative MNAR assumptions about the missing data because it is important to investigate the extent to which treatment effects are stable to departures from the MAR assumption (National Research Council, 2010).

For MNAR, we usually need a joint model of the data and the missing data mechanism called the *pattern mixture model* (Little, 1993):

$$p(\boldsymbol{y}_i, \boldsymbol{r}_i \mid \boldsymbol{\theta}, \boldsymbol{\xi}) = p(\boldsymbol{y}_i \mid \boldsymbol{r}_i, \boldsymbol{\theta}, \boldsymbol{\xi}) p(\boldsymbol{r}_i \mid \boldsymbol{\xi}), \qquad (6.9)$$

which is a product of (1) the probability distribution of the data within each missing data pattern and (2) the probability of the missing data pattern. To do this, multiple imputation methods are useful and it is recommended to specify the numerical value of sensitivity parameter δ governing the degree of departure from the MAR assumption (e.g., Molenberghs and Kenward, 2007; Carpenter and Kenward, 2013). For example, specify a pattern mixture model including δ such that $\delta = 0$ corresponds to the untestable assumption made in the primary analysis and $\delta \neq 0$ corresponds to plausible departures from that assumption. Then estimate the treatment effect over a plausible range of values of δ. Regarding the details of methods for multiple imputations associated with sensitivity analyses under MNAR, please consult other papers or textbooks (e.g., Schafer, 1997; Verbeke and Molenberghs, 2001; Diggle et al., 2002; Fitzmaurice et al., 2011; White et al., 2011; van Buuren, 2012; Carpenter and Kenward, 2013). Regarding the statistical software to perform the pattern-mixture model, the recently implemented `MNAR` statement in the SAS procedure `PROC MI` could be useful.

On the other hand, there are some ad hoc graphical procedures for assessing the missing data mechanism in longitudinal study. Especially, the procedure suggested by Carpenter et al. (2002) is very simple and just plot the repeated measurements at each time point, differentiating between two groups of patients: those who do and those who do not come in to their next scheduled visit. If you find any clear difference between the distributions of observed data for these two groups, it will be reasonable to assume that the missing data mechanism is *not* MCAR.

6.5 The Growth Data

In the previous chapter, we could conduct *complete case analysis* in that we have no missing data in the *Growth Data* shown in Table 5.1. In here, we illustrate the use of the *likelihood-based ignorable analysis*, which can be used when there are missing data assumed to be *missing at random* in the data set.

Table 6.1 is an incomplete version of the *Growth Data* where *eight* data were changed to be "missing" at random. Let us apply the *random intercept model* (5.2) and the *random intercept plus slope model* with $\rho_B = 0$ (5.7) to

TABLE 6.1
Hypothetical growth data: Eight data of Table 5.1 are set as "missing" (coded as NA) randomly.

	Weeks				
Rat No.	8	15	22	29	36
1	151.0	199.0	246.0	283.0	320.0
2	145.0	199.0	249.0	293.0	354.0
3	147.0	214.0	263.0	312.0	328.0
4	155.0	200.0	237.0	NA	NA
5	135.0	188.0	230.0	280.0	323.0
6	159.0	210.0	252.0	298.0	331.0
7	141.0	189.0	231.0	275.0	305.0
8	159.0	201.0	248.0	297.0	338.0
9	177.0	236.0	285.0	350.0	376.0
10	134.0	182.0	220.0	260.0	296.0
11	160.0	208.0	NA	313.0	352.0
12	143.0	188.0	220.0	273.0	314.0
13	154.0	200.0	244.0	289.0	325.0
14	171.0	221.0	270.0	326.0	358.0
15	163.0	216.0	242.0	281.0	312.0
16	160.0	207.0	248.0	288.0	324.0
17	142.0	187.0	234.0	280.0	316.0
18	156.0	203.0	243.0	283.0	317.0
19	157.0	212.0	259.0	307.0	336.0
20	152.0	203.0	246.0	286.0	321.0
21	154.0	205.0	253.0	298.0	334.0
22	139.0	190.0	225.0	267.0	302.0
23	146.0	191.0	NA	NA	NA
24	157.0	211.0	250.0	285.0	323.0
25	132.0	185.0	237.0	286.0	331.0
26	160.0	NA	257.0	NA	345.0
27	169.0	216.0	261.0	295.0	333.0
28	157.0	205.0	248.0	289.0	316.0
29	137.0	180.0	219.0	258.0	291.0
30	153.0	200.0	244.0	286.0	324.0

the incomplete data. You need not change the SAS program at all and have only to execute the same programs (Program and Output 5.2. and Program and Output 5.3). These results are shown in Output 6.1 and Output 6.2, respectively. Estimated results seem to be quite similar to those of the same analyses applied to the original data without missing data (Table 5.1).

Output 6.1. The model (5.2) for incomplete data in Table 6.1.

```
<Program>: the same as Program 5.2

<Output>
Covariance Parameter Estimates
Cov Parm Subject    Estimate   S.E.  Z value Pr > Z
Intercept  id        188.33   52.9284 3.56 0.0002
Residual   id         62.9778  8.4439 7.46 <.0001

Fit Statistics
-2 Res Log Likelihood 1070.2
AIC (smaller is better) 1074.2

Solution for Fixed Effects
Effect   Estimate    S.E.    DF    t Value Pr>|t| Alpha Lower Upper
Intercept 105.82  2.9733    48.9   35.59 <.0001 0.05 99.8477 111.80
day          6.241 0.06758 112     92.34 <.0001 0.05  6.1070  6.3748
```

Output 6.2. The model (5.7) with $\rho_B = 0$ for incomplete data in Table 6.1.

```
<Program>: the same as Program 5.3

<Output>
Covariance Parameter Estimates
Cov Parm Subject   Estimate S.E.   Z value Pr > Z
Intercept id       107.10   37.4757  2.86 0.0021
day       id         0.2047 0.07027 2.91 0.0018
Residual  id        37.2246 5.6936   6.54 <.0001

Fit Statistics
-2 Res Log Likelihood 1037.3
AIC (smaller is better) 1043.3

Solution for Fixed Effects
Effect   Estimate    S.E. DF t Value Pr>|t| Alpha Lower Upper
Intercept 105.89  2.2634 33.9 46.78 <.0001 0.05 101.29 110.49
day         6.24  0.0990 33.4 62.98 <.0001 0.05 6.0338 6.4365
```

TABLE 6.2
Rat Data with missing data: two randomly selected data in Table 2.1 were changed to be "missing" and coded as "NA."

	Experimental group weeks after treatment					Control group weeks after treatment			
No.	0	1	2	3	No.	0	1	2	3
1	7.5	8.6	6.9	0.8	7	13.3	13.3	12.9	11.1
2	10.6	11.7	8.8	1.6	8	10.7	10.8	10.7	NA
3	12.4	13.0	11.0	5.6	9	12.5	12.7	12.0	10.1
4	11.5	12.6	11.1	7.5	10	8.4	8.7	8.1	5.7
5	8.3	8.9	NA	0.5	11	9.4	9.6	8.0	3.8
6	9.2	10.1	8.6	3.8	12	11.3	11.7	10.0	8.5

6.6 The Rat Data

Here also, we shall illustrate the use of the *likelihood-based ignorable analysis.* Table 6.2 contains two missing data which are randomly selected from Table 2.1 and changed to be "missing." Let us apply the *random intercept plus slope model with slopes varying over time* (5.23) or the model with the *unstructured* covariance to the incomplete data. You need not change the SAS program at all and have only to execute the same program (see Section 5.3.3). Part of the SAS output is shown in Output 6.3.

Output 6.3: The model (5.23) with unstructured covariance for incomplete data in Table 6.2.

```
Fit Statistics
-2 Res Log Likelihood 85.4
AIC (smaller is better) 105.4
BIC (smaller is better) 110.2

Estimated R Matrix for id 2 (Common Covariance)
Row Col1 Col2   Col3   Col4
1 3.5122 3.4202 3.3830 4.4224
2 3.4202 3.3682 3.2832 4.3511
3 3.3830 3.2832 3.5688 4.9968
4 4.4224 4.3511 4.9968 7.9060

Solution for Fixed Effects
Effect     week Estimate S.E.  DF   t Value Pr>|t| Alpha Lower    Upper
group*week 2  -0.7000 0.1155 10    -6.06 0.0001 0.05 -0.9573 -0.4427
group*week 3   0.3013 0.3271 10.2   0.92 0.3781 0.05 -0.4251  1.0278
group*week 4   3.7376 0.9342  9.91 4.00 0.0026 0.05  1.6533  5.8220
group*week 1   0 . . . . . . .
```

Output 6.3 shows that the treatment effects at weeks 2 and 3 seem to be quite similar to those applied to the original data with no missing data. Especially, since there is no missing data at week 1, the estimated treatment effect at week 1 is shown to be equivalent to the estimate obtained for the original *Rat Data* with no missing data or to the result of Student's two-sample t-test for the difference in means of CFB (change from baseline) between groups using only the data necessary for the analysis (see Table 2.3). As I emphasized at the end of Chapter 5, this is the property of the linear mixed-effects model with the *unstructured* covariance.

6.7 MMRM vs. LOCF

In this section, let us assume that (1) the *Rat Data* comes from a randomized clinical trial, (2) the primary endpoint is the CFB at week 3 and the primary statistical method is Student's two-sample t-test. In handling missing data, the most frequently used method in the past was LOCF. In the LOCF analysis of the *Rat Data* shown in Table 6.2, the missing data at week 3 for subject No. 8 is replaced by the data 10.7 at week 2. However, the LOCF-based Student's two-sample t-test for the difference in means of CFB can be reasonably replaced by the linear mixed-effects model (5.23). Estimated treatment effects are

1. -3.77 ± 0.93, ($p = 0.0023$) from the mixed-effects model for the original data set without missing data;

2. -3.74 ± 0.93, ($p = 0.0026$) from the mixed-effects model for the data set with missing data; and

3. -4.00 ± 1.02 ($p = 0.0029$) from the LOCF-based Student's two-sample t-test.

By the same token, if the analysis of covariance adjusting for the baseline data is defined as the primary statistical method in the trial protocol, then the traditional LOCF-based ANCOVA analysis can be reasonably replaced by one of the ANCOVA-type mixed-effects models (3.34, 3.35, 4.16). The SAS program for the model (3.35) with the baseline effects changing across time modified to the style introduced in Section 5.3 is shown in Program 6.4 and part of the results are shown in Output 6.4.

Program 6.4: The ANCOVA-type mixed-effects model (3.35) with unstructured covariance for the incomplete data set in Table 6.2.

```
data d4;
  infile 'c:\book\RepeatedMeasure\experimentRatPre.dat' missover;
  input id group week y ybase;
  group=group-1;

proc mixed data = d4 method=reml covtest;
class id  week / ref=first ;
  model y = ybase ybase*week group week group*week / s ddfm=sat;
  repeated / type = un subject = id r  rcorr ;
  estimate 'CFB at week 3'
  group  1 group*week  0 1 0 / divisor=1 cl alpha=0.05;
run;
```

Output 6.4: The ANCOVA-type mixed-effects model (3.35) with unstructured covariance for the incomplete data set in Table 6.2.

```
Solution for Fixed Effects
Effect    week Estimate S.E. DF  t Value Pr>|t| Alpha Lower   Upper
CFB at week 3 -3.4730 0.9811 8.82 -3.54 0.0065 0.05 -5.6992 -1.2469
```

Then the estimated treatment effects from three kinds of methods are summarized as follows:

1. -3.50 ± 0.97 ($p = 0.0057$) from the analysis of covariance (see Section 2.4) or the ANCOVA-type mixed-effects model (3.35) (see Output 3.3) applied to the original data set without missing data

2. -3.47 ± 0.98, ($p = 0.0065$) from the ANCOVA-type mixed-effects model for the data set with missing data

3. -3.74 ± 1.09 ($p = 0.0073$) from the LOCF-based analysis of covariance

These approaches (based on some linear mixed-effects models) for handling missing data have recently been called *MMRM (mixed-effects model with repeated measures) analysis* in the literature related to clinical trials and the superiority of MMRM over LOCF and/or multiple imputation methods have been discussed (e.g., Mallinckrodt et al., 2008; Siddiqui et al., 2009; Siddiqui , 2011). However, in the framework of *S:T repeated measures design* advocated in this book, it is quite natural and not unusual to use the (generalized linear) mixed-effects model for handling missing data under the MAR assumption.

7

Mixed-effects normal linear regression models

Mixed-effects models with Gaussian errors are generally called *linear mixed-effects models* in the literature. In this book, however, they are called *mixed-effects normal regression models* in consideration of the fact that it is a member of the generalized linear mixed-effects models. In this chapter, we shall introduce the following three practical and important types of statistical analysis plans or statistical models that you frequently encounter in many randomized controlled trials:

◇ models for the treatment effect at each scheduled visit,
◇ models for the average treatment effect, and
◇ models for the treatment by linear time interaction.

These models are illustrated with real data from a randomized controlled trial called *Beat the Blues Data*. It should be noted that the problem of *which model should be used in our trial* largely depends on the purpose of the trial. Furthermore, to contrast the traditional analysis of covariance (ANCOVA) frequently used in the pre-post design (*1:1* design), where the baseline measurement is used as a covariate, we shall introduce

◇ANCOVA-type models adjusting for baseline measurement

for the *1:T* design. Finally, sample size calculations needed for some models with *S:T* repeated measures design are presented and illustrated with real data.

7.1 Example: The Beat the Blues Data with *1:4* design

Data introduced and analyzed here are from a randomized controlled trial of an interactive, multimedia program known as "Beat the Blues" designed to deliver CBT (cognitive behavioral therapy) to depressed patients via a computer terminal (see Proudfoot et al. 2003 for details), which are introduced and analyzed in Everitt and Hothorn (2010). "Beat the Blues" is an interactive program using multimedia techniques, in particular video vignettes.

TABLE 7.1
Beat the Blues Data: from a randomized controlled trial of an interactive, multimedia program known as "Beat the Blues" designed to deliver CBT (cognitive behavioral therapy) to depressed patients via a computer terminal. Data for the first fifteen patients are shown.

Subject	drug	length	treatment	bdi.pre	bdi.2m	bdi.3m	bdi.5m	bdi.8m
1	No	>6m	TAU	29	2	2	NA	NA
2	Yes	>6m	BtheB	32	16	24	17	20
3	Yes	<6m	TAU	25	20	NA	NA	NA
4	No	>6m	BtheB	21	17	16	10	9
5	Yes	>6m	BtheB	26	23	NA	NA	NA
6	Yes	<6m	BtheB	7	0	0	0	0
7	Yes	<6m	TAU	17	7	7	3	7
8	No	>6m	TAU	20	20	21	19	13
9	Yes	<6m	BtheB	18	13	14	20	11
10	Yes	>6m	BtheB	20	5	5	8	12
11	No	>6m	TAU	30	32	24	12	2
12	Yes	<6m	BtheB	49	35	NA	NA	NA
13	No	>6m	TAU	26	27	23	NA	NA
14	Yes	>6m	TAU	30	26	36	27	22
15	Yes	>6m	BtheB	23	13	13	12	23

In this trial, patients with depression recruited in the primary care setting were randomized to either the "Beat the Blues" program (BtheB group) or to treatment as usual (TAU group). The data to be analyzed here are a subset of $N = 100$ patients, $n_1 = 48$ for the TAU group and $n_2 = N - n_1 = 52$ for the BtheB group. The primary endpoint is the Beck Depression Inventory II (BDI) score. Measurements of this endpoint were made on five occasions: prior to treatment, and two, three, five, and eight months after treatment began ($S = 1, T = 4$). The mean response profile of the BDI score by treatment group with the sample size available at each occasion of visit is shown in Figure 1.1 in Chapter 1. There are two covariates, antidepressant drugs (yes or no) and length of the current episode of depression (less or more than six months). Table 7.1 shows a part of the data which is called *wide format* where missing data is coded as "missing."[1]

[1]The data is available as the data frame `BtheB` in the `R` system for statistical computing using the following code: data("BtheB", package = "HSAUR2")

7.2 Checking the missing data mechanism via a graphical procedure

As shown in Table 7.1, the *Beat the Blues Data* set includes a lot of missing data due to dropouts. As described in Chapter 6, if the missing data can be assumed to be MCAR or MAR, we can apply the *likelihood-based ignorable analysis* by simply ignoring the records that include missing data. Although we cannot judge from the observed data at hand whether the missing data are MCAR, MAR or MNAR, we can apply some ad hoc graphical procedures for assessing the missing data mechanism to a certain extent in longitudinal study. So, let us apply here the procedure suggested by Carpenter et al. (2002). It involves just plotting the repeated measurements at each time point, differentiating between two groups of subjects; those who come in ($\circ$) and those who do not come in ($\times$) to their next scheduled visit. Figure 7.1 shows such a plot for all the subjects combined. This figure indicates that there is no obvious difference between the distributions of the observed BDI scores for these two groups ($\circ$ vs. $\times$) at each visit. This observation can be expressed as the following equations:

$$\Pr\{BDI_j \mid r_{BDI_{j+1}} = 0\} \quad = \quad \Pr\{BDI_j \mid r_{BDI_{j+1}} = 1\}. \tag{7.1}$$

Namely, we have

$$\frac{\Pr\{r_{BDI_{j+1}} = 0 \mid BDI_j\}}{\Pr\{r_{BDI_{j+1}} = 0\}} \quad = \quad \frac{\Pr\{r_{BDI_{j+1}} = 1 \mid BDI_j\}}{\Pr\{r_{BDI_{j+1}} = 1\}}. \tag{7.2}$$

This means that, given the value of BDI_j, the conditional probability of the observation at the next scheduled visit being missing, the probability of an observation being missing does not depend on the observed data at a previous scheduled visit, i.e.,

$$\Pr\{r_{BDI_{j+1}} = \delta \mid BDI_j\} = \Pr\{r_{BDI_{j+1}} = \delta\}, \ (\delta = 0, 1). \tag{7.3}$$

On the other hand, MCAR requires the following condition (by replacing BDI_j with BDI_{j+1})

$$\Pr\{r_{BDI_{j+1}} = \delta \mid BDI_{j+1}\} = \Pr\{r_{BDI_{j+1}} = \delta\}, \ (\delta = 0, 1). \tag{7.4}$$

However, in the context of repeated measures design, it may not be unreasonable to assume that the missing data mechanism is MCAR. So, in the analysis

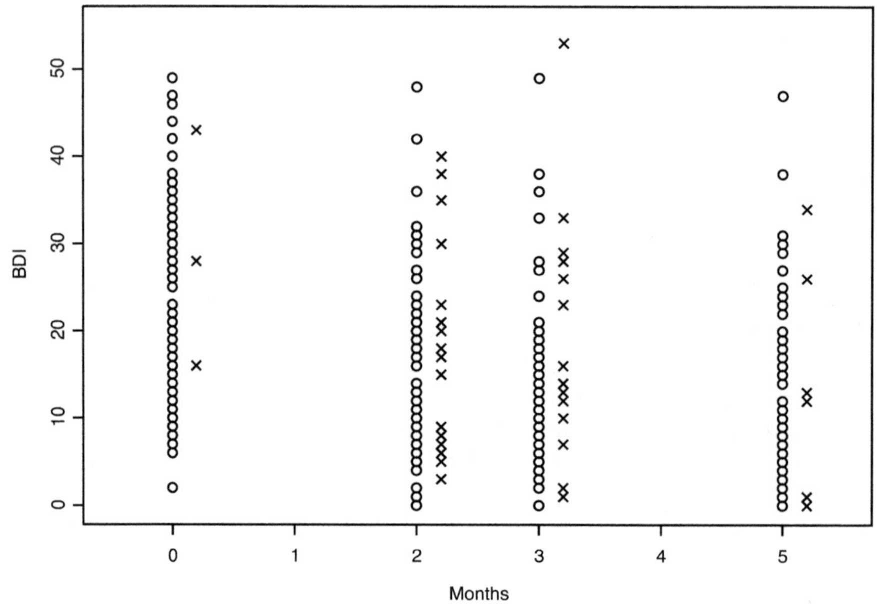

FIGURE 7.1
Distribution of the BDI scores for subjects that attend (circles) and do not attend (×) the next scheduled visit.

of the *Beat the Blues Data*, we shall apply the *likelihood-based ignorable analysis* by simply ignoring the records that include missing data.

7.3 Data format for analysis using SAS

Figure 7.2 shows the subject-specific response profile of the BDI score over time by treatment group. But to analyze these data using the SAS procedure `PROC MIXED`, we have to rearrange the data structure from the wide format into the long format structure in which each separate repeated measurement and associated covariate value appear as a separate row in the data set. The rearranged data set is shown in Table 7.2, which includes seven variables:

1. `subject`: a numeric factor indicating the subject ID.

2. `drug`: a binary variable indicating the use of antidepressant drugs (yes=1 or no=0).

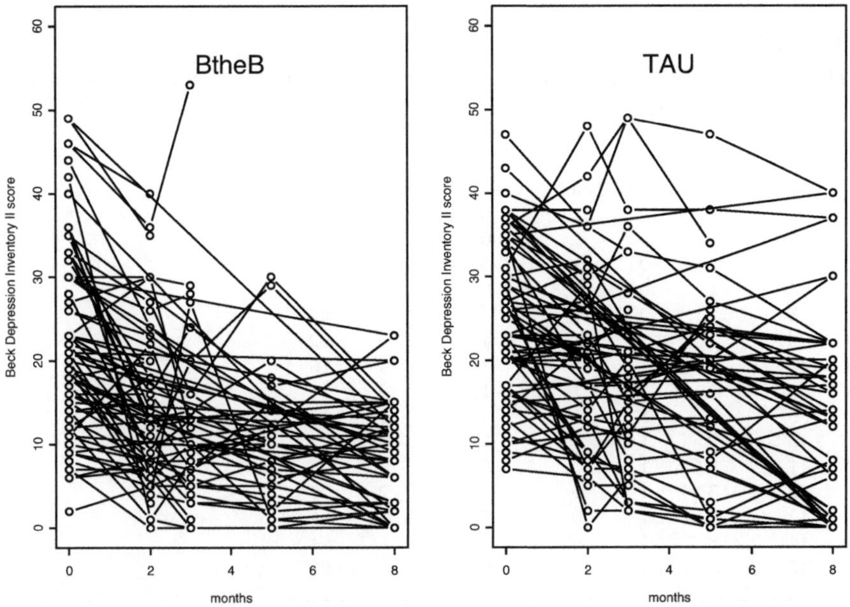

FIGURE 7.2
Subject-specific response profiles of the BDI score over time by treatment group.

3. `length`: a continuous variable indicating the length of the current episode of depression (less than six months = 0; six months or more = 1).

4. `treatment`: a binary variable indicating the treatment group (BtheB = 1, TAU = 0).

5. `visit`: a numeric factor indicating the month of visit: takes 0(baseline), 2, 3, 5, 8.

6. `bdi`: a continuous variable indicating the Beck Depression Inventory II Score.

7.4 Models for the treatment effect at each scheduled visit

Figure 7.3 shows the subject-specific changes from baseline of the BDI score by treatment group. In exploratory trials in the early phases of drug develop-

TABLE 7.2
Beat the Blues Data: Data set with long format. Data for the first three patients are shown.

No.	subject	drug	length	treatment	visit	bdi
1	1	0	1	0	0	29
2	1	0	1	0	2	2
3	1	0	1	0	3	2
4	1	0	1	0	5	NA
5	1	0	1	0	8	NA
6	2	1	1	1	0	32
7	2	1	1	1	2	16
8	2	1	1	1	3	24
9	2	1	1	1	5	17
10	2	1	1	1	8	20
11	3	1	0	0	0	25
12	3	1	0	0	2	20
13	3	1	0	0	3	NA
14	3	1	0	0	5	NA
15	3	1	0	0	8	NA

ment, statistical analyses of interest will be mainly to **estimate the time-dependent mean profile** for each treatment group and to test whether there is any treatment-by-time interaction. So, we shall here introduce three mixed-effects models to estimate the treatment effect at each scheduled visit, i.e., (1) a random intercept model, (2) a random intercept plus slope model with constant slope, and (3) a random intercept plus slope model with slopes varying over time.

7.4.1 Model I: Random intercept model

First, a *random intercept model* with a random intercept b_{0i} reflecting the inter-subject variability at month 0 (baseline) can be given as

$$
\begin{aligned}
E(y_{i0} \mid b_{0i}) &= \begin{cases} \beta_0 + b_{0i} + \boldsymbol{w}_i^t \boldsymbol{\xi}, \ i = 1, ..., n_1 \text{ (TAU group)} \\ \beta_0 + b_{0i} + \beta_1 + \boldsymbol{w}_i^t \boldsymbol{\xi}, \ i = n_1 + 1, ..., N \text{ (BtheB group)} \end{cases} \\
E(y_{ij} \mid b_{0i}) &= \begin{cases} \beta_0 + b_{0i} + \beta_{2j} + \boldsymbol{w}_i^t \boldsymbol{\xi}, \ i = 1, ..., n_1 \text{ (TAU group)} \\ \beta_0 + b_{0i} + \beta_1 + \beta_{2j} + \beta_{3j} + \boldsymbol{w}_i^t \boldsymbol{\xi}, i = n_1 + 1, ..., N \\ \qquad \text{(BtheB group)} \end{cases} \\
& \quad j = 1, ..., 4,
\end{aligned}
$$

where:

1. β_0 denotes the mean BDI score at the baseline period in the TAU group.

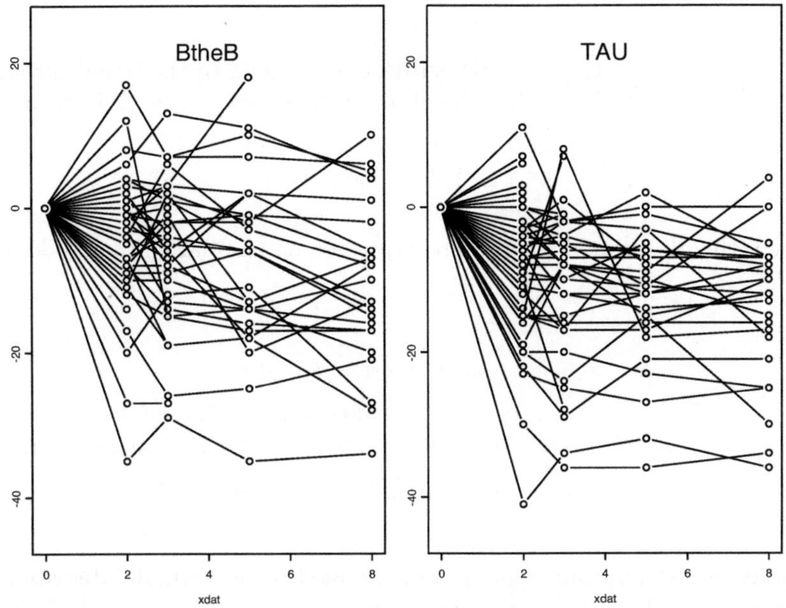

FIGURE 7.3
Subject-specific changes from baseline of the BDI score by treatment group.

2. $\beta_0 + b_{i0}$ denotes the subject-specific mean BDI score at the baseline period in the TAU group.

3. β_1 denotes the difference in means of the BDI score between the two treatment groups at the baseline period.

4. β_{2j} denotes the mean change from baseline at the $j(= 1, ..., T)$th visit in the TAU group.

5. $\beta_{2j} + \beta_{3j}$ denotes the same quantity in the BtheB group.

6. β_{3j} denotes the difference in these two means at the jth visit or the effect for the treatment-by-time interaction at the jth visit. In other words, it means the treatment effect of BtheB compared with TAU at the jth visit.

7. $\boldsymbol{w}_i^t = (w_{1i}, ..., w_{qi})$ is a vector of covariates.

8. $\boldsymbol{\xi}^t = (\xi_1, ..., \xi_q)$ is a vector of coefficients for covariates.

Needless to say, we should add the phrase "adjusted for covariates" to the interpretations of fixed-effects parameters β, but we omit the phrase in what follows. As in Section 5.3, let us introduce the two dummy variables x_{1i}, x_{2ij}:

$$x_{1i} = \begin{cases} 1, & \text{if the } i\text{th subject is assigned to the BtheB group} \\ 0, & \text{if the } i\text{th subject is assigned to the TAU group} \end{cases} \quad (7.5)$$

$$x_{2ij} = \begin{cases} 1, & \text{for } j \geq 1 \text{ (evaluation period)} \\ 0, & \text{for } j \leq 0 \text{ (baseline period)} \end{cases} \quad (7.6)$$

Then, the above model can be re-expressed as (similar to the model (5.14)):

$$\begin{aligned} y_{ij} \mid b_{0i} &= \beta_0 + b_{0i} + \beta_1 x_{1i} + \beta_{2j} x_{2ij} \\ &\qquad + \beta_{3j} x_{1i} x_{2ij} + \boldsymbol{w}_i^t \boldsymbol{\xi} + \epsilon_{ij} \\ & i = 1, ..., N; \ j = 0, 1, 2, 3, 4; \ \beta_{20} = 0, \ \beta_{30} = 0 \\ & b_{0i} \sim N(0, \sigma_{B0}^2), \ \ \epsilon_{ij} \sim N(0, \sigma_E^2), \end{aligned} \quad (7.7)$$

where the random intercept b_{0i} are assumed to be normally distributed with zero mean and variance σ_{B0}^2 and the residuals ϵ_{ij} are assumed to be normally distributed with zero mean and variance σ_E^2. The b_{0i} and ϵ_{ij} are assumed to be independent of each other. It should be noted that an important assumption is, given the random intercept b_{0i}, the subject-specific repeated measures $(y_{i0}, ..., y_{i4})$ are *mutually independent.*

7.4.2 Model II: Random intercept plus slope model

As the second model, consider a *random intercept plus slope model* by simply adding the *random slope* b_{1i} taking account of the inter-subject variability of the response to the treatment assumed to be constant during the treatment period, which is given by

$$E(y_{i0} \mid b_{0i}) \sim \begin{cases} \beta_0 + b_{0i} + \boldsymbol{w}_i^t \boldsymbol{\xi}, \ i = 1, ..., n_1 \text{ (TAU group)} \\ \beta_0 + b_{0i} + \beta_1 + \boldsymbol{w}_i^t \boldsymbol{\xi}, \ i = n_1 + 1, ..., N \text{ (BtheB group)} \end{cases}$$

$$E(y_{ij} \mid b_{0i}, b_{1i}) \sim \begin{cases} \beta_0 + b_{0i} + b_{1i} + \beta_{2j} + \boldsymbol{w}_i^t \boldsymbol{\xi}, i = 1, ..., n_1 \text{ (TAU group)} \\ \beta_0 + b_{0i} + b_{1i} + \beta_1 + \beta_{2j} + \beta_{3j} + \boldsymbol{w}_i^t \boldsymbol{\xi}, \\ \qquad\qquad i = n_1 + 1, ..., N \text{ (BtheB group)} \end{cases}$$

$$j = 1, ..., 4.$$

It should be noted that the *random slope* introduced in the above model does not mean the *slope* on the time or a linear time trend, which will be considered in Section 7.6. Interpretation of the fixed-effects parameters is the same as the random intercept model and the re-expressed mixed-effects model is shown below:

$$\begin{aligned} y_{ij} \mid (b_{0i}, b_{1i}) &= \beta_0 + b_{0i} + b_{1i}x_{2ij} + \beta_1 x_{1i} + \beta_{2j}x_{2ij} \\ &\qquad + \beta_{3j}x_{1i}x_{2ij} + \boldsymbol{w}_i^t \boldsymbol{\xi} + \epsilon_{ij} \\ &\quad i = 1, ..., N;\ j = 0, 1, 2, 3, 4;\ \beta_{20} = 0,\ \beta_{30} = 0 \\ \boldsymbol{b}_i &= (b_{0i}, b_{1i}) \sim N(0, \Phi),\quad \epsilon_{ij} \sim N(0, \sigma_E^2), \end{aligned} \tag{7.8}$$

where the $\boldsymbol{b}_i$ and ϵ_{ij} are assumed to be independent of each other and

$$\boldsymbol{\Phi} = \begin{pmatrix} \sigma_{B0}^2 & \rho_B \sigma_{B0} \sigma_{B1} \\ \rho_B \sigma_{B0} \sigma_{B1} & \sigma_{B1}^2 \end{pmatrix}. \tag{7.9}$$

In this book, we shall call Model II with $\rho_B = 0$, Model IIa, and the one with $\rho_B \neq 0$, Model IIb.

7.4.3 Model III: Random intercept plus slope model with slopes varying over time

As the third model, consider another *random intercept plus slope model* where the *random slopes* $(b_{1i1}, ..., b_{1iT})$ may vary over time, which is given by

$$\begin{aligned} y_{ij} \mid \boldsymbol{b}_i &= \beta_0 + b_{0i} + \beta_1 x_{1i} + (\beta_{2j} + b_{1ij}) x_{2ij} \\ &\qquad + \beta_{3j}x_{1i}x_{2ij} + \boldsymbol{w}_i^t \boldsymbol{\xi} + \epsilon_{ij} \\ &\quad i = 1, ..., N;\ j = 0, 1, 2, 3, 4;\ \beta_{20} = 0,\ \beta_{30} = 0 \\ \boldsymbol{b}_i &= (b_{0i}, b_{1i1}, ..., b_{1i4}) \sim N(0, \Phi),\quad \epsilon_{ij} \sim N(0, \sigma_E^2), \end{aligned} \tag{7.10}$$

where the $\boldsymbol{b}_i$ and ϵ_{ij} are assumed to be independent of each other.

7.4.4 Analysis using SAS

Now, let us apply these models to the *Beat the Blues Data* using `PROC MIXED`. Although the SAS programs to be used for the *Beat the Blues Data* are quite similar to those used in Chapter 5, the following considerations are required for coding the SAS program (some of them have already been described in Sections 3.5 and 5.3):

1. A binary variable `treatment` indicates x_{1i}.

2. We have to create a binary variable post indicating x_{2ij} in the DATA step as

```
if visit=0 then post=0; else post=1;
```

3. The fixed effects β_{2j} can be expressed via the variable visit (main factor), which must be specified as a numeric factor by the CLASS statement.

4. The fixed effects β_{3j} can be expressed via the treatment * visit interaction.

5. The CLASS statement needs the option /ref=first to specify the first category as the reference category.

6. The option "method=reml" specifies the REML estimation. In this book we usually specify REML.

7. The option "ddfm=sat" specifies the Satterthwaite method (see (B.42) for details) for estimating the degrees of freedom in the t-test and F-test for the fixed-effects estimates.

8. Model I is specified by the following RANDOM statement

```
random intercept / subject=id, g, gcorr;
```

   where intercept denotes the random intercept b_{0i} at baseline.

9. The random slope b_{1i} assumed to be constant during the evaluation period can be expressed by the binary variable post. So, to fit Model IIa, you have to use the following RANDOM statement

```
random intercept post /type=simple subject=id g gcorr ;
```

   where the option type=simple can be omitted. To fit Model IIb (the model with $\rho_B \neq 0$), you use the option type=un:

```
random intercept post /type=un subject=id g gcorr ;
```

10. To fit Model III, create the four binary variables (w1, w2, w3, w4) representing the random slopes $(b_{1i1}, b_{1i2}, b_{1i3}, b_{1i4})$ in the DATA step as

```
if visit=2 then w1=1; else w1=0;
if visit=3 then w2=1; else w2=0;
if visit=5 then w3=1; else w3=0;
if visit=8 then w4=1; else w4=0;
```

   and include these four variables in the RANDOM statement as

```
random intercept w1 w2 w3 w4 / type=un subject=id g gcorr;
```

11. Finally, let us examine residual plots. Residual plots are usually done to examine model assumptions such as peculiar patterns of residuals, normality, and detecting outliers. In the mixed model, there are two types of residuals, i.e., *marginal residuals* or *population-averaged residuals* and *conditional residuals* or *subject-specific residuals*, which are defined as

$$\begin{aligned} \text{marginal} &: \quad r_{ij,mar} = y_{ij} - E_{\boldsymbol{b}}[\hat{y}_{ij}(\hat{\boldsymbol{\beta}}, \boldsymbol{b})] \\ \text{conditional} &: \quad r_{ij,con} = y_{ij} - \hat{y}_{ij}(\hat{\boldsymbol{\beta}}, \hat{\boldsymbol{b}}). \end{aligned}$$

The latter is useful to examine whether the subject-specific model is adequate. However, these *raw* residuals are not adequate for the case of unequal variance. To account for the unequal variance of the residuals, several standardizations are carried out. Among other things, the so-called *studentized conditional residual* is often used:

$$r_{ij,con}^{(student)} = \frac{y_{ij} - \hat{y}_{ij}(\hat{\boldsymbol{\beta}}, \hat{\boldsymbol{b}})}{\sqrt{\hat{\text{Var}}(r_{ij,con})}}, \tag{7.11}$$

where $\hat{\boldsymbol{b}}$ is the estimated BLUP (best linear unbiased predictor) of the random effects $\boldsymbol{b}$ included in the mixed model. To perform residual diagnostics of the fitted model, `PROC MIXED` provides several kinds of panels of residual diagnostics. Each panel consists of a plot of residuals versus predicted values, a histogram with normal density overlaid, a Q-Q plot, and summary residual and fit statistics. To do this, "ODS Graphics" must be enabled in advance by specifying

```
ods graphics on;
```

Then, use the following `PLOTS` option in the `PROC MIXED` statement

```
plots=studentpanel( conditional blup )
```

which produces the studentized conditional residual plots. Regarding other panels of residual diagnostics, please consult the SAS/STAT User's Guide or Little et al. (2006).

The respective sets of SAS programs are shown in Program 7.1 and part of the results for Model IIa ($\rho_B = 0$) are shown in Output 7.1. To compare the goodness-of-fit of these two models, you can use an information criterion such as AIC and BIC.

Program 7.1. SAS procedure `PROC MIXED` for Model I, IIa, IIb, III

```
data dbb;
  infile 'c:\book\RepeatedMeasure\BBlong.txt' missover;
  input no subject drug length treatment visit bdi;
  if visit=0 then post=0; else post=1;
  if visit=2 then w1=1; else w1=0;
  if visit=3 then w2=1; else w2=0;
  if visit=5 then w3=1; else w3=0;
  if visit=8 then w4=1; else w4=0;

ods graphics on;
proc mixed data=dbb method=reml covtest
  plots=studentpanel( conditional blup) ;
  class subject  visit /ref=first  ;
  model bdi = drug length treatment visit treatment*visit /s cl ddfm=sat ;

/* Model I  */
  random intercept / subject= subject g gcorr ;
/* Model IIa  */
  random intercept post / type=simple subject= subject g gcorr ;
/* Model IIb */
  random intercept post / type=un subject= subject g gcorr ;
/* Model III */
  random intercept w1 w2 w3 w4 / type=un subject= subject g gcorr ;

  repeated visit / type = simple subject = subject r  rcorr ;
```

Output 7.1. SAS procedure PROC MIXED for Model IIa

```
Covariance Parameter Estimates
Cov Parm Subject  Estimate S.E.   Z value Pr > Z
Intercept subject 75.3160 13.5585 5.55 <.0001
post subject      36.5600 10.1924 3.59 0.0002
visit subject     26.4381  2.7871 9.49 <.0001

Fit statistics
-2 Res Log Likelihood 2598.1
AIC (smaller is better) 2604.1
BIC (smaller is better) 2611.9

Solution for Fixed Effects
Effect          visit Estimate S.E. DF t Value Pr>|t| Alpha Lower Upper
Intercept             21.0883 1.9147 106 11.01 <.0001 0.05 17.2921 24.8845
drug                   3.9216 2.0451 94.2 1.92 0.0582 0.05 -0.1389   7.9820
length                 3.7543 1.9450 94.1 1.93 0.0566 0.05 -0.1075   7.6162
treatment             -2.6895 2.1005 113 -1.28 0.2030 0.05 -6.8511   1.4721
visit               2 -4.4918 1.4065 158 -3.19 0.0017 0.05 -7.2698  -1.7137
visit               3 -6.1078 1.4919 181 -4.09 <.0001 0.05 -9.0515  -3.1641
visit               5 -7.6757 1.5731 204 -4.88 <.0001 0.05 -10.7773 -4.5740
visit               8 -10.4716 1.6317 219 -6.42 <.0001 0.05 -13.6875 -7.2557
visit               0  0 . . . . . . .
treatment*visit 2  -3.3352 1.9231 158 -1.73 0.0848 0.05 -7.1334 0.4631
treatment*visit 3  -3.0006 2.0717 187 -1.45 0.1492 0.05 -7.0874 1.0862
treatment*visit 5  -2.2943 2.1949 211 -1.05 0.2971 0.05 -6.6211 2.0324
treatment*visit 8  -0.2770 2.2566 222 -0.12 0.9024 0.05 -4.7241 4.1701
treatment*visit 0   0 . . . . .
```

In Model IIa, we have the following estimates on the variance components:

$$\hat{\sigma}_{B0}^2 = 75.3160, \ \hat{\sigma}_{B1}^2 = 36.5600, \ \hat{\sigma}_E^2 = 26.4381.$$

The estimated treatment effect at months 2, 3, 5 and 8 after randomization are $-3.34(s.e. = 1.92), -3.00(2.07), -2.29(2.19)$, and $-0.28(2.26)$, respectively. Although the "Beat the Blues" program tends to decrease the value of the BDI score as compared with the TAU (treatment as usual) program, all these treatment effects are not statistically significant at a significance level of 5%. The values of AIC and BIC are 2604.1 and 2611.9, respectively. The estimated mean response profile by Model IIa is given by

$$\begin{aligned}\hat{y}_{+j} &= \hat{\beta}_0 + \hat{\beta}_1 x_{1i} + \hat{\beta}_{2j} x_{2ij} + \hat{\beta}_{3j} x_{1i} x_{2ij} + \hat{\xi}_1 \text{drug} + \hat{\xi}_2 \text{length} \\ &= 21.0883 - 2.6895 \times \text{treatment} + \text{visit}[j] \\ &\qquad + \text{treatment*visit}[j] + 3.9216 \times \text{drug} + 3.7543 \times \text{length}.\end{aligned}$$

Figure 7.4 shows the estimated mean response profile of the BDI score by

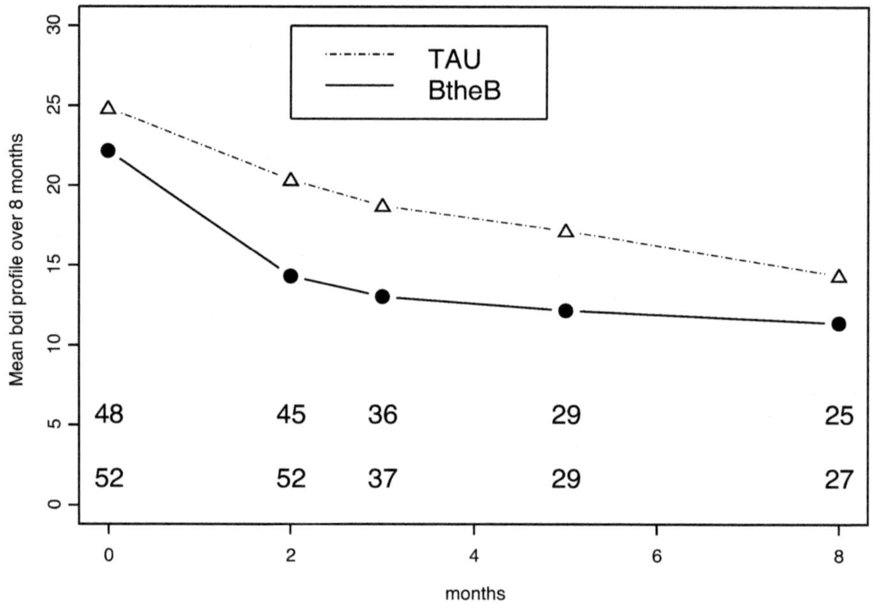

FIGURE 7.4
Estimated mean response profile (Model IIa) of the BDI score by treatment group for the subjects with `drug=0` (do not take antidepressant drugs), `length=1` (six months or more).

treatment group for the subjects with `drug=0` (do not take antidepressant drugs), `length=1` (six months or more). Table 7.3 shows the treatment effect at month 5 and month 8 for each of four models. According to AIC and BIC, the best model is Model IIa. The panel of graphics of the studentized conditional residuals of Model IIa is shown in Figure 7.5 which shows that there seem to be two outlying residuals having about 4.0 but that there seems to be no specific alarming patterns of residuals and the residuals have a mean of zero.

Table 7.3 also includes the results of the unstructured covariance model to check the closeness of the estimated treatment effects between Model III and the unstructured covariance model. To fit the unstructured covariance model, we have only to use the `REPEATED` statement with the option `type=un` without using the `RANDOM` statement. In Section 4.2, the structure of the covariance matrix of Model III is theoretically shown to be quite close to "*unstructured*" (3.32). Model III produces $\hat{\sigma}_E^2 = 13.786$ and $\mathbf{\Phi}$ is estimated as

TABLE 7.3
Estimated treatment effects $\hat{\beta}_{3j}$ at month 5 and month 8. The asterisk (*) indicates the best model. The model "un" denotes the unstructured covariance model.

Model	Month 5		Month 8		AIC	BIC
	$\hat{\beta}_{33}$ (s.e.)	Two-tailed p-value	$\hat{\beta}_{34}$ (s.e.)	Two-tailed p-value		
I	-3.21 (2.09)	0.13	-1.13 (2.17)	0.61	2626	2632
IIa*	-2.29 (2.19)	0.30	-0.28 (2.26)	0.90	2604	2612
IIb	-2.24 (2.24)	0.32	-0.23 (2.29)	0.92	2604	2614
III	-1.93 (2.29)	0.40	-0.70 (2.38)	0.77	2616	2657
"un"	-1.93 (2.29)	0.40	-0.70 (2.38)	0.77	2614	2653

$$\hat{\mathbf{\Phi}} = \begin{pmatrix} 96.4041 & -27.9861 & -17.6562 & -21.5175 & -49.6971 \\ -27.9861 & 60.2461 & 53.2449 & 55.7466 & 54.1286 \\ -17.6562 & 53.2449 & 73.0758 & 63.5810 & 57.7124 \\ -21.5175 & 55.7466 & 63.5810 & 73.3537 & 67.5982 \\ -49.6971 & 54.1286 & 57.7124 & 67.5982 & 78.9813 \end{pmatrix}.$$

From (B.33), $\Sigma = \hat{\sigma}_E^2 \boldsymbol{I} + \boldsymbol{Z}\hat{\mathbf{\Phi}}\boldsymbol{Z}^t$ is estimated as

$$\hat{\mathbf{\Sigma}} = \begin{pmatrix} 110.1901 & 68.4180 & 78.7479 & 74.8866 & 46.7070 \\ 68.4180 & 114.4640 & 104.0067 & 102.6471 & 72.8495 \\ 78.7479 & 104.0067 & 147.9535 & 120.8114 & 86.7632 \\ 74.8866 & 102.6471 & 120.8114 & 140.5088 & 92.7877 \\ 46.7070 & 72.8495 & 86.7632 & 92.7877 & 89.7772 \end{pmatrix},$$

where the matrix $\boldsymbol{Z}$ is

$$\boldsymbol{Z} = \begin{pmatrix} 1 & 0 & 0 & 0 & 0 \\ 1 & 1 & 0 & 0 & 0 \\ 1 & 0 & 1 & 0 & 0 \\ 1 & 0 & 0 & 1 & 0 \\ 1 & 0 & 0 & 0 & 1 \end{pmatrix}.$$

The estimates $\hat{\Sigma}$ are almost identical to that estimated by the unstructured model (not shown here). Therefore, the estimated treatment effects are also shown to be almost identical for the *Beat the Blues Data*.

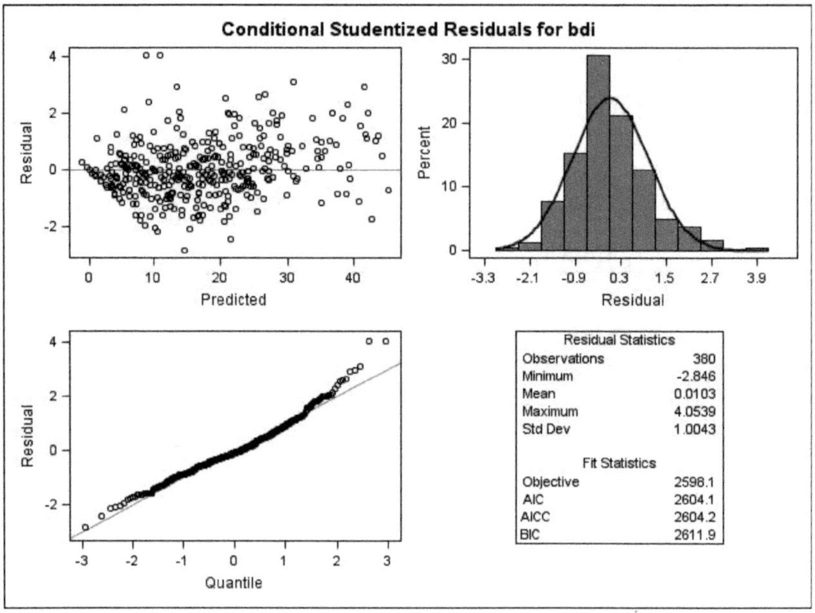

FIGURE 7.5
The panel of graphics of studentized conditional residuals of Model IIa consisting of a plot of residuals versus predicted values, a histogram with normal density overlaid, a Q-Q plot, and summary residual and fit statistics

7.5 Models for the average treatment effect

In Chapter 1 we introduced a new *S:T* repeated measures design both as an extension of the *1:1* design or pre-post design, and as a formal confirmatory trial design for randomized controlled trials. The primary interest in this design is to estimate the overall or average treatment effect during the evaluation period. So, in the trial protocol, it is important to select the evaluation period during which the treatment effect could be expected to be stable to a certain extent. So, in this section, let us assume that **the primary interest of the *Beat the Blues Trial* with the *1:4* design is to estimate the average treatment effect over eight months after randomization (evaluation period)** although many readers may not think it reasonable for the real situation of the *Beat the Blues Trial*. In this case, as already described in Section 1.2.2, we can introduce two models, a *random intercept* model and a *random intercept plus slope* model.

7.5.1 Model IV: Random intercept model

The *random intercept model* with a random intercept b_{0i} is expressed as

$$
E(y_{i0} \mid b_{0i}) \sim \begin{cases} \beta_0 + b_{0i} + \boldsymbol{w}_i^t \boldsymbol{\xi}, \ i = 1, ..., n_1 \text{ (TAU group)} \\ \beta_0 + b_{0i} + \beta_1 + \boldsymbol{w}_i^t \boldsymbol{\xi}, \ i = n_1 + 1, ..., N \text{ (BtheB group)} \end{cases}
$$

$$
E(y_{ij} \mid b_{0i}) \sim \begin{cases} \beta_0 + b_{0i} + \beta_2 + \boldsymbol{w}_i^t \boldsymbol{\xi}, \ i = 1, ..., n_1 \text{ (TAU group)} \\ \beta_0 + b_{0i} + \beta_1 + \beta_2 + \beta_3 + \boldsymbol{w}_i^t \boldsymbol{\xi}, i = n_1 + 1, ..., N \\ \qquad \text{(BtheB group)} \end{cases}
$$

$$
j = 1, ..., 4,
$$

which can be re-expressed as

$$
\begin{aligned}
y_{ij} \mid b_{0i} &= \beta_0 + b_{0i} + \beta_1 x_{1i} + \beta_2 x_{2ij} \\
&\qquad + \beta_3 x_{1i} x_{2ij} + \boldsymbol{w}_i^t \boldsymbol{\xi} + \epsilon_{ij} \\
& \quad i = 1, ..., N; \ j = 0, 1, ..., 4 \\
b_{0i} &\sim N(0, \sigma_{B0}^2), \ \ \epsilon_{ij} \sim N(0, \sigma_E^2),
\end{aligned} \tag{7.12}
$$

where the b_{0i} and ϵ_{ij} are assumed to be independent of each other and the meanings of the fixed-effects parameters are as follows:

1. β_0 denotes the mean BDI score at the baseline period in the TAU group.
2. $\beta_0 + \beta_1$ denotes the mean BDI score at the baseline period in the BtheB group.
3. $\beta_0 + \beta_2$ denotes the mean BDI score during the evaluation period in the TAU group.
4. $\beta_0 + \beta_1 + \beta_2 + \beta_3$ denotes the mean BDI score during the evaluation period in the BtheB group.
5. β_2 denotes the mean change from the baseline period to the evaluation period in the TAU group.
6. $\beta_2 + \beta_3$ denotes the same quantity in the BtheB group.
7. β_3 denotes the difference in these two mean changes from the baseline period to the evaluation period, i.e., or the effect for treatment-by-time interaction. In other words, it denotes the **average treatment effect of the new treatment** compared with the control.

7.5.2 Model V: Random intercept plus slope model

The random intercept plus slope model with random slope b_{1i} is expressed as

$$
\begin{aligned}
E(y_{i0} \mid b_{0i}) &\sim \begin{cases} \beta_0 + b_{0i} + \boldsymbol{w}_i^t \boldsymbol{\xi}, \ i = 1, ..., n_1 \text{ (TAU group)} \\ \beta_0 + b_{0i} + \beta_1 + \boldsymbol{w}_i^t \boldsymbol{\xi}, \ i = n_1 + 1, ..., N \text{ (BtheB group)} \end{cases} \\
E(y_{ij} \mid b_{0i}, b_{1i}) &\sim \begin{cases} \beta_0 + b_{0i} + b_{1i} + \beta_2 + \boldsymbol{w}_i^t \boldsymbol{\xi}, \ i = 1, ..., n_1 \text{ (TAU group)} \\ \beta_0 + b_{0i} + b_{1i} + \beta_1 + \beta_2 + \beta_3 + \boldsymbol{w}_i^t \boldsymbol{\xi}, i = n_1 + 1, ..., N \\ \qquad \text{(BtheB group)} \end{cases} \\
& j = 1, ..., 4,
\end{aligned}
$$

which is re-expressed as

$$
\begin{aligned}
y_{ij} \mid (b_{0i}, b_{1i}) &= \beta_0 + b_{0i} + \beta_1 x_{1i} + (\beta_2 + b_{1i}) x_{2ij} \\
& \qquad + \beta_3 x_{1i} x_{2ij} + \boldsymbol{w}_i^t \boldsymbol{\xi} + \epsilon_{ij} \qquad (7.13) \\
& \boldsymbol{b}_i = (b_{0i}, b_{1i}) \sim N(0, \Phi), \quad \epsilon_{ij} \sim N(0, \sigma_E^2) \\
\boldsymbol{\Phi} &= \begin{pmatrix} \sigma_{B0}^2 & \rho_B \sigma_{B0} \sigma_{B1} \\ \rho_B \sigma_{B0} \sigma_{B1} & \sigma_{B1}^2 \end{pmatrix} \\
& i = 1, ..., N; j = 0, 1, ..., 4,
\end{aligned}
$$

where the $\boldsymbol{b}_i$ and ϵ_{ij} are assumed to be independent of each other. Here also, we shall call the Model V with $\rho_B = 0$ Model Va and the one with $\rho_B \neq 0$ Model Vb.

7.5.3 Analysis using SAS

Now, let us apply three Models IV, Va, and Vb to the *Beat the Blues Data* using `PROC MIXED`. The following considerations are required for coding the SAS program.

1. The fixed effects β_2 can be expressed via the binary variable `post` (main factor).

2. The fixed effects β_3 can be expressed via the `treatment * post` interaction.

3. The `RANDOM` statement for Model IV is the same as that for Model I.

4. The `RANDOM` statements for Models Va and Vb are the same as those for Model IIa and Model IIb.

The respective sets of SAS programs and the results for Model Va ($\rho_B = 0$) are shown in Program 7.2 and Output 7.2, respectively.

Program 7.2: SAS procedure PROC MIXED for Models IV, Va, Vb

```
  proc mixed data=dbb method=reml covtest;
  class subject  visit/ ref=first ;
  model bdi = drug length treatment post treatment*post /s cl ddfm=sat ;

/* Model IV */
  random intercept / type=simple subject= subject g gcorr ;
/* Model Va  */
  random intercept post / type=simple subject= subject g gcorr ;
/* Model Vb */
  random intercept post / type=un subject= subject g gcorr ;

  repeated visit / type = simple subject = subject r  rcorr ;
 run ;
```

Output 7.2: SAS procedure PROC MIXED for Models IV, Va, Vb

```
<A part of the results for Model Va>

Covariance Parameter Estimates
Cov Parm Subject   Estimate S.E.   Z value Pr > Z
Intercept subject 74.8286 13.6362 5.49 <.0001
post subject      37.4802 10.5601 3.55 0.0002
visit subject     28.4974  2.9230 9.75 <.0001

Fit statistics
-2 Res Log Likelihood 2636.1
AIC (smaller is better) 2642.1
BIC (smaller is better) 2650.0

Solution for Fixed Effects
Effect     Estimate S.E. DF t Value Pr>|t| Alpha Lower Upper
Intercept          21.1860 1.9257 107 11.00 <.0001 0.05 17.3683 25.0036
drug                3.8048 2.0519 94.5 1.85 0.0668 0.05 -0.2690  7.8786
length              3.6322 1.9513 94.4 1.86 0.0658 0.05 -0.2418  7.5063
treatment          -2.6587 2.1160 114 -1.26 0.2115 0.05 -6.8504  1.5330
post               -6.3736 1.3114 114 -4.86 <.0001 0.05 -8.9716 -3.7756
treatment*post     -2.5138 1.8017 116 -1.40 0.1656 0.05 -6.0824  1.0548
```

In Model Va, we have the following estimates of the variance components:

$$\hat{\sigma}_{B0}^2 = 74.8286, \ \hat{\sigma}_{B1}^2 = 37.4802, \ \hat{\sigma}_E^2 = 28.4974,$$

which are quite similar to those of Model IIa. The average treatment effect during the eight-month evaluation period is estimated as -2.51 (s.e. = 1.80)

TABLE 7.4
Estimated treatment effect $\hat{\beta}_3$ for each of three models, IV, Va and Vb. The asterisk (*) indicates the best model.

Model	$\hat{\beta}_3$	s.e.	95%CI	Two-tailed p-value	AIC	BIC
IV	-2.88	1.49	(-5.82, 0.06)	0.05	2663.7	2669.0
Va*	-2.51	1.80	(-6.08, 1.05)	0.17	2642.1	2650.0
Vb	-2.47	1.86	(-6.16, 1.22)	0.19	2642.6	2653.1

with two-tailed $p = 0.17$ based on the Satterthwaite method. Table 7.4 shows the treatment effect with 95% confidence interval for each of three models. According to AIC and BIC, the best model is Model Va.

7.5.4 Heteroscedastic models

So far, we have considered the homoscedastic model (4.7)

$$\boldsymbol{\Sigma}_i = \sigma_E^2 \boldsymbol{I} + \boldsymbol{Z}\boldsymbol{\Phi}\boldsymbol{Z}^t,$$

where it is assumed that

1. the residuals ϵ_{ij} are independent and identically normally distributed with mean 0 and variance σ_E^2 common to all the treatment groups and

2. the random effects $\boldsymbol{b}_i$ are normally distributed with mean 0 and covariance $\boldsymbol{\Phi}$ common to all the treatment groups.

In this section, let us check these homoscedastic assumptions for Model Vb. To do this in `PROC MIXED`, first, we have to define `treatment` as a numeric factor as follows:

```
class subject visit treatment/ref=first ;
```

Then, change the `RANDOM` statements and/or the `REPEATED` statements shown in Program 7.2 by adding the option `group = treatment` as follows (some of them have already been introduced in Section 3.6):

1. For the model with the heteroscedastic covariance $\boldsymbol{\Phi}$:
```
random intercept post/ type=un subject= subject g gcorr
group=treatment ;
```

TABLE 7.5
Estimated treatment effect $\hat{\beta}_3$ for each of five models.

Model	$\hat{\beta}_3$	95%CI	Two-tailed p-value	AIC	BIC
Homoscedastic $\mathbf{\Sigma}$	-2.51	(-6.08, 1.05)	0.17	2642.1	2650.0
Heteroscedastic $\mathbf{\Phi}$	-2.56	(-6.15, 1.04)	0.16	2645.4	2658.4
Heteroscedastic σ_{B1}^2	-2.58	(-6.16, 1.01)	0.16	2643.8	2654.1
Heteroscedastic σ_{B0}^2	-2.49	(-6.07, 1.09)	0.17	2643.8	2654.2
Heteroscedastic σ_E^2	-2.44	(-6.04, 1.16)	0.18	2642.0	2652.4

2. For the model with the heteroscedastic variance σ_{B0}^2 and homoscedastic σ_{B1}^2:
```
random intercept/subject=subject g gcorr group=treatment;
random post /subject=subject g gcorr ;
```
3. For the model with the homoscedastic variance σ_{B0}^2 and heteroscedastic σ_{B1}^2:
```
random intercept/subject=subject g gcorr;
random post/subject= subject g gcorr group=treatment ;
```
4. For the model with the heteroscedastic σ_E^2:
```
repeated visit / type = simple subject = subject r rcorr
group=treatment ;
```

For example, the SAS program and the results for Model Va where the random effects b_{1i} have the heteroscedastic variance σ_{B1}^2 are shown in Program and Output 7.3. Model Va with heteroscedastic variance σ_{B1}^2 has the following estimates on the variance components:

$$\hat{\sigma}_{B0}^2 = 73.9,\ \hat{\sigma}_{B1}^2 = 30.7(\text{for BtheB}), 44.3(\text{for TAU})\ \hat{\sigma}_E^2 = 28.7,$$

Two estimates of the variance of the random slope are similar and both AIC (= 2643.8) and BIC (= 2654.1) are larger than those of the model with the homoscedastic variance. Table 7.5 shows the treatment effect with 95% confidence interval for each of five models. According to AIC and BIC, the best model is Model Va with the homoscedastic $\mathbf{\Sigma}$.

Program and Output 7.3: SAS procedure PROC MIXED for Model Va with heteroscedastic σ^2_{B1}

```
<SAS program>
proc mixed data=dbb method=reml covtest;
  class subject  visit treatment /ref=first  ;
  model bdi = drug length treatment post treatment*post  / s cl ddfm=sat ;
  random intercept / type=simple subject= subject g gcorr ;
  random post / type=simple subject= subject g gcorr group=treatment ;
  repeated visit / type = simple subject = subject r  rcorr ;
 run ;

<A part of the results >
Covariance Parameter Estimates
Cov Parm   Subject   Group        Estimate S.E.   Z value Pr > Z
Intercept  subject                73.9000 13.5594 5.45 <.0001
post       subject treatment 1 30.6573 13.3763 2.29 0.0110
post       subject treatment 0 44.3149 16.1667 2.74 0.0031
visit      subject                28.6760  2.9654 9.67 <.0001

Fit statistics
-2 Res Log Likelihood 2635.7
AIC (smaller is better) 2643.8
BIC (smaller is better) 2654.1

Solution for Fixed Effects
Effect     treatment  Estimate S.E.   DF t Value Pr>|t| Alpha Lower Upper
Intercept             21.2316 1.9174 106 11.07 <.0001 0.05 17.4303 25.0329
drug                   3.8250 2.0402  93  1.87 0.0640 0.05 -0.2265  7.8765
length                 3.5333 1.9410 93.2 1.82 0.0719 0.05 -0.3210  7.3876
treatment        1    -2.6665 2.1080 114 -1.26 0.2085 0.05 -6.8423  1.5092
treatment        0     0 . . . . . . .
post                  -6.3640 1.3706  54 -4.64 <.0001 0.05 -9.1118 -3.6161
post*treatment 1      -2.5755 1.8101 111 -1.42 0.1576 0.05 -6.1625  1.0115
post*treatment 0       0 . . . . . . .
```

7.6 Models for the treatment by linear time interaction

In the previous section, we focused on the mixed-effects models where we are primarily interested in comparing the average treatment effect during the evaluation period. In this section, we shall consider the situation where the primary interest is testing the treatment by *linear* time interaction, i.e., testing whether the differences between treatment groups are *linearly* increasing over time (Hedeker and Gibbons, 2006; Bhumik et al., 2008). So, in this section, let us assume that **the primary interest of the *Beat the Blues Trial* with the *1:4* design is to estimate the difference in average rates of change or improvement of the BDI score over time.** To do this, we shall consider the *random intercept* model and the *random intercept plus slope* model.

7.6.1 Model VI: Random intercept model

The *random intercept model* with a random intercept b_{0i} is expressed as

$$
\begin{aligned}
E(y_{i0} \mid b_{0i}) &\sim \begin{cases} \beta_0 + b_{0i} + \boldsymbol{w}_i^t \boldsymbol{\xi}, \ i = 1, ..., n_1 \ (\text{ TAU group}) \\ \beta_0 + b_{0i} + \beta_1 + \boldsymbol{w}_i^t \boldsymbol{\xi}, \ i = n_1 + 1, ..., N \ (\text{BtheB group}) \end{cases} \\
E(y_{ij} \mid b_{0i}) &\sim \begin{cases} \beta_0 + b_{0i} + \beta_2 t_j + \boldsymbol{w}_i^t \boldsymbol{\xi}, \ i = 1, ..., n_1 \ (\text{ TAU group}) \\ \beta_0 + b_{0i} + \beta_1 + (\beta_2 + \beta_3) t_j + \boldsymbol{w}_i^t \boldsymbol{\xi}, i = n_1 + 1, ..., N \\ \qquad\qquad\qquad\qquad (\text{BtheB group}) \end{cases} \\
& \quad j = 1, ..., 4,
\end{aligned}
$$

where:

1. t_j denotes the jth measurement time, i.e., $t_0 = 0, t_1 = 2, t_2 = 3, t_3 = 5$ and $t_4 = 8$.
2. β_0 denotes the mean BDI score at the baseline period in the TAU group.
3. $\beta_0 + b_{i0}$ denotes the subject-specific mean BDI score at the baseline period in the TAU group.
4. β_1 denotes the difference in means of the BDI score between the two treatment groups at the baseline period.
5. β_2 denotes the average rate of change of the BDI score per month during the evaluation period in the TAU group.
6. $\beta_2 + \beta_3$ denotes the average rate of change of the BDI score per month during the evaluation period in the BtheB group.
7. β_3 denotes the difference in average rates of change per month, i.e., the effect size of the treatment by linear time interaction.

The above model can be re-expressed as

$$
\begin{aligned}
y_{ij} \mid b_{0i} &= \beta_0 + b_{0i} + \beta_1 x_{1i} + (\beta_2 + \beta_3 x_{1i}) t_j + \boldsymbol{w}_i^t \boldsymbol{\xi} + \epsilon_{ij} \qquad (7.14) \\
b_{0i} &\sim N(\mathbf{0}, \sigma_{B0}^2), \quad \epsilon_{ij} \sim N(0, \sigma_E^2) \\
& \quad i = 1, ..., N; j = 0, \ 1, ..., 4,
\end{aligned}
$$

where the b_{0i} and ϵ_{ij} are assumed to be independent of each other.

7.6.2 Model VII: Random intercept plus slope model

The *random intercept plus slope* model with a random slope b_{i1} on the time is expressed as

$$\begin{aligned} y_{ij} \mid \boldsymbol{b}_i &= b_{0i} + \beta_0 + \beta_1 x_{1i} + (\beta_2 + \beta_3 x_{1i} + b_{1i}) t_j + \boldsymbol{w}_i^t \boldsymbol{\xi} + \epsilon_{ij} \quad (7.15) \\ \boldsymbol{b}_i &= (b_{0i}, b_{1i}) \sim N(\mathbf{0}, \boldsymbol{\Phi}) \\ \boldsymbol{\Phi} &= \begin{pmatrix} \sigma_{B0}^2 & \rho_B \sigma_{B0} \sigma_{B1} \\ \rho_B \sigma_{B0} \sigma_{B1} & \sigma_{B1}^2 \end{pmatrix} \\ \epsilon_{ij} &\sim N(0, \sigma_E^2) \\ & i = 1, ..., N; j = 0, \ 1, ..., 4, \end{aligned}$$

where the $\boldsymbol{b}_i$ and ϵ_{ij} are assumed to be independent of each other. Here also, we shall call the Model VII with $\rho_B = 0$, Model VIIa, and the one with $\rho_B \neq 0$, Model VIIb.

7.6.3 Analysis using SAS

Now, let us apply three Models VI, VIIa and VIIb to the *Beat the Blues Data* using `PROC MIXED`. The respective sets of SAS programs and the results for Model VI are shown in Program and Output 7.4. In this program, we need to create the continuous variable `xvisit` indicating t_j in the `DATA` step and the `MODEL` statement should be

```
model bdi = drug length treatment xvisit treatment*xvisit
                                            /s cl ddfm=sat;
```

To fit Model VIIa, for example, you have to use the following `RANDOM` statement

```
random intercept xvisit /type=simple subject= subject g gcorr;
```

where `xvisit` denotes the random slope b_{1i}.

Program and Output 7.4: SAS procedure `PROC MIXED` for Model VI, VIIa, VIIb

```
<SAS program>
data dbb;
  infile 'c:\book\RepeatedMeasure\BBlong.txt' missover;
  input no subject drug length treatment visit bdi;
  if visit=0 then post=0; else post=1;
  xvisit=visit;

  proc mixed data=dbb method=reml covtest;
  class subject  visit/ref=first  ;
  model bdi = drug length treatment xvisit treatment*xvisit/s cl ddfm=sat ;

 /* model VI */
   random intercept /  subject= subject g gcorr ;
 /* model VIIa */
   random intercept xvisit/  subject= subject g gcorr ;
 /* model VIIb */
   random intercept xvisit/ type=un subject= subject g gcorr ;

  repeated visit / type = simple subject = subject r  rcorr ;
 run ;

<A part of the results for Model VI>
Covariance Parameter Estimates
Cov Parm    Subject  Estimate S.E.  Z value Pr > Z
Intercept   subject    80.3571 13.6537  5.89  <.0001
visit       subject    40.2083  3.4278 11.73  <.0001

Fit statistics
-2 Res Log Likelihood 2676.7
AIC (smaller is better) 2680.7
BIC (smaller is better) 2685.9

Solution for Fixed Effects
Effect                Estimate S.E.  DF t Value Pr>|t| Alpha Lower Upper
Intercept            20.7228 1.9343 107 10.71 <.0001 0.05 16.8882 24.5574
drug                  2.0496 2.0457 92.3 1.00 0.3190 0.05 -2.0131  6.1123
length                3.4205 1.9461 92.4 1.76 0.0821 0.05 -0.4445  7.2855
treatment            -3.8827 2.1338 117 -1.82 0.0714 0.05 -8.1086  0.3433
xvisit               -1.3067 0.1947 290 -6.71 <.0001 0.05 -1.6898 -0.9235
treatment*xvisit     -0.1587 0.2711 290 -0.59 0.5588 0.05 -0.6923  0.3749
```

In Model VIIa, we have the following estimates of the variance components:

$$\hat{\sigma}_{B0}^2 = 80.3571,\ \hat{\sigma}_E^2 = 40.2083.$$

The difference in average rates of change per month is estimated as -0.1587 (s.e $= 0.27$) with two-tailed $p = 0.56$. The interpretation seems to be that the average rate of improvement of the BDI score tends to be more rapid for the BtheB group compared with the TAU group, but the difference is not statistically significant. Table 7.6 shows the treatment effect with 95%

TABLE 7.6
Estimated treatment effect $\hat{\beta}_3$ for each of the Models, IV, Va and Vb. The asterisk (*) indicates the best model.

Model	$\hat{\beta}_3$	s.e.	95%CI	Two-tailed p-value	AIC	BIC
VI*	-0.16	0.27	(-0.69, 0.37)	0.56	2680.7	2685.9
VIIa	-0.15	0.30	(-0.74, 0.44)	0.61	2681.1	2688.9
VIIb	-0.15	0.30	(-0.75, 0.44)	0.61	2683.1	2693.5

confidence interval for each of three models. According to AIC and BIC, the best model is Model VI.

7.6.4 Checking the goodness-of-fit of linearity

However, we should be cautious about the goodness-of-fit of the models for the treatment by *linear* time interaction because the *linear trend model* has a very strong assumption on linearity. So, whenever the treatment by linear time interaction is defined as the primary interest of the statistical analysis, we should check the goodness-of-fit. To do this, we can apply the following *random intercept* model and the *random intercept plus slope* model including the treatment by quadratic time interaction.

Another important issue to remember here is that neither AIC nor BIC based on the REML estimators can be used to compare models including non-linear terms on time t_j with the above three models including only a linear term, as explained in Section 3.5. So, here we have to use AIC and BIC based on the maximum likelihood estimators for such comparisons.

1. Model VIQ: Random intercept model

$$\begin{aligned} y_{ij} \mid b_{0i} &= \beta_0 + b_{0i} + \beta_1 x_{1i} + (\beta_2 + \beta_3 x_{1i}) t_j + \\ &\quad (\beta_4 + \beta_5 x_{1i}) t_j^2 + \boldsymbol{w}_i^t \boldsymbol{\xi} + \epsilon_{ij} \\ b_{0i} &\sim N(\mathbf{0}, \sigma_{B0}^2) \quad \epsilon_{ij} \sim N(0, \sigma_E^2) \\ &\quad i = 1, ..., N; j = 0,\ 1, ..., 4, \end{aligned} \tag{7.16}$$

where the b_{0i} and ϵ_{ij} are assumed to be independent of each other.

2. Model VIIQ: Random intercept plus slope model

The random intercept plus slope model with a random intercept b_{0i}, random slopes b_{1i} on the linear term, and b_{2i} on the quadratic term is expressed by:

$$\begin{aligned}
y_{ij} \mid b_{0i}, b_{1i}, b_{2i} &= \beta_0 + b_{0i} + \beta_1 x_{1i} + (\beta_2 + \beta_3 x_{1i} + b_{1i}) t_j + \\
&\quad (\beta_4 + \beta_5 x_{1i} + b_{2i}) t_j^2 + \boldsymbol{w}_i^t \boldsymbol{\xi} + \epsilon_{ij} \qquad (7.17)\\
\boldsymbol{b}_i &= (b_{0i}, b_{1i}, b_{2i}) \sim N(\mathbf{0}, \boldsymbol{\Phi}) \\
\boldsymbol{\Phi} &= \begin{pmatrix} \sigma_{B0}^2 & \rho_{01}\sigma_{B0}\sigma_{B1} & \rho_{02}\sigma_{B0}\sigma_{B2} \\ \rho_{01}\sigma_{B0}\sigma_{B1} & \sigma_{B1}^2 & \rho_{12}\sigma_{B1}\sigma_{B2} \\ \rho_{02}\sigma_{B0}\sigma_{B2} & \rho_{12}\sigma_{B1}\sigma_{B2} & \sigma_{B2}^2 \end{pmatrix} \\
\epsilon_{ij} &\sim N(0, \sigma_E^2) \\
& \quad i = 1, ..., N; j = 0,\ 1, ..., 4,
\end{aligned}$$

where the $\boldsymbol{b}_i$ and ϵ_{ij} are assumed to be independent of each other. Now, let us apply two Models VIQ and VIIQ to the *Beat the Blues Data* using `PROC MIXED`. The respective sets of SAS programs and the results for Model VIIQ are shown in Program and Output 7.5. In this program, we need to create the continuous variable `xvisit2` indicating the quadratic term (here we used $t_j^2/8$) in the `DATA` step. Then, the `MODEL` statement should be

```
model bdi = drug length treatment xvisit xvisit2
         treatment*xvisit  treatment*xvisit2 /s cl ddfm=sat;
```

and the `RANDOM` statement for Model VIIQ should be

```
random intercept xvisit xvist2/type=un subject= subject g gcorr;
```

Program and Output 7.5: SAS procedure PROC MIXED for Model VIIQ

```
<SAS program>
data dbb;
  infile 'c:\book\RepeatedMeasure\BBlong.txt' missover;
  input no subject drug length treatment visit bdi;
 if visit=0 then post=0; else post=1;
 xvisit=visit;
 xvisit2=visit*visit/8;

 /* model VIIQ (quadratic trend )  */
proc mixed data=dbb method=reml covtest;
  class subject  visit/ref=first  ;
  model bdi = drug length treatment xvisit xvisit2 treatment*xvisit
                             treatment*xvisit2/s cl ddfm=sat ;
  random intercept xvisit xvisit2/ type=un subject= subject g gcorr ;
  repeated visit / type = simple subject = subject r  rcorr ;
 run ;

<A part of the results >
Covariance Parameter Estimates
Cov Parm  Subject Estimate S.E.  Z value Pr > Z
UN(1,1) subject 78.5341  15.2934  5.14   <.0001
UN(2,1) subject -1.0748   5.2603 -0.20   0.8381
UN(2,2) subject  7.7681   2.8280  2.75   0.0030
UN(3,1) subject -2.5723   4.5870 -0.56   0.5750
UN(3,2) subject -5.5188   2.3684 -2.33   0.0198
UN(3,3) subject  3.9485   2.0907  1.89   0.0295
visit subject   27.1872   3.2589  8.34   <.0001

Fit statistics
-2 Res Log Likelihood 2618.3
AIC (smaller is better) 2632.3
BIC (smaller is better) 2650.6

Solution for Fixed Effects
Effect            Estimate S.E.  DF t Value Pr>|t| Alpha Lower Upper
Intercept          20.5989 1.8683 103  11.03 <.0001 0.05 16.8936 24.3041
drug                3.9664 1.9069 79.1  2.08 0.0408 0.05  0.1710  7.7618
length              4.3919 1.8195 81.2  2.41 0.0180 0.05  0.7719  8.0119
treatment          -3.0075 2.1087 98   -1.43 0.1570 0.05 -7.1921  1.1771
xvisit             -2.3133 0.6379 92.7 -3.63 0.0005 0.05 -3.5802 -1.0464
xvisit2             1.0114 0.5489 90    1.84 0.0687 0.05 -0.07901 2.1019
treatment*xvisit  -1.5184 0.8814 94.8 -1.72 0.0882 0.05 -3.2683  0.2315
treatment*xvisit2  1.4967 0.7577 91.7  1.98 0.0512 0.05 -0.00821 3.0016
```

In Model VIIQ, we have $\hat{\sigma}_E^2 = 27.1872$ and

$$\hat{\mathbf{\Phi}} = \begin{pmatrix} 74.8623 & -0.8005 & -2.7651 \\ -0.8005 & 7.4067 & -5.2246 \\ -2.7651 & -5.2246 & 3.6867 \end{pmatrix}.$$

According to AIC and BIC, Model VIIQ is better than Model VIQ (AIC =

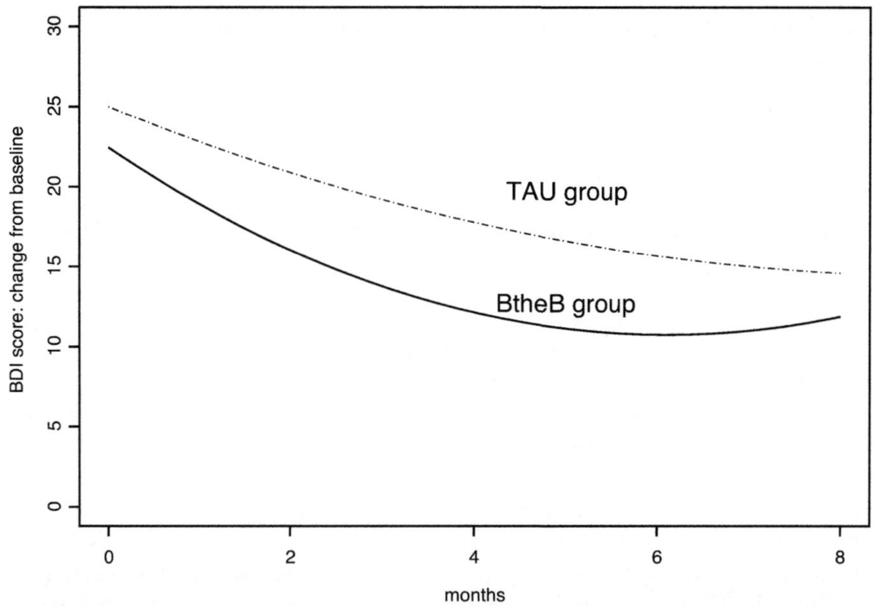

FIGURE 7.6
Estimated mean quadratic trend (Model VIIQ-1) of the BDI score by treatment group for the subjects with `drug=0` (do not take antidepressant drugs), `length=1` (six months or more).

2647.6, BIC = 2655.5). To compare Model VIIQ with Model VI, as explained above, we have to use AIC and BIC based on the maximum likelihood estimators. To do this using SAS, we have only to replace the option `method=reml` with `method=ml`. The resultant values of (AIC, BIC) are (2701.0, 2721.8) for Model VI and (2657.2, 2696.3) for Model VIIQ, indicating that Model VIIQ is better than Model VI. The estimated mean quadratic trend by the treatment group for the subject with `drug=0` (no use of drug) and `length=1` (six months or more) is

$$\hat{y}(t) = \begin{cases} \hat{\beta}_0 + \hat{\beta}_2 t + \hat{\beta}_4 t^2 + \boldsymbol{w}_i^t \hat{\boldsymbol{\xi}}, & (\text{ TAU group}) \\ \hat{\beta}_0 + \hat{\beta}_1 + (\hat{\beta}_2 + \hat{\beta}_3) t + (\hat{\beta}_4 + \hat{\beta}_5) t^2 + \boldsymbol{w}_i^t \hat{\boldsymbol{\xi}}, & (\text{BtheB group}) \end{cases}$$
$$= \begin{cases} 24.99 - 2.31t + 1.01t^2, & (\text{ TAU group}) \\ 22.44 - 3.83t + 2.51t^2, & (\text{BtheB group}). \end{cases}$$

These two quadratic lines are plotted in Figure 7.6, which seems to be quite similar to the estimated mean response profile by treatment group via Model IIa (Figure 7.4). These results suggest that the results derived by Model VI, the best model for the treatment by linear time interaction, may not be acceptable.

7.7 ANCOVA-type models adjusting for baseline measurement

As described in Chapter 1, in many confirmatory trials in the later phases of drug development, we need a simple and clinically meaningful effect size of the new treatment. So, many RCTs tend to try to narrow the evaluation period down to one time point (ex., the last Tth measurement), leading to the so-called the *pre-post* design or the *1:1* design. Some other RCTs define a summary statistic such as the mean $\bar{y}_i$ of repeated measures during the evaluation period (ex., mean of $y_{i(T-1)}$ and y_{iT}), which also leads to a *1:1* design. In these simple *1:1* designs, traditional analysis of covariance (ANCOVA) has been used to analyze data where the baseline measurement is used as a covariate. In Chapter 4, it is shown that the mixed-effects repeated measures models (4.5) and (4.11) are shown to be more natural than the ANCOVA-type models (4.16) within the framework of the *S:T* design.

In this section, we shall apply some ANCOVA-type models to the *Beat the Blues Data* with *1:4* repeated measures design and compare the results with those of the corresponding repeated measures models.

7.7.1 Model VIII: Random intercept model for the treatment effect at each visit

Let us consider here the following two models: Model VIIIa and Model VIIIb.

Model VIIIa: A random slope constant over time

Consider first the compound symmetry model where the random intercept $b_{i(Ancova)}$ is assumed to be constant during the evaluation period:

$$E(y_{ij} \mid b_{i(Ancova)}) = \begin{cases} b_{i(Ancova)} + \beta_0 + \beta_{2j} + \theta y_{i0} + \boldsymbol{w}_i^t \boldsymbol{\xi}, & \text{(TAU group)} \\ b_{i(Ancova)} + \beta_0 + \beta_1 + \beta_{2j} + \beta_{3j} + \theta y_{i0} + \boldsymbol{w}_i^t \boldsymbol{\xi}, & \\ & \text{(BtheB group)} \end{cases}$$
$$j = 1, ..., 4,$$

where:

1. β_0 denotes the mean BDI score at the 1st visit in the TAU group.

2. $b_{i(Ancova)} + \beta_0$ denotes the subject-specific mean BDI score at the 1st visit in the TAU group.

3. $\beta_0 + \beta_1$ denotes the mean BDI score at the 1st visit in the BtheB group.

4. $b_{i(Ancova)} + \beta_0 + \beta_1$ denotes the subject-specific mean BDI score at the 1st visit in the BtheB group.

5. β_1 denotes the difference in means of the BDI score at the 1st visit between the two treatment groups.

6. θ denotes the coefficient for the baseline measurement y_{i0}.

7. $\beta_0 + \beta_{2j}$ denotes the mean BDI score at the jth visit in the TAU group.

8. $\beta_0 + \beta_1 + \beta_{2j} + \beta_{3j}$ denotes the mean BDI score at the jth visit in the BtheB group.

9. $\beta_1 + \beta_{3j}$ denotes the difference in means of the BDI score at the jth visit or the effect for the treatment-by-time interaction at the jth visit. In other words, it means the treatment effect of BtheB compared with TAU at jth visit.

This model is re-expressed as follows:

$$
\begin{aligned}
y_{ij} \mid b_{i(Ancova)} &= \beta_0 + b_{i(Ancova)} + \theta y_{i0} + \beta_1 x_{1i} + \beta_{2j} \\
&\qquad + \beta_{3j} x_{1i} + \boldsymbol{w}_i^t \boldsymbol{\xi} + \epsilon_{ij} \qquad (7.18) \\
&\quad i = 1, ..., N,\ j = 1, 2, 3, 4;\ \beta_{21} = 0,\ \beta_{31} = 0 \\
b_{i(Ancova)} &\sim N(0, \sigma^2_{B(Ancova)}),\quad \epsilon_{ij} \sim N(0, \sigma^2_E),
\end{aligned}
$$

where the $b_{i(Ancova)}$ and ϵ_{ij} are assumed to be independent of each other.

Model VIIIb: Random slopes varying over time

Second, let us consider here the *random intercept* model where the random slopes $b_{ij(Ancova)}$ may change over time, and let

$$\boldsymbol{b}_{i(Ancova)} = (b_{i1(Ancova)}, ..., b_{i4(Ancova)}).$$

In this case, the model is expressed by

$$\begin{aligned} y_{ij} \mid \boldsymbol{b}_{i(Ancova)} &= \beta_0 + b_{ij(Ancova)} + \theta y_{i0} + \beta_1 x_{1i} + \beta_{2j} \\ &\qquad + \beta_{3j} x_{1i} + \boldsymbol{w}_i^t \boldsymbol{\xi} + \epsilon_{ij} \qquad (7.19) \\ &\quad i = 1, ..., N,\ j = 1,2,3,4;\ \beta_{21} = 0,\ \beta_{31} = 0 \\ \boldsymbol{b}_{i(Ancova)} &= (b_{i1(Ancova)}, ..., b_{i4(Ancova)}) \sim N(0, \Phi), \\ \epsilon_{ij} &\sim N(0, \sigma_E^2), \end{aligned}$$

where the $\boldsymbol{b}_{i(Ancova)}$ and ϵ_{ij} are assumed to be independent of each other.

In the above two models, the treatment effect at time j can be expressed via some linear contrast (see (3.39) and (3.40)). For example, the treatment effect at month 8 ($j = 4$) can be expressed as

$$\begin{aligned} \tau_{21}^{(4)} &= \beta_1 + \beta_{34} \\ &= (1)\beta_1 + (0,0,0,1)(\beta_{31}, \beta_{32}, \beta_{33}, \beta_{34})^t. \qquad (7.20) \end{aligned}$$

7.7.2 Model IX: Random intercept model for the average treatment effect

In this section, we shall consider Model IX in which the treatment effect is assumed to be constant during the evaluation period.

$$\begin{aligned} y_{ij} \mid b_{i(Ancova)} &= \beta_0 + b_{i(Ancova)} + \theta y_{i0} + \beta_3 x_{1i} + \boldsymbol{w}_i^t \boldsymbol{\xi} + \epsilon_{ij} \qquad (7.21) \\ &\quad i = 1, ..., N,\ j = 1,2,3,4 \\ &\quad b_{i(Ancova)} \sim N(0, \sigma_{B(Ancova)}^2) \\ &\quad \epsilon_{ij} \sim N(0, \sigma_E^2), \end{aligned}$$

where β_3 denotes the average treatment effect during the evaluation period and $b_{i(Ancova)}$ and ϵ_{ij} are assumed to be independent of each other.

7.7.3 Analysis using SAS

Now, let us apply Models VIIIa, VIIIb, and IX to the *Beat the Blues Data* using `PROC MIXED`. But, as is shown in Table 3.7, the first step for the analysis is to rearrange the data structure from the long format shown in Table 7.2 into another long format shown in Table 7.7 where the baseline records were deleted and the new variable `bdi0` indicating baseline data was created.

The respective sets of SAS programs are shown in Program 7.7. Here also,

TABLE 7.7
A part of the long format *Beat the Blues Data* set for the ANCOVA-type model. The variable `bdi0` indicates the baseline measurement. (Data for the first three patients are shown.)

No.	Subject	drug	length	treatment	visit	bdi	bdi0
1	1	0	1	0	2	2	29
2	1	0	1	0	3	2	29
3	1	0	1	0	5	NA	29
4	1	0	1	0	8	NA	29
5	2	1	1	1	2	16	32
6	2	1	1	1	3	24	32
7	2	1	1	1	5	17	32
8	2	1	1	1	8	20	32
9	3	1	0	0	2	20	25
10	3	1	0	0	3	NA	25
11	3	1	0	0	5	NA	25
12	3	1	0	0	8	NA	25

due to the option `/ref=first` used in the `CLASS` statement, the coefficients of the linear contrast for the `treatment*visit` interaction needs the order change (e.g., see Sections 3.5 and 5.3). For example, according to the equation (7.20), the linear contrast for the treatment effect at month 8 ($j = 4$) can be expressed in SAS as

```
estimate 'CFB: 8m' treatment 1 treatment*visit  0 0 0 1
```

However, due to the option `/ref=first`, the following change should be made for the `treatment*visit` interaction:

```
estimate 'CFB: 8m' treatment 1 treatment*visit  0 0 1 0
```

Furthermore, the fixed effects β_3 in Model IX can be expressed by the variable `treatment` and the `MODEL` statement and the `RANDOM` statement should be

```
model bdi = drug length bdi0 treatment  / s cl ddfm=sat ;
random intercept /  subject= subject g gcorr ;
```

Program 7.7: SAS procedure PROC MIXED for Models VIIIa, VIIIb and IX

```
data dbb2;
  infile 'c:\book\RepeatedMeasure\BBlongAncova.txt' missover;
  input no subject drug length treatment visit bdi bdi0;
  if visit=3 then w2=1; else w2=0;
  if visit=5 then w3=1; else w3=0;
  if visit=8 then w4=1; else w4=0;

proc mixed data=dbb2 method=reml covtest;
   class subject visit /ref=first  ;
   model bdi = drug length bdi0 visit treatment treatment*visit
                                    / s cl ddfm=sat ;
<Model VIIIa>
   random intercept /  subject= subject g gcorr ;
<Model VIIIb>
   random intercept w2 w3 w4/  subject= subject g gcorr ;

   repeated visit/ type =simple subject = subject r  rcorr ;
    estimate 'CFB:   2m   '
      treatment  1  treatment*visit  0 0 0 1/ divisor=1 cl alpha=0.05;
    estimate 'CFB:   3m   '
      treatment  1  treatment*visit  1 0 0 0 / divisor=1 cl alpha=0.05;
    estimate 'CFB:   5m   '
      treatment  1  treatment*visit  0 1 0 0 / divisor=1 cl alpha=0.05;
    estimate 'CFB:   8m   '
      treatment  1  treatment*visit  0 0 1 0 / divisor=1 cl alpha=0.05;

<Model IX>
proc mixed data=dbb2 method=reml covtest;
   class subject visit ;
   model bdi = drug length bdi0 treatment  / s cl ddfm=sat ;
   random intercept /  subject= subject g gcorr ;
   repeated visit / type = simple subject = subject r  rcorr ;
```

The results of Model Vllla are shown in Output 7.7 and those of Model IV are shown in Output 7.8. The results of Model VIIIb are omitted here.

Output 7.7: SAS procedure `PROC MIXED` for Model VIIIa

```
Covariance Parameter Estimates
Cov Parm   Subject  Estimate S.E.   Z value Pr > Z
Intercept  subject   52.3498 9.3601 5.59    <.0001
visit      subject   25.3580 2.6804 9.46    <.0001

Fit statistics
-2 Res Log Likelihood 1848.5
AIC (smaller is better) 1852.5
BIC (smaller is better) 1857.7

Solution for Fixed Effects
Effect           visit  Estimate S.E. DF t Value Pr>|t| Alpha Lower Upper
Intercept                4.7949 2.3116 103    2.07 0.0405 0.05  0.2104  9.3793
drug                    -2.7681 1.7795 92.3 -1.56 0.1232 0.05 -6.3023  0.7660
length                   0.2545 1.6891 94.4  0.15 0.8805 0.05 -3.0991  3.6082
bdi0                     0.6397 0.0802 97.7  7.98 <.0001 0.05  0.4806  0.7989
visit               3  -1.5905 1.1684 188   -1.36 0.1751 0.05 -3.8953  0.7144
visit               5  -3.1347 1.2668 190   -2.47 0.0142 0.05 -5.6335 -0.6358
visit               8  -5.9190 1.3358 191   -4.43 <.0001 0.05 -8.5539 -3.2842
visit               2   0 . . . . . . .
treatment              -3.0325 1.8849 131   -1.61 0.1101 0.05 -6.7613  0.6963
treatment*visit     3   0.3239 1.6342 191    0.20 0.8431 0.05 -2.8995  3.5473
treatment*visit     5   0.9724 1.7817 193    0.55 0.5859 0.05 -2.5418  4.4866
treatment*visit     8   2.9925 1.8539 193    1.61 0.1081 0.05 -0.6641  6.6491
treatment*visit     2   0 . .

Estimates
Label          Estimate S.E.   DF t Value Pr>|t| Alpha Lower Upper
CFB:   2m      -3.0325  1.8849 131 -1.61 0.1101 0.05 -6.7613 0.6963
CFB:   3m      -2.7085  2.0299 159 -1.33 0.1840 0.05 -6.7176 1.3005
CFB:   5m      -2.0601  2.1482 183 -0.96 0.3388 0.05 -6.2983 2.1782
CFB:   8m      -0.03996 2.2085 196 -0.02 0.9856 0.05 -4.3955 4.3155
```

In Section 4.4, we compared the estimates $\hat{\beta}_{3j}$ with the estimates $\hat{\beta}_{3j,Ancova}$ in the *1:1* design and concluded that (1) $\hat{\beta}_{3j}$ is unbiased and $\hat{\beta}_{3j,Ancova}$ is biased and (2) $\hat{\beta}_{3j,Ancova}$ is more precise than $\hat{\beta}_{3j}$. However, the gain in efficiency by using $\hat{\beta}_{3j,Ancova}$ seems to be small in many cases. So, here, it will be interesting to compare the estimates of treatment effect obtained from the ANCOVA-type models VIIIa (IX) with those from the repeated measures models VIIa (Va), which are shown in Table 7.8. In the *Beat the Blues Data*, both Model VIIa (Va) and Model VIIIa (IX) gave similar estimates, but the repeated measures models tend to give smaller p-values although all estimates are statistically non-significant at 5% significance level.

TABLE 7.8
Comparison of estimated treatment effects between repeated measures models and ANCOVA-type models.

Treatment effect	Repeated measures models Models IIa, Va		ANCOVA-type models Models VIIIa, IX	
	Estimate (s.e.)	Two-tailed p-value	Estimate (s.e.)	Two-tailed p-value
Model IIa vs. Model VIIIa				
$\hat{\beta}_{31}$: month 2	-3.3352 (1.9231)	0.0848	-3.0325 (1.8849)	0.1101
$\hat{\beta}_{32}$: month 3	-3.0006 (2.0717)	0.1492	-2.7085 (2.0299)	0.1840
$\hat{\beta}_{33}$: month 5	-2.2943 (2.1949)	0.2971	-2.0601 (2.1482)	0.3388
$\hat{\beta}_{34}$: month 8	-0.2770 (2.2566)	0.9024	-0.0400 (2.2085)	0.9856
Model Va vs. Model IX				
$\hat{\beta}_3$: Average	-2.5138 (1.8017)	0.1656	-2.1827 (1.7623)	0.2187

Output 7.8: SAS procedure `PROC MIXED` for Model IX

```
Covariance Parameter Estimates
Cov Parm   Subject   Estimate S.E.   Z value Pr > Z
Intercept  subject   54.4812 9.7725   5.57 <.0001
visit      subject   27.5797 2.8643   9.63 <.0001

Fit statistics
-2 Res Log Likelihood 1886.8
AIC (smaller is better) 1890.8
BIC (smaller is better) 1896.1

Solution for Fixed Effects
Effect    Estimate S.E. DF t Value Pr>|t| Alpha Lower Upper
Intercept  3.0264  2.2985  91.8  1.32 0.1912 0.05 -1.5387 7.5916
drug      -3.0083  1.8216  92.8 -1.65 0.1020 0.05 -6.6258 0.6092
length    -0.09467 1.7274  94.6 -0.05 0.9564 0.05 -3.5242 3.3349
bdi0       0.6473  0.08215 98.3  7.88 <.0001 0.05  0.4843 0.8104
treatment -2.1827  1.7623  91.9 -1.24 0.2187 0.05 -5.6829 1.3174
```

7.8 Sample size

In this chapter, various mixed-effects models were illustrated with the *Beat the Blues Data* which has *1:4* repeated measures design. In this section, we shall consider the sample size determination. The sample size determinations for longitudinal data analysis in the literature (for example, see Diggle et al., 2002; Hedeker and Gibbons, 2006; Fitzmaurice, Laird and Ware, 2011) are based on the *basic 1:T design* where the baseline data is used as a covariate. In other words, this design is essentially the *0:T design.* In this section, we shall consider the sample size (number of subjects) needed for the *S:T design* with $S > 0$, which is different from what appears in the literature. For technical details of derivation of sample size formula, see Appendix A (Tango, 2016a, 2016b).

7.8.1 Sample size for the average treatment effect

We first consider a typical situation where investigators are interested in estimating the average treatment effect during the evaluation period. To do this, let us consider Model V or the *random intercept plus slope* model (12.13) within the framework of *S:T* design. Namely, the model is expressed as

$$\begin{aligned} y_{ij} \mid (b_{0i}, b_{1i}) &= \beta_0 + b_{0i} + \beta_1 x_{1i} + (\beta_2 + b_{1i}) x_{2ij} \\ &\qquad + \beta_3 x_{1i} x_{2ij} + \epsilon_{ij} \qquad (7.22) \\ \epsilon_{ij} &\sim N(0, \sigma_E^2) \\ \boldsymbol{b}_i &= (b_{0i}, b_{1i}) \sim N(0, \boldsymbol{\Phi}) \\ \boldsymbol{\Phi} &= \begin{pmatrix} \sigma_{B0}^2 & \rho_B \sigma_{B0} \sigma_{B1} \\ \rho_B \sigma_{B0} \sigma_{B1} & \sigma_{B1}^2 \end{pmatrix} \\ i &= 1, ..., n_1 \text{ (the control group);} \\ &= n_1 + 1, ..., n_1 + n_2 = N \text{ (the new treatment group)} \\ j &= -(S-1), -(S-2), ..., 0, 1, ..., T, \end{aligned}$$

7.8.1.1 Sample size assuming no missing data

When there is no missing data, given the covariance matrix $\boldsymbol{\Sigma}$,

$$\boldsymbol{\Sigma} = \sigma_E^2 \boldsymbol{I} + \boldsymbol{Z} \boldsymbol{\Phi} \boldsymbol{Z}^t, \quad (\boldsymbol{I} \text{ denotes the identity matrix}) \qquad (7.23)$$

the maximum likelihood estimator $\hat{\boldsymbol{\beta}} = (\hat{\beta}_0, \hat{\beta}_1, \hat{\beta}_2, \hat{\beta}_3)^t$ for Model V is expressed by the general form

$$\hat{\boldsymbol{\beta}} = \left(\sum_{i=1}^{N} \boldsymbol{X}_i^t \boldsymbol{\Sigma}^{-1} \boldsymbol{X}_i\right)^{-1} \sum_{i=1}^{N} \boldsymbol{X}_i^t \boldsymbol{\Sigma}^{-1} \boldsymbol{y}_i \tag{7.24}$$

and its covariance matrix is given by

$$\mathrm{Var}(\hat{\boldsymbol{\beta}}) = \left(\sum_{i=1}^{N} \boldsymbol{X}_i^t \boldsymbol{\Sigma}^{-1} \boldsymbol{X}_i\right)^{-1} \tag{7.25}$$

where

$$\boldsymbol{X}_i = \begin{pmatrix} 1 & x_{1i} & x_{2i(1-S)} & x_{1i}x_{2i(1-S)} \\ \vdots & \vdots & \vdots & \vdots \\ 1 & x_{1i} & x_{2i0} & x_{1i}x_{2i0} \\ 1 & x_{1i} & x_{2i1} & x_{1i}x_{2i1} \\ \vdots & \vdots & \vdots & \vdots \\ 1 & x_{1i} & x_{2iT} & x_{1i}x_{2iT} \end{pmatrix} = \begin{pmatrix} 1 & x_{1i} & 0 & 0 \\ \vdots & \vdots & \vdots & \vdots \\ 1 & x_{1i} & 0 & 0 \\ 1 & x_{1i} & 1 & x_{1i} \\ \vdots & \vdots & \vdots & \vdots \\ 1 & x_{1i} & 1 & x_{1i} \end{pmatrix} \tag{7.26}$$

$$\boldsymbol{Z} = \begin{pmatrix} 1 & x_{2i(1-S)} \\ \vdots & \vdots \\ 1 & x_{2i0} \\ 1 & x_{2i1} \\ \vdots & \vdots \\ 1 & x_{2iT} \end{pmatrix} = \begin{pmatrix} 1 & 0 \\ \vdots & \vdots \\ 1 & 0 \\ 1 & 1 \\ \vdots & \vdots \\ 1 & 1 \end{pmatrix} \tag{7.27}$$

and the unknown variance components (Φ, σ_E^2) of covariance matrix $\boldsymbol{\Sigma}$ is estimated by the restricted maximum likelihood method (B.38). Especially, the maximum likelihood estimator $\hat{\beta}_3$ is given by the difference in means of change from baseline, i.e.,

$$\hat{\beta}_3 = \frac{1}{n_2} \sum_{i=1}^{N} d_i(S,T)x_{1i} - \frac{1}{n_1} \sum_{i=1}^{N} d_i(S,T)(1 - x_{1i}) \tag{7.28}$$

where

$$d_i(S,T) = \bar{y}_{i+(post)} - \bar{y}_{i+(pre)} \quad (7.29)$$

$$\bar{y}_{i+(post)} = \frac{1}{T}\sum_{j=1}^{T} y_{ij}, \quad (7.30)$$

$$\bar{y}_{i+(pre)} = \frac{1}{S}\sum_{j=-S+1}^{0} y_{ij} \quad (7.31)$$

and its variance is given by

$$\text{Var}(\hat{\beta}_3) = \frac{n_1+n_2}{n_1 n_2}\left\{\sigma_{B1}^2 + \left(\frac{S+T}{ST}\right)\sigma_E^2\right\}. \quad (7.32)$$

As the parameter β_3 denotes the treatment effect (*average* here) of the new treatment compared with the control treatment, the null and alternative hypotheses of interest will be one of the following three sets of hypotheses as discussed in Section 1.3:

1. Test for superiority: If a negative β_3 indicates benefits as in the BDI example, the superiority hypotheses are given by

$$H_0 : \beta_3 \geq 0, \text{ versus } H_1 : \beta_3 < 0. \quad (7.33)$$

If a positive β_3 indicates benefits, then they are

$$H_0 : \beta_3 \leq 0, \text{ versus } H_1 : \beta_3 > 0. \quad (7.34)$$

2. Test for non-inferiority : If a negative β_3 indicates benefits as in the BDI example, the non-inferiority hypotheses are given by

$$H_0 : \beta_3 \geq \Delta, \text{ versus } H_1 : \beta_3 < \Delta. \quad (7.35)$$

where $\Delta(>0)$ denotes the non-inferiority margin. If a positive β_3 indicates benefits, then they are

$$H_0 : \beta_3 \leq -\Delta, \text{ versus } H_1 : \beta_3 > -\Delta. \quad (7.36)$$

3. Test for *substantial superiority*: If a negative β_3 indicates benefits as in the BDI example, the substantial superiority hypotheses are given by

$$H_0 : \beta_3 \geq -\Delta, \text{ versus } H_1 : \beta_3 < -\Delta. \quad (7.37)$$

where $\Delta(>0)$ denotes the *substantial* superiority margin. If a positive β_3 indicates benefits, then they are

$$H_0 : \beta_3 \leq \Delta, \text{ versus } H_1 : \beta_3 > \Delta. \quad (7.38)$$

Then, the sample size (number of subjects) formula with two equally sized groups ($n_1 = n_2 = n$) with an effect size β_3 for the *superiority test* under the *random intercept plus slope* model with two-sided significance level α and power $100(1-\phi)\%$ for the *1:1 design* is given by

$$n_{S=1,T=1} \quad = \quad 2(Z_{\alpha/2}+Z_{\phi})^2 \times \frac{\sigma_{B1}^2 + 2\sigma_E^2}{\beta_3^2}, \tag{7.39}$$

where Z_γ denotes the upper $100\gamma\%$ percentile of the standard normal distribution. Then, we have the following sample size $n_{S,T}$ for the *superiority test* under the *S:T design*:

$$n_{S,T} \quad = \quad 2(Z_{\alpha/2}+Z_{\phi})^2 \times \frac{\sigma_{B1}^2 + \left(\frac{S+T}{ST}\right)\sigma_E^2}{\beta_3^2}. \tag{7.40}$$

Namely, compared with the *1:1 design*, the reduction percent $r_{S,T}$ in sample size is given by

$$r_{S,T} = 1 - \frac{n_{S,T}}{n_{S=1,T=1}} = \frac{\left(2-\frac{S+T}{ST}\right)\sigma_E^2}{\sigma_{B1}^2 + 2\sigma_E^2}. \tag{7.41}$$

The corresponding sample size formula $n_{S,T}^{(NI)}$ for the *non-inferiority test* (7.35) or (7.36) is given by

$$n_{S,T}^{(NI)} \quad = \quad 2(Z_{\alpha/2}+Z_{\phi})^2 \times \frac{\sigma_{B1}^2 + \left(\frac{S+T}{ST}\right)\sigma_E^2}{(\beta_3+\Delta\text{sign}(\beta_3))^2}, \tag{7.42}$$

where

$$\text{sign}(x) \quad = \quad \begin{cases} 1, & x>0 \\ -1, & x<0. \end{cases}$$

Furthermore, the corresponding sample size formula $n_{S,T}^{(SS)}$ for the *substantial superiority test* (7.37) or (7.38) is given by

$$n_{S,T}^{(SS)} \quad = \quad 2(Z_{\alpha/2}+Z_{\phi})^2 \times \frac{\sigma_{B1}^2 + \left(\frac{S+T}{ST}\right)\sigma_E^2}{(\beta_3-\Delta\text{sign}(\beta_3))^2}. \tag{7.43}$$

It should be noted that the sample size formulas for the *superiority test* in longitudinal data analysis described in the literature (Diggle et al., 2002; Fitzmaurice, Laird and Ware, 2011) are different from those above and are based on the following repeated measures model for the *0:T design* where the baseline data is usually used as a covariate:

$$\begin{aligned} y_{ij} \mid b_{2i} &= \beta_0 + b_{2i} + \beta_3^* x_{1i} + \epsilon_{ij},\ j = 1, ..., T \\ b_{2i} = b_{0i} + b_{1i} &\sim N(0, \sigma_{B2}^2),\ \sigma_{B2}^2 = \sigma_{B0}^2 + \sigma_{B1}^2 + 2\rho_B \sigma_{B0} \sigma_{B1} \\ \epsilon_{ij} &\sim N(0, \sigma_E^2), \end{aligned}$$

where β_3^* denote the difference in means of average treatment effect during the evaluation period, which is expected to be equal to β_3 in RCT, i.e.,

$$\hat{\beta}_3^* = \frac{1}{n_2} \sum_{i=1}^{N} \bar{y}_{i+(post)} x_{1i} - \frac{1}{n_1} \sum_{i=1}^{N} \bar{y}_{i+(post)} (1 - x_{1i})$$

and

$$\mathrm{Var}(\hat{\beta}_3^*) = \frac{n_1 + n_2}{n_1 n_2} \left(\sigma_{B0}^2 + \sigma_{B1}^2 + 2\rho_B \sigma_{B0} \sigma_{B1} + \frac{1}{T} \sigma_E^2 \right).$$

Namely, the sample size formula is

$$\begin{aligned} n_T &= 2(Z_{\alpha/2} + Z_\beta)^2 \times \frac{\sigma_{B2}^2 + \sigma_E^2 / T}{\beta_3^2} \\ &= \frac{2(Z_{\alpha/2} + Z_\beta)^2 \sigma^2}{\beta_3^2} \cdot \frac{1 + (T-1)\rho}{T}, \end{aligned} \tag{7.44}$$

where $\sigma^2 = \mathrm{Var}(y_{ij}) = \sigma_{B2}^2 + \sigma_E^2$ and covariance $\mathrm{Cov}(y_{ij}, y_{ij'})$ has a compound symmetry with a correlation coefficient ρ given by

$$\rho = \frac{\sigma_{B2}^2}{\sigma_{B2}^2 + \sigma_E^2} = \frac{\sigma_{B0}^2 + \sigma_{B1}^2 + 2\rho_B \sigma_{B0} \sigma_{B1}}{\sigma_{B0}^2 + \sigma_{B1}^2 + 2\rho_B \sigma_{B0} \sigma_{B1} + \sigma_E^2}. \tag{7.45}$$

Example:

In the *random intercept plus slope* model (Model Va), when applied to the *Beat the Blues Data*, the variances of random effects (b_{0i}, b_{1i}) are estimated as nearly $\hat{\sigma}_{B1}^2 = 40$, $\hat{\sigma}_E^2 = 30$. Using these variance estimates, let us calculate

TABLE 7.9
Reduction percent $r_{S,T}$ in the sample size of the *S:T design* compared with the *1:1 design* under the *random intercept plus slope* normal regression model for the case of $\hat{\sigma}^2_{B1} = 40$, $\hat{\sigma}^2_E = 30$.

S	T				
	1	2	3	4	5
1	.	0.150	0.200	0.225	0.240
2	0.150	0.300	0.350	0.375	0.390
3	0.200	0.350	0.400	0.425	0.440
4	0.225	0.375	0.425	0.450	0.465
5	0.240	0.390	0.440	0.465	0.480

the sample size (7.40) for the *superiority test* (7.33) or (7.34) needed to detect an effect size of $\beta_3 = 2.5$ (BDI score), an estimate from the model, with 80% power at $\alpha = 0.05$. For example, for the *1:4* design, the sample size (equal number of subjects per group) is calculated to be

$$n_{S=1,T=4} = 2 \times (1.96 + 0.84)^2 \times \left(40 + \frac{1+4}{1 \times 4} \times 30\right) / (2.5^2) = 194.4.$$

Thus, we need 195 subjects per group and need to enroll 390 subjects in total. However, if we plan *2:4* design, the sample size is

$$n_{S=2,T=4} = 2 \times (1.96 + 0.84)^2 \times \left(40 + \frac{2+4}{2 \times 4} \times 30\right) / (2.5^2) = 156.8.$$

Thus, we need a total of $157 \times 2 = 314$ subjects, which is a reduction of 19.5% compared with the *1:4* design. Furthermore, if we plan *3:4* design, we need a total of 290 subjects, indicating a reduction of 25.6% compared with the *1:4* design.

Using estimates $\hat{\sigma}^2_{B1} = 40$, $\hat{\sigma}^2_E = 30$, the reduction percent $r_{S,T}$ (7.41) of the sample size required for the *S:T design* compared with that of the *1:1 design* is shown for several combination of values of (S, T) in Table 7.9.

7.8.1.2 Sample size allowing for missing data

In longitudinal repeated measures studies, missing data are said to be *the rule*, not *the exception* (Fitzmaurice et al., 2011). Consequently, it is often recommended to calculate the sample size *conservatively* to adjust for the potential loss of power due to the occurrence of missing data.

The sample size calculations for longitudinal data analysis in the literature (for example, Diggle et al., 2002; Hedeker and Gibbons, 2006; Fitzmaurice, Laird and Ware, 2011) consider formulas for sample size estimation and assessment of statistical power allowing for subject attrition and a variety of covariance structures for the repeated measurements. However, it seems that they do not consider the *baseline data* in their longitudinal design and consider the *0:T* design in the comparison of two groups across all time points including the first time point.

Much of the literature on the modeling of missing data has been restricted to dropout or attrition, that is, to the missing patterns in which missing data are always only followed by missing data (for example, see Verbeke and Molenberghs, 2001; Diggle et al., 2002). The main reason for this is that it is easier to formulate models for patterns with dropouts than those with intermittent missing data because the latter includes a wider variety of patterns that are more difficult to handle. In such a modeling approach, however, there occurs inevitable difficulty because the same pattern of dropout might have different meanings and/or reasons depending on the subject, i.e., one might be informative but another non-informative.

In this section, we do not undertake any complex modeling approach but only assume that any patterns of missing data occur as MAR (missing at random) or as MCAR (missing completely at random) according to the Rubin's definition (1976). Then, under at least the MAR assumption, we shall calculate the power of the sample size $n_{S,T}$ and modify the sample size formula (7.40) for the superiority test to allow for the *distribution of the number of missing data* to be expected at the stage of statistical analysis (Tango, 2017).

A. Number of subjects eligible and missing distribution

Let us assume here that, at the design stage, the sample size $n_{S,T}(= n_1 = n_2)$ is determined by formula (7.40) with a two-sided significance level α and power $100(1-\phi)\%$. At the stage of statistical analysis of data, let $s_i(= 0, 1, ..., S-1)$ and $t_i(= 0, 1, ..., T)$ denote the number of missing data for the ith subject during the baseline period and during the evaluation period, respectively. Needless to say, the number of missing data during the baseline period could be zero in a well-controlled clinical trial, but here we shall consider the possibility of "missing" due to some inevitable reasons which are obviously *missing completely at random* (MCAR). Assume further here that the ith subject with $t_i = T$ (all data are missing during the evaluation period) is defined as *ineligible* and is excluded from the statistical analysis. Let π denote the probability of being *ineligible* and

$$x_{3ij} = \begin{cases} 0, & \text{if the } j\text{th measurement is missing for the } i\text{th subject} \\ 1, & \text{otherwise} \end{cases} \quad (7.46)$$

$$\delta_{a,b} = \begin{cases} 0, & \text{if } a = b \\ 1, & \text{otherwise.} \end{cases} \quad (7.47)$$

Then, the number of subjects eligible for the statistical analysis, m_1 for the control group and m_2 for the new treatment group, are given by

$$m_1 = \sum_{i=1}^{n_1} \delta_{T,t_i}, \ m_2 = \sum_{i=n_1+1}^{n_1+n_2} \delta_{T,t_i}. \quad (7.48)$$

Let m_{1kl} and m_{2kl} denote the frequency distribution of subjects eligible for statistical analysis that have $k(\leq S-1)$ missing data during the baseline period and $l(\leq T-1)$ missing data during the evaluation period in the control group and the new treatment group, respectively. Letting $p_{1kl} = m_{1kl}/m_1$ and $p_{2kl} = m_{2kl}/m_2$, i.e., we have

$$\sum_{k=0}^{S-1}\sum_{l=0}^{T-1} p_{1kl} = \sum_{k=0}^{S-1}\sum_{l=0}^{T-1} p_{2kl} = 1. \quad (7.49)$$

We shall call p_{1kl} and p_{2kl} *the missing distribution* among eligible subjects in the control group and the new treatment group, respectively.

B. Maximum likelihood estimator allowing for missing data

Let $\boldsymbol{y}_i^{(kl)}$ denote the $(S+T-k-l)\times 1$ vector of *the observed data rearranged to the origin* in $\boldsymbol{y}_i$. To illustrate this, let us consider several examples for the case of $S=2, T=3$ where y_{miss} denotes the missing data:

$$\boldsymbol{y}_i = (y_{i(-1)}, y_{i0}, y_{i1}, y_{miss}, y_{miss}) \Rightarrow \boldsymbol{y}_i^{(02)} = (y_{i(-1)}, y_{i0}, y_{i1})$$

$$\boldsymbol{y}_i = (y_{i(-1)}, y_{i0}, y_{i1}, y_{miss}, y_{i3}) \Rightarrow \boldsymbol{y}_i^{(01)} = (y_{i(-1)}, y_{i0}, y_{i1}, y_{i2}^*) \text{ with } y_{i2}^* = y_{i3}$$

$$\boldsymbol{y}_i = (y_{i(-1)}, y_{miss}, y_{miss}, y_{i2}, y_{i3}) \Rightarrow \boldsymbol{y}_i^{(11)} = (y_{i0}^*, y_{i1}^*, y_{i2}^*) \text{ with } y_{i0}^* = y_{i(-1)}, \ y_{i1}^* = y_{i2}, \ y_{i2}^* = y_{i3}$$

Needless to say, we have $\boldsymbol{y}_i^{(00)} = \boldsymbol{y}_i$. Then let

$$\boldsymbol{s}_{1kl} = \sum_{i=1}^{n_1} \boldsymbol{y}_i^{(kl)}, \ \boldsymbol{s}_{2kl} = \sum_{i=n_1+1}^{n_1+n_2} \boldsymbol{y}_i^{(kl)}. \tag{7.50}$$

Furthermore, we shall define three types of matrices. Let $\boldsymbol{W}_{1kl}$ and $\boldsymbol{W}_{2kl}$ denote the $(S+T-k-l) \times 4$ segment of the $(S+T) \times 4$ matrix $\boldsymbol{X}_i$ with $x_{1i} = 0$ (for the control group) and $x_{1i} = 1$ (for the new treatment group), respectively, i.e.,

$$\boldsymbol{W}_{1kl} = \left(\begin{array}{cccc} 1 & 0 & 0 & 0 \\ \vdots & \vdots & \vdots & \vdots \\ 1 & 0 & 0 & 0 \\ \hline 1 & 0 & 1 & 0 \\ \vdots & \vdots & \vdots & \vdots \\ 1 & 0 & 1 & 0 \end{array}\right) \begin{array}{l} S-k \\ \\ T-l \end{array} \tag{7.51}$$

$$\boldsymbol{W}_{2kl} = \left(\begin{array}{cccc} 1 & 1 & 0 & 0 \\ \vdots & \vdots & \vdots & \vdots \\ 1 & 1 & 0 & 0 \\ \hline 1 & 1 & 1 & 1 \\ \vdots & \vdots & \vdots & \vdots \\ 1 & 1 & 1 & 1 \end{array}\right) \begin{array}{l} S-k \\ \\ T-l. \end{array} \tag{7.52}$$

Let $\boldsymbol{\Psi}_{kl}$ denote the $(S+T-k-l) \times (S+T-k-l)$ matrix such that

$$\boldsymbol{\Psi}_{kl} = C \times \begin{array}{c} \quad S-k \qquad\qquad T-l \\ \left(\begin{array}{cccc|cccc} \rho_2 & \rho_1 & \cdots & \rho_1 & \rho_3 & \rho_3 & \cdots & \rho_3 \\ \rho_1 & \rho_2 & \cdots & \rho_1 & \rho_3 & \rho_3 & \cdots & \rho_3 \\ \vdots & \vdots & \ddots & \vdots & \vdots & \vdots & \vdots & \vdots \\ \rho_1 & \rho_1 & \cdots & \rho_2 & \rho_3 & \rho_3 & \cdots & \rho_3 \\ \hline \rho_3 & \rho_3 & \cdots & \rho_3 & 1 & \rho_4 & \cdots & \rho_4 \\ \rho_3 & \rho_3 & \cdots & \rho_3 & \rho_4 & 1 & \cdots & \rho_4 \\ \vdots & \vdots & \vdots & \vdots & \vdots & \vdots & \ddots & \vdots \\ \rho_3 & \rho_3 & \cdots & \rho_3 & \rho_4 & \rho_4 & \cdots & 1 \end{array}\right) \end{array} \begin{array}{l} S-k \\ \\ T-l \end{array} \tag{7.53}$$

where

$$\begin{aligned}
C &= \sigma_{B0}^2 + 2\rho_B\sigma_{B0}\sigma_{B1} + \sigma_{B1}^2 + \sigma_E^2 \\
\rho_1 &= \frac{\sigma_{B0}^2}{\sigma_{B0}^2 + 2\rho_B\sigma_{B0}\sigma_{B1} + \sigma_{B1}^2 + \sigma_E^2} \\
\rho_2 &= \frac{\sigma_{B0}^2 + \sigma_E^2}{\sigma_{B0}^2 + 2\rho_B\sigma_{B0}\sigma_{B1} + \sigma_{B1}^2 + \sigma_E^2} \\
\rho_3 &= \frac{\sigma_{B0}^2 + \rho_B\sigma_{B0}\sigma_{B1}}{\sigma_{B0}^2 + 2\rho_B\sigma_{B0}\sigma_{B1} + \sigma_{B1}^2 + \sigma_E^2} \\
\rho_4 &= \frac{\sigma_{B0}^2 + 2\rho_B\sigma_{B0}\sigma_{B1} + \sigma_{B1}^2}{\sigma_{B0}^2 + 2\rho_B\sigma_{B0}\sigma_{B1} + \sigma_{B1}^2 + \sigma_E^2}.
\end{aligned}$$

Then the maximum likelihood estimator for $\boldsymbol{\beta}$ *ignoring the missing data*, say $\hat{\boldsymbol{\beta}}^{(m)}$, can be expressed by the following special form

$$\begin{aligned}
\hat{\boldsymbol{\beta}}^{(m)} &= \left(\sum_{k=0}^{S-1}\sum_{l=0}^{T-1}(m_1p_{1kl}\boldsymbol{W}_{1kl}^t\boldsymbol{\Psi}_{kl}^{-1}\boldsymbol{W}_{1kl} + m_2p_{2kl}\boldsymbol{W}_{2kl}^t\boldsymbol{\Psi}_{kl}^{-1}\boldsymbol{W}_{2kl})\right)^{-1} \\
&\cdot \sum_{k=0}^{S-1}\sum_{l=0}^{T-1}(m_1p_{1kl}\boldsymbol{W}_{1kl}^t\boldsymbol{\Psi}_{kl}^{-1}\boldsymbol{s}_{1kl} + m_2p_{2kl}\boldsymbol{W}_{2kl}^t\boldsymbol{\Psi}_{kl}^{-1}\boldsymbol{s}_{2kl}) \qquad (7.54)
\end{aligned}$$

and its covariance matrix is given by

$$\begin{aligned}
\mathrm{Var}(\hat{\boldsymbol{\beta}}^{(m)}) &= \left(\sum_{k=0}^{S-1}\sum_{l=0}^{T-1}(m_1p_{1kl}\boldsymbol{W}_{1kl}^t\boldsymbol{\Psi}_{kl}^{-1}\boldsymbol{W}_{1kl} + m_2p_{2kl}\boldsymbol{W}_{2kl}^t\boldsymbol{\Psi}_{kl}^{-1}\boldsymbol{W}_{2kl})\right)^{-1} \\
&= \boldsymbol{V}_1. \qquad (7.55)
\end{aligned}$$

It should be noted that when there is no missing data, the variance of $\hat{\beta}_3$ (7.32) does not depend on the value of variance σ_{B0}^2, but when there are missing data, the variance (7.55) does depend on σ_{B0}^2. Its dependency, however, is quite small and could be negligible as shown later in examples.

C. Sample size formula allowing for missing data

Then the power $100(1-\phi')\%$ of the sample size $n_{S,T}$ (the number of actually randomized patients) that has (i) $2n_{S,T} - m_1 - m_2$ ineligible subjects and (ii) the missing distributions among eligible subjects, which could be expected in the design stage, is given by asymptotically

$$\begin{aligned}
1-\phi' &= \Pr\left\{\frac{\hat{\beta}_3}{\sqrt{(\boldsymbol{V}_1)_{44}}} > Z_{\alpha/2} \mid H_1\right\} \\
&= \Pr\left\{\frac{\hat{\beta}_3-\beta_3}{\sqrt{(\boldsymbol{V}_1)_{44}}} > Z_{\alpha/2} - \frac{\beta_3}{\sqrt{(\boldsymbol{V}_1)_{44}}} \mid H_1\right\} \\
&= G\left((Z_{\alpha/2}+Z_\phi)\sqrt{\frac{\frac{2}{n_{S,T}}\{\sigma_{B1}^2 + \left(\frac{S+T}{ST}\right)\sigma_E^2\}}{(\boldsymbol{V}_1)_{44}}} - Z_{\alpha/2}\right), \quad (7.56)
\end{aligned}$$

where $G(.)$ denotes the cumulative distribution function of the standard normal distribution and $(\boldsymbol{V}_1)_{44}$ is the (4,4) element of the covariance matrix $\boldsymbol{V}_1$. When $m_1 = m_2 = n_{S,T}$, i.e., all subjects are eligible, the above power is

$$1-\phi' = G\left((Z_{\alpha/2}+Z_\phi)\sqrt{\frac{2\{\sigma_{B1}^2 + \left(\frac{S+T}{ST}\right)\sigma_E^2\}}{(\boldsymbol{V}_2)_{44}}} - Z_{\alpha/2}\right), \quad (7.57)$$

where $\boldsymbol{V}_2$ is given by

$$\boldsymbol{V}_2 = \left(\sum_{k=0}^{S-1}\sum_{l=0}^{T-1}(p_{1kl}\boldsymbol{W}_{1kl}^t\boldsymbol{\Psi}_{kl}^{-1}\boldsymbol{W}_{1kl} + p_{2kl}\boldsymbol{W}_{2kl}^t\boldsymbol{\Psi}_{kl}^{-1}\boldsymbol{W}_{2kl})\right)^{-1}. \quad (7.58)$$

Needless to say, when there are no missing data, i.e., $m_1 = m_2 = n_{S,T}$, $p_{100} = 1$, $p_{200} = 1$, we have $1-\phi' = 1-\phi$. Furthermore, the sample size formula to allow for (a) the proportion π (its estimate will be $(2n_{S,T} - m_1 - m_2)/2n_{S,T}$ assuming to be equal for both groups) of the number of subjects with no data during the evaluation period and (b) the missing distribution among eligible subjects which could be expected in the design stage can be

$$n_{S,T}^{(mis)} = \frac{(Z_{\alpha/2}+Z_\phi)^2}{(1-\pi)\beta_3^2} \times (\boldsymbol{V}_2)_{44}, \quad (7.59)$$

where the number of eligible subjects are assumed to be equal for both treatment groups, i.e., $m_1 = m_2$.

D. Examples

To illustrate use of the formulas (7.40), (7.56) and (7.59), we shall use the *Beat the Blues Data* where we assume that the evaluation period is the first eight months after treatment began. So the repeated measures design will be a *1:4* design.

Using the SAS procedure `PROC MIXED`, we applied Model V (7.22) to the *Beat the Blues Data* without missing data ($n_1 = 25$ and $n_2 = 27$) and to the full dataset with missing data. For the latter dataset, we used the likelihood-based ignorable analysis by ignoring missing data under the MAR assumption. Judging from the value of AIC, Model V with $\rho_B = 0$ fit better than that with $\rho_B \neq 0$ for the full dataset. For the complete case analysis, we have the following estimates (s.e.)

$$\hat{\beta}_3 = -4.86(2.4),\ \hat{\sigma}^2_{B0} = 33.5(10.8),\ \hat{\sigma}^2_{B1} = 39.8(13.4),\ \hat{\sigma}^2_E = 29.6(3.4)$$

and the corresponding estimates for the full dataset are

$$\hat{\beta}_3 = -2.51(1.8),\ \hat{\sigma}^2_{B0} = 74.8(13.6),\ \hat{\sigma}^2_{B1} = 37.5(10.6),\ \hat{\sigma}^2_E = 28.5(2.9).$$

These estimates tell us that the true effect size β_3 could be between 2.5 and 5.0 and the variance components $(\sigma^2_{B1}, \sigma^2_E)$ are estimated as nearly $\hat{\sigma}^2_{B1} = 40$, $\hat{\sigma}^2_E = 30$ with and without missing data. Furthermore, the full dataset tells us that the number of missing data at baseline is zero and the number of ineligible (all data are missing during evaluation period) is 3 only for the TAU group, leading to $m_1 = 45, m_2 = 52$. The frequency distributions of the missing data are $(m_{100}, m_{101}, m_{102}, m_{103}) = (25, 4, 7, 9)$ for the TAU group and $(m_{200}, m_{201}, m_{202}, m_{203}) = (27, 2, 8, 15)$ for the BtheB group. Then the missing distributions are

$$\begin{array}{ll} \text{TAU group:} & \boldsymbol{p}_1 = (p_{100}, p_{101}, p_{102}, p_{103}) = (0.55, 0.09, 0.16, 0.20) \\ \text{BtheB group:} & \boldsymbol{p}_2 = (p_{200}, p_{201}, p_{202}, p_{203}) = (0.52, 0.04, 0.15, 0.29). \end{array}$$

Needless to say, these missing data are assumed to be *missing at random* here for illustration.

To examine the power $1 - \phi'$ of the sample size $n_{S,T}$ calculated to detect an effect size β_3 with 80% power at $\alpha = 0.05$ assuming no missing data and the sample size $n^{(mis)}_{S,T}$ to allow for ineligible percent π and the missing distributions $\{(p_{1kl}, p_{2kl}), k = 0, ..., (S-1); l = 0, ..., (T-1)\}$, we considered the following settings:

1. The true effect size is considered to be $\beta_3 = 3.0$.
2. Regarding the covariance of random effects, we considered $\sigma^2_{B0} = 70$, $\sigma^2_{B1} = 40$, $\rho_B = 0$, $\sigma^2_E = 30$ similar to those of the "Beat the Blues" RCT. However, to examine the dependency of the covariances $\boldsymbol{V}_1$ or $\boldsymbol{V}_2$ on σ^2_{B0}, we shall consider the two other values, i.e., $\sigma^2_{B0} = 20,\ 150$.

3. Regarding the probability of being ineligible, two cases $\pi = 0.00$ and $\pi = 0.05$ are considered.

4. Two repeated measures designs, the *1:4* design and the *2:4* design, are considered.

5. For the *1:4* design, "no missing data at baseline" is assumed (because subjects with no baseline data cannot be randomized) and three types of missing distributions during the evaluation period are considered, i.e.,

(1-1) No missing data, i.e., $p_{100} = p_{200} = 1.0$.

(1-2) Type A: similar to the missing distribution of the "Beat the Blues" RCT:

$$\begin{array}{ll} \text{TAU group:} & \boldsymbol{p}_1 = (0.5, 0.1, 0.2, 0.2) \\ \text{BtheB group:} & \boldsymbol{p}_2 = (0.5, 0.05, 0.15, 0.3) \end{array}$$

(1-3) Type B: Shift all the subjects' number of missing data in type A to the largest three, a bit extreme, to examine the effect on power and sample size.

$$\begin{array}{ll} \text{TAU group:} & \boldsymbol{p}_1 = (0.5, 0.0, 0.0, 0.5) \\ \text{BtheB group:} & \boldsymbol{p}_2 = (0.5, 0.0, 0.0, 0.5) \end{array}$$

6. For the *2:4* design, we considered six types of missing distributions, i.e.,

(2-1) No missing data at all, i.e., $p_{100} = p_{200} = 1$.

(2-2) No missing data during the baseline period and the type A missing distribution during the evaluation period:

$$\begin{aligned} \text{TAU group: } \boldsymbol{p}_1 &= \begin{pmatrix} p_{100} & p_{101} & p_{102} & p_{103} \\ p_{110} & p_{111} & p_{112} & p_{113} \end{pmatrix} \\ &= \begin{pmatrix} 0.5 & 0.1 & 0.2 & 0.2 \\ 0.0 & 0.0 & 0.0 & 0.0 \end{pmatrix} \\ \text{BtheB group: } \boldsymbol{p}_2 &= \begin{pmatrix} p_{200} & p_{201} & p_{202} & p_{203} \\ p_{210} & p_{211} & p_{212} & p_{213} \end{pmatrix} \\ &= \begin{pmatrix} 0.5 & 0.05 & 0.15 & 0.3 \\ 0.0 & 0.00 & 0.00 & 0.0 \end{pmatrix}. \end{aligned}$$

(2-3) No missing data during the baseline period and the type B missing distribution during the evaluation period:

$$\begin{aligned}\text{TAU group: } \boldsymbol{p}_1 &= \begin{pmatrix} 0.5 & 0.0 & 0.0 & 0.5 \\ 0.0 & 0.0 & 0.0 & 0.0 \end{pmatrix} \\ \text{BtheB group: } \boldsymbol{p}_2 &= \begin{pmatrix} 0.5 & 0.0 & 0.0 & 0.5 \\ 0.0 & 0.0 & 0.0 & 0.0 \end{pmatrix}.\end{aligned}$$

(3-1) 10% missing during the baseline period and no missing data during the evaluation period, i.e., $p_{100} = p_{200} = 0.9, p_{110} = p_{210} = 0.1$.

(3-2) 10% missing during the baseline period and the type A missing distribution during the evaluation period:

$$\begin{aligned}\text{TAU group: } \boldsymbol{p}_1 &= \begin{pmatrix} 0.45 & 0.09 & 0.18 & 0.18 \\ 0.05 & 0.01 & 0.02 & 0.02 \end{pmatrix} \\ \text{BtheB group: } \boldsymbol{p}_2 &= \begin{pmatrix} 0.45 & 0.04 & 0.13 & 0.27 \\ 0.05 & 0.01 & 0.02 & 0.03 \end{pmatrix}.\end{aligned}$$

(3-3) 10% missing during the baseline period and the type B missing distribution during the evaluation period:

$$\begin{aligned}\text{TAU group: } \boldsymbol{p}_1 &= \begin{pmatrix} 0.45 & 0.0 & 0.0 & 0.45 \\ 0.05 & 0.0 & 0.0 & 0.05 \end{pmatrix} \\ \text{BtheB group: } \boldsymbol{p}_2 &= \begin{pmatrix} 0.45 & 0.0 & 0.0 & 0.45 \\ 0.05 & 0.0 & 0.0 & 0.05 \end{pmatrix}.\end{aligned}$$

Results are shown in Table 7.10. For example, the sample size $n_{S,T}$ assuming no ineligible subjects and no missing data is calculated as 135.2 for the *1:4* design and 109.0 for the *2:4* design, respectively, indicating that the *2:4* design has a 19.4% reduction in sample size compared with the *1:4* design. It should be noted that the sample size $n_{S,T}$ (indicated in bold numbers in Table 7.10) does not depend on σ^2_{B0}. For the *1:4* design with $\pi = 5\%$, no missing data at baseline, and the type A missing distribution during the evaluation period, the power decreases to 75.1% and the required sample size $m_{1,4}$ increases to 153.5. On the other hand, for the *2:4* design with $\pi = 5\%$, no missing data during the baseline period, and the missing type B during the evaluation period, the power decreases to 72.1% and the required sample size $m_{2,4}$ increases

TABLE 7.10

Power $1-\phi'$ of sample size $n_{S,T}$ to detect an effect size $\beta_3 = 3.0$ ($\sigma^2_{B1} = 40, \sigma^2_E = 30$) with 80% power at $\alpha = 0.05$ and sample size $n^{(mis)}_{S,T}$ with 80% power at $\alpha = 0.05$ to allow for missing data for various combinations of repeated measures designs, probability of being ineligible π, value of σ^2_{B0}, missing distribution during baseline and evaluation period $\{(p_{1kl}, p_{2kl}), k = 0, ..., (S-1); l = 0, ..., (T-1)\}$. Bold numbers indicate $n^{(mis)}_{S,T} = n_{S,T}$.

π	Missing distribution	Power of $n_{S,T}$			$n^{(mis)}_{S,T}$		
		Value of σ^2_{B0}			Value of σ^2_{B0}		
		20	70	150	20	70	150
(1) 1 : 4 design with no missing data at baseline							
0.00	None	0.800	0.800	0.800	**135.2**	**135.2**	**135.2**
	Type A	0.770	0.770	0.769	145.6	145.8	145.9
	Type B	0.753	0.752	0.752	151.7	152.0	152.2
0.05	None	0.782	0.782	0.782	142.3	142.3	142.3
	Type A	0.751	0.751	0.751	153.3	153.5	153.6
	Type B	0.734	0.733	0.733	159.7	160.0	160.2
(2) 2 : 4 design with no missing data during the baseline period							
0.00	None	0.800	0.800	0.800	**109.0**	**109.0**	**109.0**
	Type A	0.764	0.763	0.763	119.3	119.5	119.5
	Type B	0.743	0.742	0.742	125.4	125.5	125.5
0.05	None	0.780	0.780	0.780	114.7	114.7	114.7
	Type A	0.742	0.742	0.742	125.6	125.7	125.8
	Type B	0.721	0.721	0.720	132.0	132.1	132.2
(3) 2 : 4 design with 10% missing data during the baseline period							
0.00	None	0.790	0.790	0.789	111.9	111.9	112.0
	Type A	0.757	0.756	0.755	121.2	121.6	121.7
	Type B	0.737	0.736	0.735	127.2	127.6	127.7
0.05	None	0.753	0.752	0.752	117.8	117.8	117.9
	Type A	0.735	0.734	0.734	127.6	128.0	128.1
	Type B	0.715	0.714	0.713	133.9	134.3	134.4

Regarding missing distribution during evaluation period,

#:None means that $p_{1+0} = p_{2+0} = 1$.

#:Type A: Close to the missing distributions during the evaluation period of the BDI example.

#:Type B: $p_{1+0} = p_{1+3} = p_{2+0} = p_{2+3} = 0.5$ for both treatment groups.

to 132.1, which is close to $n_{1,4} = 135.2$. For all the combinations examined here, the effects of the value of variance σ_{B0}^2 on the power $1 - \phi'$ and $n_{S,T}^{(mis)}$ are shown to be negligible.

7.8.2 Sample size for the treatment by linear time interaction

In this section, we shall consider the situation where the primary interest is testing the treatment by *linear* time interaction, i.e., testing whether the differences between treatment groups are *linearly* increasing over time as discussed in Section 7.6. In other words, the treatment effect can be expressed in terms of the difference in slopes of linear trend or rates of improvement. To do this, we shall consider Model VII or the *random intercept plus slope* model within the framework of *S:T* design. Namely, the model is expressed as

$$
\begin{aligned}
y_{ij} \mid \boldsymbol{b}_i &= b_{0i} + \beta_0 + \beta_1 x_{1i} + (\beta_2 + \beta_3 x_{1i} + b_{1i}) t_j + \epsilon_{ij} \qquad (7.60)\\
\boldsymbol{b}_i &= (b_{0i}, b_{1i}) \sim N(\mathbf{0}, \boldsymbol{\Phi})\\
\boldsymbol{\Phi} &= \begin{pmatrix} \sigma_{B0}^2 & \rho_B \sigma_{B0} \sigma_{B1} \\ \rho_B \sigma_{B0} \sigma_{B1} & \sigma_{B1}^2 \end{pmatrix}\\
i &= 1, ..., n_1 \text{ (the control group);}\\
&= n_1 + 1, ..., n_1 + n_2 = N \text{ (the new treatment group)}\\
j &= -(S-1), -(S-2), ..., 0, 1, ..., T,
\end{aligned}
$$

where the $\boldsymbol{b}_i$ and ϵ_{ij} are assumed to be independent of each other and t_j denotes the jth measurement time but all the measurement times during the baseline period are set to be the same time as t_0, which is usually set to be zero, i.e.,

$$
t_{-S+1} = t_{-S+2} = \cdots = t_0 = 0. \qquad (7.61)
$$

Here also, the parameter β_3 denotes the treatment effect. Then, the null and alternative hypotheses of interest will be one of the three sets of hypotheses (7.33)–(7.38). The maximum likelihood estimator $\hat{\beta}_3$ is given by the following closed form

$$
\hat{\beta}_3 = \frac{1}{n_2} \sum_{i=n_1+1}^{n_1+n_2} \hat{\gamma}_i(S,T) - \frac{1}{n_1} \sum_{i=1}^{n_1} \hat{\gamma}_i(S,T), \qquad (7.62)
$$

where $\hat{\gamma}_i(S,T)$ is the estimate for the ith subject's slope $\gamma_i = \beta_2 + b_{1i} + \beta_3 x_{1i}$, i.e.,

$$\hat{\gamma}_i(S,T) = \frac{\sum_{j=1-S}^{T}(t_j - \bar{t}^*)(y_{ij} - \bar{y}_{i+})}{\sum_{j=1-S}^{T}(t_j - \bar{t}^*)^2} \tag{7.63}$$

$$\bar{t}^* = \frac{(S-1)t_0 + (T+1)\bar{t}}{S+T} \tag{7.64}$$

$$\bar{t} = \frac{\sum_{j=0}^{t} t_j}{T+1}, \tag{7.65}$$

and its variance is given by

$$\begin{aligned} \text{Var}(\hat{\beta}_3) &= \frac{n_1+n_2}{n_1 n_2}\left\{\sigma_{B1}^2 + \sigma_E^2\left(\sum_{j=1-S}^{T}(t_j - \bar{t}^*)^2\right)^{-1}\right\} \\ &= \frac{n_1+n_2}{n_1 n_2}(\sigma_{B1}^2 + \sigma_E^2\, Q(S,T)^{-1}), \end{aligned} \tag{7.66}$$

where

$$Q(S,T) = \sum_{j=0}^{T}(t_j - \bar{t})^2 + \frac{(S-1)(T+1)}{S+T}(t_0 - \bar{t})^2. \tag{7.67}$$

Then, the sample size (number of subjects) formula (Tango 2016b) with two equal sized groups ($n_1 = n_2 = n$) to detect an effect size β_3 for the *superiority test* (7.33) or (7.34) with two-sided significance level α and power $100(1-\phi)\%$ is given by

$$n_{S,T} = 2\frac{(Z_{\alpha/2} + Z_\phi)^2}{\beta_3^2}(\sigma_{B1}^2 + \sigma_E^2\, Q(S,T)^{-1}) \tag{7.68}$$

which is an extension of the sample size formula $n_{1,T}$ described in the literature (for example, see Fitzmaurice, Laird, and Ware (2011), Chapter 20). As an important fact, sample size $n_{S,T}$ is smaller than $n_{1,T}$ and the reduction percent $r_{S,T}$ in sample size is given by

$$\begin{aligned} r_{S,T} &= 1 - \frac{n_{S,T}}{n_{1,T}} \\ &= \sigma_E^2 \times \frac{(\sum_{j=0}^{T}(t_j - \bar{t})^2)^{-1} - Q(S,T)^{-1}}{\sigma_{B1}^2 + \sigma_E^2(\sum_{j=0}^{T}(t_j - \bar{t})^2)^{-1}}. \end{aligned} \tag{7.69}$$

The corresponding sample size formula $n_{S,T}^{(NI)}$ for the *non-inferiority test* (7.35) or (7.36) is given by

$$n_{S,T}^{(NI)} = 2\frac{(Z_{\alpha/2}+Z_{\phi})^2}{(\beta_3+\Delta\text{sign}(\beta_3))^2}(\sigma_{B1}^2+\sigma_E^2\,Q(S,T)^{-1}) \tag{7.70}$$

Furthermore, the corresponding sample size formula $n_{S,T}^{(SS)}$ for the *substantial superiority test* (7.37) or (7.38) is given by

$$n_{S,T}^{(SS)} = 2\frac{(Z_{\alpha/2}+Z_{\phi})^2}{(\beta_3-\Delta\text{sign}(\beta_3))^2}(\sigma_{B1}^2+\sigma_E^2\,Q(S,T)^{-1}) \tag{7.71}$$

However, the impact of the missing data on the sample size required for a test of treatment by linear time interaction strongly depends on the patterns of missing data and so it is not so easy to derive the general formula of the sample size allowing for missing data.

Example:

To illustrate use of the sample size formula (7.68) and the reduction percent (7.69), let us consider the same example as that used by Fitzmaurice, Laird and Ware (2011). Suppose that investigators are interested in establishing whether the new treatment is *superior* (a *superiority test*) to the control treatment regarding the rate of improvement, in other words, the difference in slopes, β_3. The response variable is continuous and assumed to have an approximate normal distribution. The investigators plan to (1) set the length of the study as two years, (2) randomize an equal number of subjects to receive either of the two treatments, and (3) take five repeated measurements of the response, one during the baseline period, and the remainder at 6-month intervals until the completion of the study. Namely, they plan the *1:4* design with five measurement times $(t_0, t_1, t_2, t_3, t_4) = (0, 0.5, 1.0, 1.5, 2.0)$.

Suppose further that the investigators want to detect a minimum treatment effect of $\beta_3 = 1.2$, that is, a difference in the annual rates of change in the new treatment and control groups of no less than 1.2. Based on the historical data from similar populations, the investigators posit that $\sigma_{B1}^2 = 2$ and $\sigma_E^2 = 7$. Then, the sample size per group $n_{1,4}$ with 90% power at $\alpha = 0.05$ is calculated to be

$$n_{1,4} = 2\,\frac{(1.96+1.28)^2}{1.2^2} \times (2 + 7/2.5) = 70.0,$$

where $\bar{t} = 1, \sum_{j=0}^{T}(t_j - \bar{t})^2 = 2.5$. If the investigators plan two ($S = 2$) measurements during the baseline period, the sample size would be

TABLE 7.11
Sample size $n_{S,T}$ and the reduction percent $r_{S,T}$ (in brackets) of the *S:T design* for the *superiority tests* of the *random intercept plus slope* model (7.60) with $\sigma_{B1}^2 = 7$, $\sigma_E^2 = 2$ and an effect size $\beta_3 = 1.2$ with 90% power at $\alpha = 0.05$ where T measurement times after randomization are assumed to be equally spaced throughout the two-year duration of the study.

S	T				
	2	3	4	5	6
1	80.3	75.2	70.0	65.7	62.0
2	66.3 (17.4)	63.0 (16.2)	60.0 (14.3)	57.1 (13.0)	54.8 (11.6)
3	61.1 (23.9)	57.9 (22.9)	55.2 (21.2)	52.9 (19.3)	51.1 (17.6)
4	58.4 (27.3)	55.1 (26.6)	52.5 (25.0)	50.5 (23.1)	48.8 (21.3)
5	56.7 (29.4)	53.4 (29.0)	50.8 (27.5)	48.8 (25.6)	47.2 (23.8)

$$
\begin{aligned}
n_{2,4} &= 2\,\frac{(1.96+1.28)^2}{1.2^2} \\
&\quad \times \left\{ 2 + 7 \times \left(2.5 + \frac{(2-1)\times(4+1)}{2+4} \times (0-1)^2 \right)^{-1} \right\} \\
&= 60.0.
\end{aligned}
$$

which leads to 14.3% reduction. Furthermore, if they plan three ($S = 3$) or four ($S = 4$) measurements during the baseline period, the sample size would be reduced to 55.1 (21.2% reduction) or 52.5 (25.0% reduction), respectively. Within the framework of a two-year study period, the sample size $n_{S,T}$ and the reduction percent $r_{S,T}$ to detect $\beta_3 = 1.2$ with 90% power at $\alpha = 0.05$ is shown in Table 7.11 for several combinations of values of (S, T) where T measurement times after randomization are assumed to be equally spaced throughout the two-year duration of the study.

7.9 Discussion

In this chapter, several mixed-effects models are introduced and are illustrated with real data from a randomized controlled trial called *Beat the Blues Data* with *1:4* design. Needless to say, selection of the appropriate model depends on the purpose of the trial and an appropriate model should be examined cautiously using data from the previous trials.

Especially, we would like to stress that the set of models for the average treatment effect within the framework of *S:T* repeated measures design should be considered as a practical and important trial design, which is a better extension of the ordinary *1:1* design combined with ANCOVA in terms of *sample size reduction* and *easier handling of missing data.* Section 7.7.3 compared the estimates of treatment effect obtained from the ANCOVA-type models VIIIa (IX) with those from the repeated measures models VIIa (Va) and both Model VIIa (Va) and Model VIIIa (IX) gave similar estimates but the repeated measures models tend to give smaller p-values, although all estimates are statistically non-significant at 5% significance level.

However, the repeated measures models can be more natural for the *S:T* repeated measures design with $S > 1$ than the ordinary ANCOVA because the latter model must additionally consider how to deal with repeated measurements made before randomization.

8

Mixed-effects logistic regression models

In this chapter, we shall introduce the following three practical and important types of statistical analysis plans or statistical models that you frequently encounter in many randomized controlled trials:

◇ models for the treatment effect at each scheduled visit,
◇ models for the average treatment effect, and
◇ models for the treatment by linear time interaction,

which are illustrated with real data from a randomized controlled trial called *Respiratory Data.* It should be noted that the problem of *which model should be used in our trial* largely depends on the purpose of the trial. Furthermore, to contrast the traditional ANCOVA-type analysis frequently used in the pre-post design (*1:1* design) where the baseline measurement is used as a covariate, we shall introduce

◇ANCOVA-type models adjusting for baseline measurement

for the *1:T* design. Finally, sample size calculations needed for some models with *S:T* repeated measures design are presented and illustrated with real data.

8.1 Example 1: The Respiratory Data with *1:4* design

The first data used in this chapter comes from a randomized controlled trial conducted in two centres to compare two treatments for a respiratory illness (see Davis 1991 for details), which are introduced and analyzed in Everitt and Hothorn (2010). The respiratory status (categorized "poor" or "good") was determined prior to randomization and at each of four monthly visits after randomization ($S = 1, T = 4$). There are three covariates, centre (1, 2), age, and gender (male, female). The trial recruited $N = 111$ patients in total ($n_1 = 57$ in the placebo group, $n_2 = N - n_1 = 54$ in the active treatment group) and there were no missing data. A part of the *Respiratory Data* in

TABLE 8.1
Respiratory Data: Data set with long format from a randomized placebo-controlled trial for patients suffering from respiratory illness. Data for the first fifteen patients are shown.

No.	centre	subject	visit	treatment	status	gender	age
1	1	1	0	placebo	poor	female	46
2	1	1	1	placebo	poor	female	46
3	1	1	2	placebo	poor	female	46
4	1	1	3	placebo	poor	female	46
5	1	1	4	placebo	poor	female	46
6	1	2	0	placebo	poor	female	28
7	1	2	1	placebo	poor	female	28
8	1	2	2	placebo	poor	female	28
9	1	2	3	placebo	poor	female	28
10	1	2	4	placebo	poor	female	28
11	1	3	0	treatment	good	female	23
12	1	3	1	treatment	good	female	23
13	1	3	2	treatment	good	female	23
14	1	3	3	treatment	good	female	23
15	1	3	4	treatment	good	female	23

the long format is shown in Table 8.1 [1] which includes the following eight variables:

1. `no`: serial number for each record within the data set.
2. `centre`: a numeric factor for the study center (1, 2).
3. `subject`: a numeric factor indicating the subject ID.
4. `visit`: a numeric factor indicating the month of visit to the center during the treatment period, which has 0 (baseline), 1, 2, 3, 4.
5. `treatment`: a binary variable for the treatment group (the new treatment = 1, placebo = 0).
6. `status`: a binary variable for the respiratory status at each visit (poor = 0, good = 1)
7. `gender`: a binary variable for gender (female = 0, male = 1).

[1]This data set is available as the data frame `respiratory` in the `R` system for statistical computing using the following code: data("respiratory", package="HSAUR2")

TABLE 8.2
Frequency distribution of the respiratory status by treatment group and visit.

Treatment group	0	1	2	3	4 months
good	24	37	38	39	34
poor	30	17	16	15	20

Placebo group	0	1	2	3	4 months
good	26	28	22	26	25
poor	31	29	35	31	32

8. **age**: a continuous variable for age.

8.2 Odds ratio

In Table 8.2, the frequency distribution of the respiratory status by treatment group and visit is shown, which seems to have some information regarding the efficacy of the new treatment compared with the placebo. In the placebo group, the proportion or probability of the respiratory status being "good" is $p_0 = 26/57 = 45.6\%$ at baseline and does not change a lot all through the period. On the other hand, in the new treatment group, the probability is $p_0 = 24/54 = 44.4\%$ at baseline but improved to $p_1 = 37/54 = 68.5\%$ at month 1 and, after that, the probability is estimated to have ranged between 63% (at month 4) and 72% (at month 3).

One typical way of illustrating this situation is to use the *odds* and the *odds ratio* among the population in each treatment group at each visit. The *odds* of being "good" is defined as the ratio of the probability of being "good" to the probability of being "poor." For example, the odds of being "good" is estimated as $p_0/(1-p_0) = 26/31$ at baseline and $p_1/(1-p_1) = 28/29$ at month 1 for the placebo group. The odds ratio of being "good" at the jth visit to the baseline is calculated as the odds of being "good" at the jth visit divided by the odds at baseline. This gives

$$OR_{10} = p_1/(1-p_1) \div p_0/(1-p_0) = (28/29) \div (26/31) = 1.15$$

as an estimate of the odds ratio at month 1 to the baseline for the placebo group. Similarly, we have

$$
\begin{aligned}
OR_{20} &= (22/35) \div (26/31) = 0.749 \\
OR_{30} &= (26/31) \div (26/31) = 1.00 \\
OR_{40} &= (25/32) \div (26/31) = 0.931.
\end{aligned}
$$

In this case, these odds and odds ratios among the population are assumed to be the same for all the subjects. So, these odds and odds ratios are called *marginal or population-averaged* odds and odds ratios. Figure 8.1 shows the change of the *population-averaged* odds ratio over time by treatment group. It should be noted that these odds ratios do not take into account the heterogeneity of the subject-specific transition of the respiratory status from time to time. In other words, these odds ratios can be estimated from the usual *fixed-effects* logistic regression models as is shown in the next section. On the other hand, the mixed-effects logistic regression model to be introduced in this chapter does take the heterogeneity of the subject-specific transition of the respiratory status into account and gives the *subject-specific* odds ratios.

8.3 Logistic regression models

Let y_{ij} denote the respiratory status of the ith subject at the jth visit and $y_{ij} = 1$ if subject i's respiratory status is "good" and $y_{ij} = 0$ if the status is "poor." In this binary response variable, the linear (normal) regression model assuming y_{ij} to be distributed with a normal distribution would not be suitable. Rather, it would be quite natural to apply the logistic regression model which models the *logarithm of odds of being "good."* Let p denote the probability of being "good" in general. As the *logarithm of odds of being "good"* is simply the *logit transformation* of p, i.e., a *fixed-effects* logistic regression model with covariates $(x_1, ..., x_q)$ is defined as

$$
\text{logit } p = \log \frac{p}{1-p} = \beta_0 + \beta_1 x_1 + \cdots + \beta_q x_q. \tag{8.1}
$$

For example, consider the following *fixed-effects* logistic model to the *Respiratory Data*:

$$
\text{logit } p_{ij} = \log \frac{p_{ij}}{1-p_{ij}} = \beta_0^{PA} + \beta_1^{PA} x_{2ij} \tag{8.2}
$$

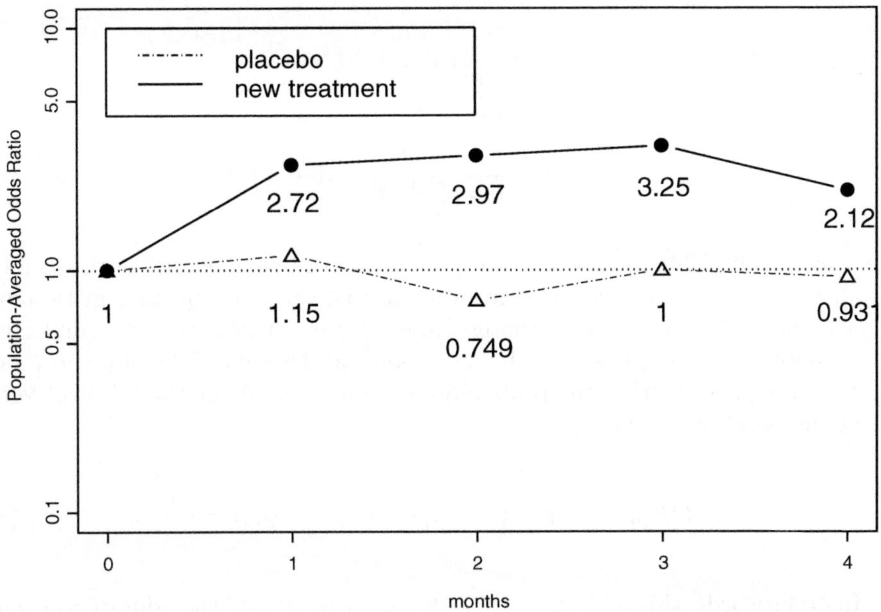

FIGURE 8.1
The response profile by treatment group based on the *population-averaged* odds ratio of being "good" at each visit versus the baseline.

where y_{ij} follows the Bernoulli distribution

$$\begin{aligned} y_{ij} &\sim \text{Bernoulli}(p_{ij}) && (8.3) \\ p_{ij} &= \Pr(y_{ij} = 1) = E(y_{ij}) && (8.4) \end{aligned}$$

and the probability function of the Bernoulli distribution is expressed as

$$f(y \mid p) = p^y(1-p)^{1-y} \tag{8.5}$$

and

$$x_{2ij} = \begin{cases} 1, & \text{for } j \geq 1 \\ 0, & \text{for } j = 0. \end{cases} \tag{8.6}$$

For the purpose of illustration, it is assumed here that all the subjects received the same new treatment. Then the probability of the respiratory status being "good" at baseline and during the treatment period is

$$p_{i0} = \frac{e^{\beta_0^{PA}}}{1 + e^{\beta_0^{PA}}}, \tag{8.7}$$

$$p_{ij} = \frac{e^{\beta_0^{PA}+\beta_1^{PA}}}{1 + e^{\beta_0^{PA}+\beta_1^{PA}}} \text{ (for } j \geq 1), \tag{8.8}$$

respectively. This means that the probability of being "good" is the same for all the subjects at each visit, in other words, the *fixed-effects* logistic model does not take into account the heterogeneity or variability of the underlying probability or propensity of being "good" at baseline. Therefore, the odds ratio OR_{j0} comparing the probability of being "good" at the jth visit versus at the baseline is given by

$$OR_{j0} = p_{ij}/(1 - p_{ij}) \div p_{i0}/(1 - p_{i0}) = e^{\beta_1^{PA}}. \tag{8.9}$$

In other words, this odds ratio (8.9) denotes the ratio of the odds of an *average subject* with "good" respiratory status at month j to the odds of an *average subject* with "good" status at baseline.

Next, let us consider the logistic regression model where subjects in the populations may differ with respect to their propensity of being "good" at baseline. To do this, we shall introduce the unobserved *random intercept* b_{0i} reflecting the heterogeneity or inter-subject variability at baseline and consider the following mixed-effects logistic regression model:

$$\text{logit } \Pr(y_{ij} = 1 \mid b_{0i}) = \beta_0^{SS} + b_{0i} + \beta_1^{SS} x_{2ij} \tag{8.10}$$

where, conditional on the random intercept b_{0i}, each y_{ij} independently follows the Bernoulli distribution

$$y_{ij} \mid b_{0i} \sim \text{Bernoulli}(p_{ij}), \tag{8.11}$$

where p_{ij} is the *conditional* expected value of y_{ij}, i.e.,

$$p_{ij} = \Pr(y_{ij} = 1 \mid b_{0i}) = E(y_{ij} \mid b_{01}). \tag{8.12}$$

Then, from the mixed-effects model (8.10), we have

$$\Pr(y_{i0} = 1 \mid b_{0i}) = \frac{e^{\beta_0^{SS} + b_{0i}}}{1 + e^{\beta_0^{SS} + b_{0i}}}, \tag{8.13}$$

$$\Pr(y_{ij} = 1 \mid b_{0i}) = \frac{e^{\beta_0^{SS} + b_{0i} + \beta_1^{SS}}}{1 + e^{\beta_0^{SS} + b_{0i} + \beta_1^{SS}}} \text{ (for } j \geq 1), \tag{8.14}$$

which shows clearly the subject-specific probability of being "good" at baseline and during the treatment period. Then, the *subject-specific* odds ratio is given by

$$\begin{aligned} OR_{j0} &= \frac{\Pr(y_{ij} = 1 \mid b_{0i})}{1 - \Pr(y_{ij} = 1 \mid b_{0i})} \div \frac{\Pr(y_{i0} = 1 \mid b_{0i})}{1 - \Pr(y_{i0} = 1 \mid b_{0i})} \\ &= e^{\beta_1^{SS}}. \end{aligned} \tag{8.15}$$

The odds ratio (8.15) denotes the ratio of the odds of a given subject with "good" respiratory status at month j to the odds of the *same subject* with "good" status at baseline. That's why the mixed-effects logistic regression model is called the *subject-specific model* or SS model, and the fixed-effects model is called the *population-averaged model* or PA model.

8.4 Models for the treatment effect at each scheduled visit

In exploratory trials in the early phases of drug development, statistical analyses of interest will be mainly to **estimate the time-dependent mean profile** for each treatment group and to test whether there is any treatment-by-time interaction. So, we shall here introduce two mixed-effects models to estimate the treatment effect at each scheduled visit, i.e., (1) a random intercept model and (2) a random intercept plus slope model with constant slope. during the evaluation period.

8.4.1 Model I: Random intercept model

First, a *random intercept model* with random intercept b_{0i} reflecting the inter-subject variability at month 0 (baseline) can be given as

$$
\begin{aligned}
\operatorname{logit} \Pr(y_{i0} = 1 \mid b_{0i}) &= \begin{cases} \beta_0 + b_{0i} + \boldsymbol{w}_i^t \boldsymbol{\xi}, & \text{(Placebo)} \\ \beta_0 + b_{0i} + \beta_1 + \boldsymbol{w}_i^t \boldsymbol{\xi}, & \text{(New treatment)} \end{cases} \\
\operatorname{logit} \Pr(y_{ij} = 1 \mid b_{0i}) &= \begin{cases} \beta_0 + b_{0i} + \beta_{2j} + \boldsymbol{w}_i^t \boldsymbol{\xi}, & \text{(Placebo)} \\ \beta_0 + b_{0i} + \beta_1 + \beta_{2j} + \beta_{3j} + \boldsymbol{w}_i^t \boldsymbol{\xi}, & \\ & \text{(New treatment)} \end{cases} \\
& \quad j = 1, ..., 4,
\end{aligned}
$$

where:

1. β_0 denotes the mean subject-specific log-odds of being "good" in the placebo group at baseline.
2. $e^{\beta_0 + b_{i0}}$ denotes the subject-specific odds of being "good" in the placebo group at baseline.
3. e^{β_1} denotes the subject-specific odds ratio comparing the odds of being "good" in the new treatment group versus in the placebo group at baseline.
4. $e^{\beta_{2j}}$ denotes the subject-specific odds ratio comparing the odds of being "good" at the jth visit versus at baseline in the placebo group.
5. $e^{\beta_{2j}+\beta_{3j}}$ denotes the same quantity in the new treatment group.
6. β_{3j} denotes the effect for the treatment-by-time interaction at the jth visit or $e^{\beta_{3j}}$ denotes a *ratio* of these two subject-specific odds ratios or the subject-specific *odds ratio ratio (ORR)*. In other words, $e^{\beta_{3j}}$ means the subject-specific treatment effect of the new treatment compared with placebo at the jth visit in terms of the *ORR*.
7. $\boldsymbol{w}_i^t = (w_{1i}, ..., w_{qi})$ is a vector of covariates.
8. $\boldsymbol{\xi}^t = (\xi_1, ..., \xi_q)$ is a vector of coefficients for covariates.

Needless to say, we should add the phrase "adjusted for covariates" to the interpretations of fixed-effects parameters β, but we omit the phrase in what follows. As in Section 7.4.1, by introducing the two dummy variables x_{1i}, x_{2ij}, the above model can be re-expressed as

$$
\begin{aligned}
\operatorname{logit} \Pr(y_{ij} = 1 \mid b_{0i}) &= \beta_0 + b_{0i} + \beta_1 x_{1i} + \beta_{2j} x_{2ij} + \beta_{3j} x_{1i} x_{2ij} + \boldsymbol{w}_i^t \boldsymbol{\xi} \quad (8.16) \\
i &= 1, ..., N; \quad j = 0, 1, 2, 3, 4; \quad \beta_{20} = 0, \quad \beta_{30} = 0 \\
b_{0i} &\sim N(0, \sigma_{B0}^2),
\end{aligned}
$$

where the random intercepts b_{0i} are assumed to be normally distributed with zero mean and variance σ_{B0}^2 and

$$
\begin{aligned}
x_{1i} &= \begin{cases} 1, & \text{if the } i\text{th subject is assigned to the new treatment} \\ 0, & \text{if the } i\text{th subject is assigned to the control} \end{cases} && (8.17)\\
x_{2ij} &= \begin{cases} 1, & \text{for } j \geq 1 \text{ (evaluation period)} \\ 0, & \text{for } j \leq 0 \text{ (baseline period).} \end{cases} && (8.18)
\end{aligned}
$$

It should be noted here also that an important assumption is, given the random intercept b_{0i}, the subject-specific repeated measures $(y_{i0}, ..., y_{i4})$ are *mutually independent.*

8.4.2 Model II: Random intercept plus slope model

As the second model, consider a *random intercept plus slope model* by simply adding the random slope b_{1i} taking account of the inter-subject variability of the response to the treatment assumed to be constant during the treatment period, which is given by

$$
\begin{aligned}
\text{logit}\,\Pr(y_{i0} = 1 \mid b_{0i}) &= \begin{cases} \beta_0 + b_{0i} + \boldsymbol{w}_i^t \boldsymbol{\xi}, & \text{(Placebo)} \\ \beta_0 + b_{0i} + \beta_1 + \boldsymbol{w}_i^t \boldsymbol{\xi}, & \text{(New treatment)} \end{cases} \\
\text{logit}\,\Pr(y_{ij} = 1 \mid b_{0i}, b_{1i}) &= \begin{cases} \beta_0 + b_{0i} + b_{1i} + \beta_{2j} + \boldsymbol{w}_i^t \boldsymbol{\xi}, & \text{(Placebo)} \\ \beta_0 + b_{0i} + b_{1i} + \beta_1 + \beta_{2j} + \beta_{3j} + \boldsymbol{w}_i^t \boldsymbol{\xi}, & \\ \qquad\qquad\qquad\qquad \text{(New treatment)} \end{cases} \\
& \quad j = 1, ..., 4.
\end{aligned}
$$

Namely, we have

$$
\begin{aligned}
\text{logit}\,\Pr(y_{ij} = 1 \mid b_{0i}, b_{1i}) &= \beta_0 + b_{0i} + b_{1i} x_{2ij} + \beta_1 x_{1i} + \beta_{2j} x_{2ij} \\
& \quad + \beta_{3j} x_{1i} x_{2ij} + \boldsymbol{w}_i^t \boldsymbol{\xi} \qquad (8.19) \\
i &= 1, ..., N; \;\; j = 0, 1, 2, 3, 4; \;\; \beta_{20} = 0, \;\; \beta_{30} = 0 \\
\boldsymbol{b}_i &= (b_{0i}, b_{1i}) \sim N(0, \Phi) \\
\boldsymbol{\Phi} &= \begin{pmatrix} \sigma_{B0}^2 & \rho_B \sigma_{B0} \sigma_{B0} \\ \rho_B \sigma_{B0} \sigma_{B1} & \sigma_{B1}^2 \end{pmatrix}.
\end{aligned}
$$

We shall call the model II with $\rho_B = 0$ Model IIa and the one with $\rho_B \neq 0$ Model IIb. It should be noted that the *random slope* introduced in the above model does not mean the *slope* on the time or a linear time trend, which will be considered in Section 8.6.

8.4.3 Analysis using SAS

Now, let us apply Models I, IIa and IIb to the *Respiratory Data* using `PROC GRIMMIX`. The following considerations are required for coding SAS programs (some of them have already been described in Sections 3.5 and 7.4.4):

1. A binary variable `treatment` indicates x_{1i}.

2. Create a new binary variable `post` indicating x_{2ij} in the `DATA` step as

```
if visit=0 then post=0; else post=1;
```

3. The fixed effects β_{2j} can be expressed via the variable `visit` (main factor), which must be specified as a numeric factor by the `CLASS` statement.

4. The fixed effects β_{3j} can be expressed via the `treatment * visit` interaction.

5. As already explained in Section 3.5, the `CLASS` statement needs the option `/ref=first` to specify that first category is the reference category.

6. The option `method=quad` specifies the adaptive Gauss–Hermite quadrature method for evaluating integrals involved in the calculation of the log-likelihood. For details on the reason why the adaptive Gauss-Hermite quadrature method is used, see Section B.3 in Appendix B.

7. The option `(qpoints=15)` specifies the number of nodes used for evaluating integrals for the likelihood. For the details to select the number of nodes, see Section B.3.3.2 in Appendix B.

8. The logistic regression model is specified as

```
model status (event="1") =
```

   because the `status` =1 for "good."

9. When you would like to fit the *random intercept and slope model* with $\rho_B = 0$, you have to use the following `RANDOM` statement:

```
random intercept post /type=simple subject=id g gcorr ;
```

   When you would like to fit the model with $\rho_B \neq 0$, you have to use the option `type=un`

```
random intercept post /type=un subject=id g gcorr ;
```

10. As in the case of the normal linear regression models, let us perform the same diagnostic based on *studentized conditional residuals*, which is useful to examine whether the subject-specific model is adequate, although `PROC GLIMMIX` provides several kinds of panels of residual diagnostics. Each panel consists of a plot of residuals versus predicted values, a histogram with normal density overlaid, a Q-Q plot, and the box plots of residuals. We can do this in the same manner as explained in Section 7.4.4.

The respective sets of SAS programs are shown in Program 8.1 and the results for Model I are shown in Output 8.1.

Program 8.1. SAS procedure `PROC GRIMMIX` for Models I, IIa, IIb

```
data resplong ;
 infile 'c:\book\RepeatedMeasure\longresp.txt' missover;
 input no centre subject visit treatment status gender age;
 if visit=0 then post=0; else post=1;

ods graphics on;
proc glimmix data=resplong method=quad (qpoints=15)
 plots=studentpanel( conditional blup) ;
 class subject centre visit/ref=first   ;
 model status (event="1") = centre gender age treatment
                            visit treatment*visit
                               / d=bin link=logit s cl ;
/* Model I  */
  random intercept / subject= subject g gcorr ;

/* Model IIa  */
  random intercept post / type=simple subject= subject g gcorr ;

/* Model IIb */
  random intercept post / type=un subject= subject g gcorr ;
```

Output 8.1. SAS procedure PROC GRIMMIX for Models I

```
Fit statistics
-2 Res Log Likelihood 565.95
AIC (smaller is better) 593.95
BIC (smaller is better) 631.88

Covariance Parameter Estimates
Cov Parm    Subject   Estimate S.E.
Intercept   subject   5.9674 1.6638

Solution for Fixed Effects
Effect     center visit Estimate S.E. DF t Value Pr>|t| Alpha Lower Upper
Intercept               -0.2810 0.8603 106 -0.33 0.7446 0.05 -1.9866 1.4246
centre       2            2.0290 0.5908 436  3.43 0.0007 0.05  0.8677 3.1902
centre       1            0 . . . . . . .
gender                  -0.4151 0.7397 436 -0.56 0.5750 0.05 -1.8689 1.0388
age                     -0.0302 0.0219 436 -1.38 0.1684 0.05 -0.0733 0.01284
treatment               -0.1789 0.7363 436 -0.24 0.8081 0.05 -1.6260 1.2681
visit              1     0.2779 0.5278 436  0.53 0.5988 0.05 -0.7595 1.3153
visit              2    -0.5593 0.5317 436 -1.05 0.2934 0.05 -1.6042 0.4856
visit              3     2.2E-6 0.5269 436  0.00 1.0000 0.05 -1.0356 1.0356
visit              4    -0.1389 0.5273 436 -0.26 0.7923 0.05 -1.1752 0.8974
visit              0     0 . . . . . . .
treatment*visit    1     1.7181 0.7918 436  2.17 0.0306 0.05 0.1619  3.2742
treatment*visit    2     2.7284 0.8082 436  3.38 0.0008 0.05 1.1401  4.3168
treatment*visit    3     2.3477 0.8080 436  2.91 0.0039 0.05 0.7596  3.9358
treatment*visit    4     1.6411 0.7781 436  2.11 0.0355 0.05 0.1119  3.1703
treatment*visit    0     0 . . . . . .
```

In Model I, the estimated variance of the random intercept is $\hat{\sigma}^2_{B0} = 5.97$ ($s.e. = 1.66$). In Figure 8.2, the response profile over time based on the estimated *subject-specific* odds ratio, $e^{\hat{\beta}_{2j}}$ (for the placebo group) or $e^{\hat{\beta}_{2j}+\hat{\beta}_{3j}}$ (for the new treatment group), is shown by group. The *ratio of odds ratios*, i.e., the subject-specific effect size of the new treatment at each of four visits after randomization $e^{\beta_{3j}}$, is estimated as

$$e^{1.72} = 5.57, \; e^{2.73} = 15.31, \; e^{2.35} = 10.46, \; e^{1.64} = 5.16,$$

respectively, and all are statistically significant at 5% level. Some readers may find that the absolute value of the *subject-specific* log odds ratios are larger than the absolute value of the *population-averaged* log odds ratios shown in Figure 8.1. Indeed, for example, the ratios of the former to the latter in the placebo group are as follows:

- At month 1: $0.2779/\log(1.15) = 1.99$
- At month 2: $\mid -0.5593 \mid / \mid \log(0.749) \mid = 1.94$
- At month 4: $\mid -0.1389 \mid / \mid \log(0.931) \mid = 1.94$

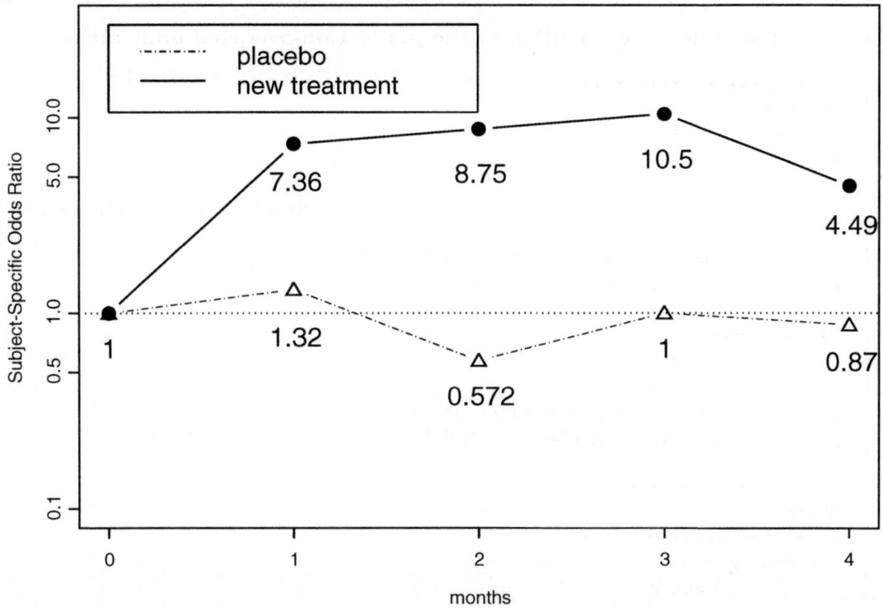

FIGURE 8.2
The response profile by treatment group based on the estimated *subject-specific* odds ratios (via Model I) of being "good" at each visit versus the baseline.

Namely, these ratios are almost constant and falling around 1.95. Theoretically, the relationship between these two kinds of fixed parameters is given by

$$\Pr\{y_{ij} = 1\} = \int_{-\infty}^{\infty} \Pr\{y_{ij} = 1 \mid b_{0i}\}\phi(b_{0i})db_{0i}, \tag{8.20}$$

where $\phi(.)$ denotes the probability density function of the random intercept b_{0i}. We will show the computation of the *population-averaged* odds ratios by visit in more detail below.

Examples of calculation of the population-averaged odds ratios

```
++++++++++++++++++++++
Month 1
++++++++++++++++++++++
New drug group                        Fig 8.1
             month
                                                  Model I (fixed-effects only)
             0   1
good        24  37  ORn = 37*30/(24*17) = 2.72
poor        30  17  ORn/ORp         = 2.36
                    log(ORn/ORp) = 0.86                   = beta_3j
Placebo group
             month
             0   1
good        26  28  ORp = 28*31/(26*29) = 1.15
poor        31  29  log(ORp)        = 0.14                = beta_2j

++++++++++++++++++++++
Month 2
++++++++++++++++++++++
New drug group
             month
             0   2
good        24  38  ORn = 38*30/(24*16) = 2.97
poor        30  16  ORn/ORp         = 3.96
                    log(ORn/ORp) = 1.38                   = beta_3j
Placebo group
             month
             0   2
good        26  22  ORp = 22*31/(26*35) = 0.75
poor        31  35  log(ORp)        = -0.29               = beta_2j

++++++++++++++++++++++
Month 3
++++++++++++++++++++++
New drug group
             month
             0   3
good        24  39   ORn = 39*30/(24*15) = 3.25
poor        30  15   ORn/ORp         = 3.25
                     log(ORn/ORp) = 1.18                  = beta_3j
Placebo group
             month
             0   3
good        26  26   ORp = 26*31/(26*31) = 1.00
poor        31  31   log(ORp)        = 0.00               = beta_2j
```

As a matter of fact, these estimates of population-averaged odds ratios can be obtained by applying Model I using the SAS procedure `PROC GRIMMIX`, where the `RANDOM` statement is deleted as shown in Program and Output 8.2.

Program and Output 8.2. SAS procedure `PROC GRIMMIX` for Model I (fixed-effects only) — deleting `RANDOM` statement —

```
<SAS program>
 proc glimmix data=resplong method=quad (qpoints=15);
   class subject centre visit/ref=first  ;
   model status (event="1")  =  treatment visit treatment*visit
                                     / d=bin link=logit s cl ;

<A part of the results>
Fit statistics
-2 Res Log Likelihood 732.44
AIC (smaller is better) 752.44
BIC (smaller is better) 795.63

Solution for Fixed Effects
Effect          visit  Estimate S.E. DF t Value Pr>|t|
Intercept               -0.1759  0.2659 545 -0.66 0.5086
treatment               -0.04725 0.3817 545 -0.12 0.9015
visit             1      0.1408  0.3754 545  0.38 0.7077
visit             2     -0.2884  0.3805 545 -0.76 0.4487
visit             3     -687E-17 0.3761 545 -0.00 1.0000
visit             4     -0.07097 0.3768 545 -0.19 0.8507
visit             0      0 . . . .
treatment*visit 1        0.8600  0.5493 545  1.57 0.1180
treatment*visit 2        1.3766  0.5555 545  2.48 0.0135
treatment*visit 3        1.1787  0.5556 545  2.12 0.0344
treatment*visit 4        0.8247  0.5444 545  1.51 0.1304
treatment*visit 0        0 . . . .
```

The fitted model assumes independence between visits. Judging from AIC (752 vs. 593) and BIC (796 vs. 632), the goodness-of-fit of this independence model is quite worse than Model I.

On the other hand, the *subject-specific* model considers the *subject-specific* transition of a respiratory status over time. To simplify the problem, let us consider the *1:1* repeated measures design and the transition from the baseline respiratory status to the status at visit $j = 1$. Table 8.3 shows the frequency distribution of the transition in general, i.e., the matched-pair, 2×2 contingency table. In this case, we have only to consider the case of $y_{i+} = y_{i0} + y_{i1} = 1$ because the case that $y_{i+} = 0$ or $y_{i+} = 2$ does not contribute to the conditional likelihood for (β_{21}, β_{31}). (Why conditional likelihood? Please see Appendix A.) Then, the conditional likelihood given $y_{i+} = 1$ is

$$L_C(\beta_{21}, \beta_{31} \mid t = 1) \quad = \quad \prod_{i:y_{i+}=1} \frac{\exp\{y_{i1}(\beta_{21} + \beta_{31} x_{1i})\}}{1 + \exp\{\beta_{21} + \beta_{31} x_{1i}\}}. \tag{8.21}$$

Then, the conditional maximum likelihood estimators of (β_{21}, β_{31}) are given by

TABLE 8.3
Matched-pair 2-by-2 contingency table for change of respiratory status from baseline period to post randomization by treatment group.

Before randomization ($j = 0$)	Post randomization ($j = 1$)		Total
	Good	Poor	
New treatment (2)			
good		$y_{gp}^{(2)}$	
poor	$y_{pg}^{(2)}$		
total			n_2
Control treatment (1)			
good		$y_{gp}^{(1)}$	
poor	$y_{pg}^{(1)}$		
total			n_1

$$\hat{\beta}_{21C} = \log\left(\frac{y_{pg}^{(1)}}{y_{gp}^{(1)}}\right) \tag{8.22}$$

$$\hat{\beta}_{31C} = \log\left\{\left(\frac{y_{pg}^{(2)}}{y_{gp}^{(2)}}\right) / \left(\frac{y_{pg}^{(1)}}{y_{gp}^{(1)}}\right)\right\} = \log\left(\frac{y_{pg}^{(2)} y_{gp}^{(1)}}{y_{gp}^{(2)} y_{pg}^{(1)}}\right), \tag{8.23}$$

where $y_{pg}^{(k)}$ and $y_{gp}^{(k)}$ denote the number of subjects whose respiratory status improved ("poor" $\rightarrow$ "good") and got worse ("good" $\rightarrow$ "poor") from baseline to month 1 in the treatment group k, respectively. Interpretations of these estimates will be that conditional maximum likelihood estimator $e^{\hat{\beta}_{21C}}$ implies the matched-pair odds ratio of improvement ("poor" $\rightarrow$ "good") in the control group and the the conditional maximum likelihood estimator $e^{\hat{\beta}_{31C}}$ of treatment effect implies the ratio of the improvement odds ratio in the new treatment group to the improvement odds ratio in the control treatment group. For more details, see Appendix A.

Concrete calculations of the *subject-specific* odds ratio are shown below. These conditional maximum likelihood estimates $(\hat{\beta}_{2jC}, \hat{\beta}_{3jC})$, $j = 1, 2, 3$ are shown to be close (not the same) to those of Model I where the full maximum likelihood estimates are obtained.

Calculations of the *subject-specific* odds ratios

```
++++++++++++++++++++++
Month 1: Matched-pair Odds ratio
++++++++++++++++++++++
New drug group                                      Model I
         month 1
       good poor
  good  24    0  ORn =13.5/0.5 = 27
  poor  13   17  ORn/ORp       = 21
                 log(ORn/ORp)= 3.04 (se=1.53),    beta_3j =1.72 (se=0.79)
Placebo group
        month 1
       good poor
  good  19    7  ORp = 9/7     = 1.29
  poor   9   22  log(ORp)      = 0.25 (se=0.53),  beta_2j =0.28 (se=0.53)
++++++++++++++++++++++
Month 2: Matched-pair Odds ratio
++++++++++++++++++++++
New drug group
         month 2
       good poor
  good  21    3  ORn   = 17/3  = 5.67
  poor  17   13  ORn/ORp       = 8.90
                 log(ORn/ORp)= 2.19 (se=0.79),    beta_3j =2.73 (se=0.80)
Placebo group
         month 2
       good poor
  good  15   11  ORp = 7/11    = 0.63
  poor   7   24  log(ORp)    = -0.45(se=0.48),  beta_2j = -0.56 (se=0.53)
++++++++++++++++++++++
Month 3: Matched-pair Odds ratio
++++++++++++++++++++++
New drug group
         month 3
       good poor
  good  23    1  ORn = 16/1    = 16
  poor  16   14  ORn/ORp       = 16
                 log(ORn/ORp)= 2.77 (se=1.15),   beta_3j = 2.35 (se=0.80)
Placebo group
         month 3
       good poor
  good  18    8  ORp = 8/8     = 1.00
  poor   8   23  log(ORp)   = 0.00 (se=0.50),  beta_2j = 0.00 (se=0.53)
```

In Table 8.4, we have shown the estimated treatment effect $\hat{\beta}_{3j}$ at each of four visits for Model I and Model IIa ($\rho_B = 0$). Although the estimates of Model IIb are omitted, its AIC and BIC are 596.6 and 639.9, respectively. Therefore, based on these information criteria, Model I fits better than Model IIa and Model IIb. The panel of graphics of the studentized conditional residuals of Model I is shown in Figure 8.3. Especially, a plot of residuals versus predicted values looks significantly different from the usual patterns seen in these kinds

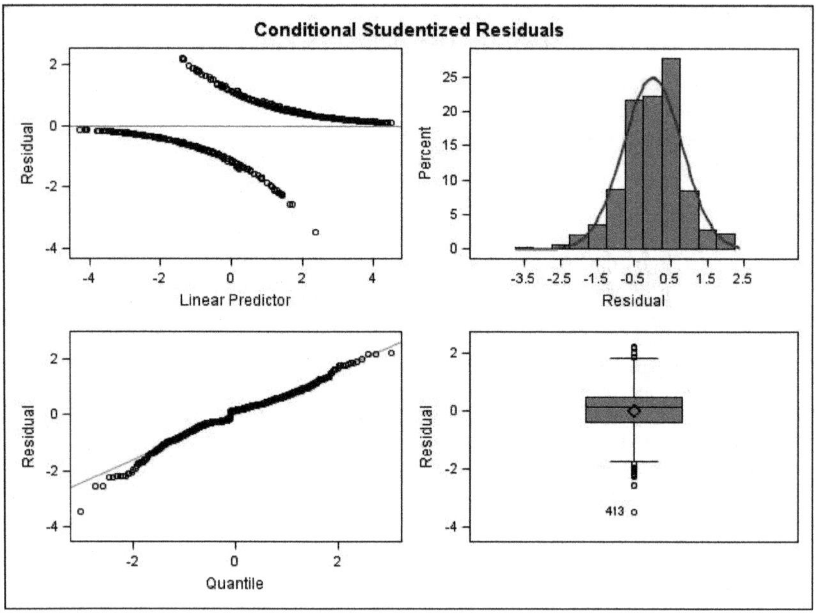

FIGURE 8.3
The panel of graphics of studentized conditional residuals of Model I consisting of a plot of residuals versus predicted values, a histogram with normal density overlaid, a Q-Q plot, and a box plot.

of plots, such as those in the case of normal regression models shown in Figure 7.5. However, since the response variable is binary, these observed patterns of studentized conditional residuals $r_{ij,con}^{(student)}$ (7.11) are logically imaginable enough by taking the following simple setting into account:

$$\text{For } y_{ij} = 1: \quad r_{ij,con}^{(student)} = \frac{1 - \hat{p}_{ij}}{\sqrt{\hat{p}_{ij}(1 - \hat{p}_{ij})}} = \sqrt{\frac{1 - \hat{p}_{ij}}{\hat{p}_{ij}}} \tag{8.24}$$

$$\text{For } y_{ij} = 0: \quad r_{ij,con}^{(student)} = \frac{0 - \hat{p}_{ij}}{\sqrt{\hat{p}_{ij}(1 - \hat{p}_{ij})}} = -\sqrt{\frac{\hat{p}_{ij}}{1 - \hat{p}_{ij}}}, \tag{8.25}$$

where $\hat{p}_{ij}$ is the predicted value. Namely, the pattern (8.24) corresponds to the curve for the positive residuals and the pattern (8.25) corresponds to the curve for the negative residuals. As a whole, there seems to be no alarming patterns of residuals.

TABLE 8.4
Estimated subject-specific treatment effect $e^{\hat{\beta}_{3j}}$ (in terms of *ORR, odds ratio ratio*) at each of four visits for Model I and Model IIa ($\rho_B = 0$).

	Model I AIC=594.0, BIC=631.9		Model IIa ($\rho_B = 0$) AIC=594.7, BIC=635.3	
Months	Estimate (95%CI)	Two-tailed p	Estimate (95%CI)	Two-tailed p
1	5.57 (1.18, 26.42)	0.0306	6.09 (1.15, 32.14)	0.0334
2	15.31 (3.12, 74.95)	0.0008	17.63 (3.19, 97.43)	0.0011
3	10.46 (2.13, 51.20)	0.0039	11.78 (2.15, 64.59)	0.0046
4	5.16 (1.12, 23.81)	0.0355	5.63 (1.09, 38.02)	0.0388

8.5 Models for the average treatment effect

In Chapter 1 we introduced a new *S:T* repeated measures design both as an extension of the *1:1* design or pre-post design and as a formal confirmatory trial design for randomized controlled trials. The primary interest in this design is to estimate the overall or average treatment effect during the evaluation period. So, in the trial protocol, it is important to select the evaluation period during which the treatment effect could be expected to be stable to a certain extent. So, in this section, let us assume that **the primary interest of the *Respiratory Trial* with the *1:4* design is to estimate the average treatment effect over four months after randomization (evaluation period)**, although many readers may not think it reasonable for the real situation of the *Respiratory Trial.* In this case, as already described in Sections 1.2.2 and 7.5, we can introduce two models, a *random intercept* model and a *random intercept plus slope* model.

8.5.1 Model IV: Random intercept model

The *random intercept model* with random intercept b_{0i} is expressed as

$$\text{logit}\Pr(y_{i0} = 1 \mid b_{0i}) = \begin{cases} \beta_0 + b_{0i} + \boldsymbol{w}_i^t\boldsymbol{\xi}, & \text{(Placebo)} \\ \beta_0 + b_{0i} + \beta_1 + \boldsymbol{w}_i^t\boldsymbol{\xi}, & \text{(New treatment)} \end{cases}$$

$$\text{logit}\Pr(y_{ij} = 1 \mid b_{0i}) = \begin{cases} \beta_0 + b_{0i} + \beta_2 + \boldsymbol{w}_i^t\boldsymbol{\xi}, & \text{(Placebo)} \\ \beta_0 + b_{0i} + \beta_1 + \beta_2 + \beta_3 + \boldsymbol{w}_i^t\boldsymbol{\xi}, & \\ & \text{(New treatment)} \end{cases}$$

$$j = 1, ..., 4,$$

which can be re-expressed as

$$\begin{aligned} \text{logit}\Pr(y_{ij}=1 \mid b_{0i}) &= \beta_0 + b_{0i} + \beta_1 x_{1i} + \beta_2 x_{2ij} \\ &\quad + \beta_3 x_{1i} x_{2ij} + \boldsymbol{w}_i^t \boldsymbol{\xi} \qquad (8.26) \\ b_{0i} &\sim N(0, \sigma_{B0}^2), \end{aligned}$$

where the interpretations of the parameters that are different from Model I are as follows:

1. $e^{\beta_0+b_{i0}}$ denotes the subject-specific odds of being "good" in the placebo group at baseline.
2. $e^{\beta_0+b_{i0}+\beta_1}$ denotes the subject-specific odds of being "good" in the new treatment group at baseline.
3. $e^{\beta_0+b_{i0}+\beta_2}$ denotes the subject-specific odds of being "good" in the placebo group in the evaluation period.
4. $e^{\beta_0+b_{i0}+\beta_1+\beta_2+\beta_3}$ denotes the subject-specific odds of being "good" in the new treatment group in the evaluation period.
5. e^{β_2} denotes the subject-specific odds ratio comparing the odds of being "good" in the evaluation period versus baseline period in the placebo group.
6. $e^{\beta_2+\beta_3}$ denotes the same quantity in the new treatment group.
7. e^{β_3} denotes the *ratio* of these two odds ratios, i.e., the subject-specific average treatment effect of the new treatment compared with placebo in terms of ORR, the *odds ratio ratio.*

8.5.2 Model V: Random intercept plus slope model

The random intercept plus slope model with random slope b_{1i} is expressed as

$$\begin{aligned} \text{logit}\Pr(y_{i0}=1 \mid b_{0i}) &= \begin{cases} \beta_0 + b_{0i} + \boldsymbol{w}_i^t \boldsymbol{\xi}, & \text{(Placebo)} \\ \beta_0 + b_{0i} + \beta_1 + \boldsymbol{w}_i^t \boldsymbol{\xi}, & \text{(New treatment)} \end{cases} \\ \text{logit}\Pr(y_{ij}=1 \mid b_{0i}, b_{1i}) &= \begin{cases} \beta_0 + b_{0i} + b_{1i} + \beta_2 + \boldsymbol{w}_i^t \boldsymbol{\xi}, & \text{(Placebo)} \\ \beta_0 + b_{0i} + b_{1i} + \beta_1 + \beta_2 + \beta_3 + \boldsymbol{w}_i^t \boldsymbol{\xi}, & \\ \qquad \text{(New treatment)} & \end{cases} \\ & j = 1, ..., 4. \end{aligned}$$

Namely, it is re-expressed as

$$\begin{aligned} \text{logit} \Pr(y_{ij} = 1 \mid b_{0i}, b_{1i}) &= \beta_0 + b_{0i} + \beta_1 x_{1i} + (\beta_2 + b_{1i}) x_{2ij} \\ &\quad + \beta_3 x_{1i} x_{2ij} + \boldsymbol{w}_i^t \boldsymbol{\xi} \qquad (8.27) \\ \boldsymbol{b}_i &= (b_{0i}, b_{1i}) \sim N(0, \Phi), \end{aligned}$$

We shall call Model V with $\rho_B = 0$, Model Va, and the model with $\rho_B \neq 0$, Model Vb.

8.5.3 Analysis using SAS

Now, let us apply Models IV, Va, and Vb to the *Respiratory Data* using the SAS procedure `PROC GLIMMIX`. The following considerations are required for coding the SAS program.

1. The fixed effects β_2 can be expressed via the binary variable `post` (main factor).

2. The fixed effects β_3 can be expressed via the `treatment * post` interaction.

3. Model IV (the random intercept model) is specified by the following `RANDOM` statement

```
random intercept / subject=id, g, gcorr;
```

   where `intercept` denotes the inter-subject variability at baseline b_{0i}.

4. The random slope b_{1i} can be expressed by the binary variable `post` indicating x_{2ij}. So, to fit Model Va (the random intercept plus slope model with $\rho_B = 0$), you have to use the following `RANDOM` statement

```
random intercept post /type=simple subject=id g gcorr ;
```

   where the option `type=simple` can be omitted. To fit Model Vb (the model with $\rho_B \neq 0$), then you use the option `type=un`:

```
random intercept post /type=un subject=id g gcorr ;
```

The respective sets of SAS programs and the results for Model Va ($\rho_B = 0$) are shown in Program and Output 8.3.

TABLE 8.5
Estimated subject-specific average treatment effect $e^{\hat{\beta}_3}$ (in terms of *ORR*, *odds ratio ratio*) for each of the Models, IV, Va, and Vb. The model with the asterisk (*) indicates the best model based on AIC and BIC.

Model	Estimate (95%CI)	Two-sided p	AIC	BIC
IV*	7.94 (2.32, 27.19)	0.0010	586.89	608.57
Va ($\rho_B = 0$)	8.72 (2.28, 33.32)	0.0016	587.82	612.21
Vb ($\rho_B \neq 0$)	8.63 (2.42, 30.77)	0.0009	589.75	616.84

Program and Ouptut 8.3. SAS procedure PROC GRIMMIX for Model IV, Va, Vb

```
<SAS program>
proc glimmix data=resplong method=quad (qpoints=15);
 class subject centre visit/ref=first  ;
 model status (event="1")  = centre gender age  treatment
                    post treatment*post / d=bin link=logit s cl ;
 /* Model IV  */
   random intercept /  subject= subject g gcorr ;
 /* Model Va */
   random intercept post / type=simple subject= subject g gcorr ;
 /* Model Vb*/
   random intercept post / type=un subject= subject g gcorr ;

<Partial results for Model IV>
Fit statistics
-2 Res Log Likelihood 570.89
AIC (smaller is better) 586.89
BIC (smaller is better) 608.57

Covariance Parameter Estimates
Cov Parm   Subject   Estimate S.E.
Intercept  subject   5.7453 1.5994

Solution for Fixed Effects
Effect   center visit Estimate S.E. DF t Value Pr>|t| Alpha Lower Upper
Intercept          -0.2755 0.8472 106 -0.33 0.7457 0.05 -1.9551 1.4042
centre           2  1.9959 0.5805 442  3.44 0.0006 0.05  0.8550 3.1368
centre           1  0 . . . . . . .
gender             -0.4082 0.7273 442 -0.56 0.5749 0.05 -1.8377 1.0213
age                -0.0298 0.0216 442 -1.38 0.1680 0.05 -0.0721 0.01259
treatment          -0.1756 0.7270 442 -0.24 0.8093 0.05 -1.6044 1.2533
post               -0.1030 0.4141 442 -0.25 0.8036 0.05 -0.9168 0.7108
treatment*post      2.0719 0.6263 442  3.31 0.0010 0.05  0.8409 3.3029
```

In Model IV, the variance of the random intercept is estimated as $\hat{\sigma}^2_{B0} = 5.7453$ ($s.e. = 1.5994$), which is not so different from the variance estimate

5.9674 (*s.e.* = 1.6638) of Model I. The values of AIC and BIC are 586.89 and 608.57, respectively. The subject-specific average treatment effect is estimated in terms of the ratio of the odds ratios, exp(2.0719) = 7.94 and the 95% confidence interval is (2.32, 27.19). On the other hand, the values of AIC and BIC for Model IIa are 587.82 and 612.21, respectively. The values of AIC and BIC for Model IIb are larger than those for Model Ia, respectively, as is shown in Table 8.5. Then, the best model is selected to be Model IV.

8.6 Models for the treatment by linear time interaction

In the previous section, we focused on the mixed-effects models where we are primarily interested in comparing the average treatment effect during the evaluation period. In this section, we shall consider the situation where the primary interest is testing the treatment by *linear* time interaction (Hedeker and Gibbons, 2006; Bhaumik et al., 2008). So let us assume here that **the primary interest of the *Respiratory Trial* with the *1:4* design is to estimate the difference in average rates of change or improvement of respiratory status over time**. To do this, we shall consider the *random intercept* model and the *random intercept plus slope* model.

8.6.1 Model VI: Random intercept model

The *random intercept model* with random intercept b_{0i} is expressed as

$$
\begin{aligned}
\text{logit}\,\Pr(y_{i0} = 1 \mid b_{0i}) &= \begin{cases} \beta_0 + b_{0i} + \boldsymbol{w}_i^t\boldsymbol{\xi}, & \text{(Placebo)} \\ \beta_0 + b_{0i} + \beta_1 + \boldsymbol{w}_i^t\boldsymbol{\xi}, & \text{(New treatment)} \end{cases} \\
\text{logit}\,\Pr(y_{ij} = 1 \mid b_{0i}) &= \begin{cases} \beta_0 + b_{0i} + \beta_2 t_j + \boldsymbol{w}_i^t\boldsymbol{\xi}, & \text{(Placebo)} \\ \beta_0 + b_{0i} + \beta_1 + (\beta_2 + \beta_3)t_j + \boldsymbol{w}_i^t\boldsymbol{\xi}, & \\ & \text{(New treatment)} \end{cases} \\
& \quad j = 1, ..., 4,
\end{aligned}
$$

where:

1. t_j denotes the jth measurement time, i.e., $t_0 = 0, t_1 = 1, t_2 = 2, t_3 = 3$ and $t_4 = 4$.

2. β_2 denotes the subject-specific change of the log odds of being "good" for an increase of one unit in t_j in the placebo group, in other words, *the subject-specific rate of change of the log odds of being "good" per month* in the placebo group. Therefore, e^{β_2} denotes the subject-specific odds ratio of being "good" per month in the placebo group.

3. $e^{\beta_2+\beta_3}$ denotes the subject-specific odds ratio of being "good" per month in the new treatment group.

4. e^{β_3} denotes the ratio of these two subject-specific odds ratios per month, i.e., the subject-specific effect size of the treatment by linear time interaction in terms of the *odds ratio ratio (ORR).*

The above model can be re-expressed as

$$\begin{aligned} \text{logit}\,\Pr(y_{ij} = 1 \mid b_{0i}) &= \beta_0 + b_{0i} + \beta_1 x_{1i} \\ &\qquad + (\beta_2 + \beta_3 x_{1i})t_j + \boldsymbol{w}_i^t \boldsymbol{\xi} \qquad (8.28) \\ b_{0i} &\sim N(\mathbf{0}, \sigma_{B0}^2), \\ &\qquad j = 0,\ 1, ..., 4. \end{aligned}$$

8.6.2 Model VII: Random intercept plus slope model

The *random intercept plus slope* model is expressed as

$$\begin{aligned} \text{logit}\,\Pr(y_{ij} = 1 \mid \boldsymbol{b}_i) &= b_{0i} + \beta_0 + \beta_1 x_{1i} \\ &\qquad + (\beta_2 + \beta_3 x_{1i} + b_{1i})t_j + \boldsymbol{w}_i^t \boldsymbol{\xi} \quad (8.29) \\ \boldsymbol{b}_i &= (b_{0i}, b_{1i}) \sim N(\mathbf{0}, \boldsymbol{\Phi}) \\ \boldsymbol{\Phi} &= \begin{pmatrix} \sigma_{B0}^2 & \rho_B \sigma_{B0} \sigma_{B1} \\ \rho_B \sigma_{B0} \sigma_{B1} & \sigma_{B1}^2 \end{pmatrix} \\ &\qquad j = 0,\ 1, ..., 4, \end{aligned}$$

We shall call the model Model VII with $\rho_B = 0$, Model VIIa, and the model with $\rho_B \neq 0$, Model VIIb.

8.6.3 Analysis using SAS

Now, let us apply Models VI, VIIa, and VIIb to the *Respiratory Data* using the SAS procedure `PROC GLIMMIX`. The respective sets of SAS programs are shown in Program 8.4 and the results for Model VI are shown in Output 8.4. In these programs, we need to create a continuous variable `xvisit` indicating t_j in the `DATA` step and the `MODEL` statement should be

```
model status (event="1")  = centre gender age
treatment xvisit treatment*xvisit /d=bin link=logit s cl ;
```

To fit Model VIIa, for example, you have to use the following `RANDOM` statement

```
random intercept xvisit / subject= subject g gcorr ;
```

where `xvisit` denotes the random slope b_{1i}.

Program 8.4: SAS procedure `PROC GLIMMIX` for Model VI

```
data resplong ;
 infile 'c:\book\RepeatedMeasure\longresp.txt' missover;
 input no centre subject visit treatment status gender age;
 if visit=0 then post=0; else post=1;
 xvisit=visit;

proc glimmix data=resplong method=quad (qpoints=15);
   class subject centre visit/ref=first  ;
   model status (event="1")  = centre gender age
            treatment xvisit treatment*xvisit/d=bin link=logit s cl ;
 /* model VI */
   random intercept /  subject= subject g gcorr ;
 /* model VIIa */
   random intercept xvisit/  subject= subject g gcorr ;
 /* model VIIb */
   random intercept xvisit/ type=un subject= subject g gcorr ;
run;
```

Output 8.4: SAS procedure `PROC GLIMMIX` for Model VI

```
Covariance Parameter Estimates
Cov Parm  Subject  Estimate S.E.
Intercept  subject   5.2135 1.4418

Fit statistics
-2 Res Log Likelihood 583.39
AIC (smaller is better) 599.39
BIC (smaller is better) 621.07

Solution for Fixed Effects
Effect      centre    Estimate S.E.   DF t Value Pr>|t| Alpha Lower Upper
Intercept             -0.2118 0.7814 106 -0.27 0.7868 0.05 -1.7610  1.3373
centre         2       1.9101 0.5544 442  3.45 0.0006 0.05  0.8206  2.9996
centre         1       0 . . . . . . .
gender                -0.3912 0.6964 442 -0.56 0.5745 0.05 -1.7598  0.9774
age                   -0.0293 0.0206 442 -1.42 0.1564 0.05 -0.06985 0.01126
treatment              0.6290 0.6280 442  1.00 0.3171 0.05 -0.6052  1.8631
xvisit                -0.0539 0.1162 442 -0.46 0.6430 0.05 -0.2822  0.1744
treatment*xvisit       0.3877 0.1727 442  2.24 0.0253 0.05  0.04824 0.7272
```

In Model VI, the variance of the random intercept is estimated as $\hat{\sigma}^2_{B0} = 5.21$ ($s.e. = 1.44$). The subject-specific rate of change of the log odds of being "good" per month is estimated as $\hat{\beta}_2 = -0.054$ ($s.e. = 0.12$) in the placebo group and $\hat{\beta}_2 + \hat{\beta}_3 = -0.054 + 0.388 = 0.334$ in the new treatment group, respectively. The difference in these two changes is estimated as $\hat{\beta}_3 = 0.388$ ($s.e. = 0.17$), $p = 0.025$. Namely, the estimated subject-specific odds ratio per month is $e^{-0.054} = 0.947$ in the placebo group and $e^{0.334} = 1.37$ in

TABLE 8.6
Estimated subject-specific treatment effect $e^{\hat{\beta}_3}$ (in terms of *ORR, the odds ratio ratio*) for Models, VI, VIIa and VIIb. The model with the asterisk (*) indicates the best model.

Model	$e^{\hat{\beta}_3}$	95%CI	Two-tailed p-value	AIC	BIC
VI*	1.47	(1.04, 2.06)	0.025	599.39	621.07
VIIa	1.66	(1.05, 2.62)	0.029	598.02	622.41
VIIb	1.70	(1.07, 2.72)	0.026	599.86	626.96

the new treatment group, respectively. These results indicate that for every increase of one month, the chance of being "good" increases 0.947 times in the placebo group and 1.37 times in the new treatment group in terms of odds ratio. Therefore, the subject-specific treatment effect of the new treatment compared with placebo is expressed as the ratio of these two odds ratios, i.e., $e^{\hat{\beta}_3} = e^{0.388} = 1.37/0.947 = 1.47$ in terms of ORR, the odds ratio ratio, indicating that the speed of improvement of the respiratory status in the new treatment group is 1.37 times faster than that in the placebo group.

Table 8.6 shows the subject-specific treatment effect with 95% confidence interval for each of three models. According to the values of AIC and BIC, the best model will be Model VI.

8.6.4 Checking the goodness-of-fit of linearity

However, as discussed and illustrated in Section 7.6.4, we should be cautious about the goodness-of-fit of the models for treatment by *linear* time interaction because the *linear trend model* has very strong assumptions concerning linearity. So, whenever the treatment by linear time interaction is defined as the primary interest of the statistical analysis, we should check the goodness-of-fit. To do this, we can apply the following *random intercept* model and the *random intercept plus slope* model including the treatment by quadratic time interaction.

1. Model VIQ: Random intercept model

$$\begin{aligned} \text{logit}\,\Pr(y_{ij} = 1 \mid b_{0i}) &= \beta_0 + b_{0i} + \beta_1 x_{1i} + (\beta_2 + \beta_3 x_{1i})t_j + \\ &\quad (\beta_4 + \beta_5 x_{1i})t_j^2 + \boldsymbol{w}_i^t \boldsymbol{\xi} \qquad (8.30) \\ b_{0i} &\sim N(\mathbf{0}, \sigma_{B0}^2) \\ &\quad i = 1, ..., N; j = 0,\ 1, ..., 4 \end{aligned}$$

2. Model VIIQ: Random intercept plus slope model

The random intercept plus slope model with a random intercept b_{0i}, random slopes b_{1i} on the linear term, and b_{2i} on the quadratic term is expressed by

$$\begin{aligned} \text{logit}\,\Pr(y_{ij} = 1 \mid b_{0i}, b_{1i}, b_{2i}) &= \beta_0 + b_{0i} + \beta_1 x_{1i} + (\beta_2 + \beta_3 x_{1i} + b_{1i})t_j + \\ &\quad (\beta_4 + \beta_5 x_{1i} + b_{2i})t_j^2 + \boldsymbol{w}_i^t \boldsymbol{\xi} \qquad (8.31) \\ \boldsymbol{b}_i &= (b_{0i}, b_{1i}, b_{2i}) \sim N(\mathbf{0}, \boldsymbol{\Phi}) \\ \boldsymbol{\Phi} &= \begin{pmatrix} \sigma_{B0}^2 & \rho_{01}\sigma_{B0}\sigma_{B1} & \rho_{02}\sigma_{B0}\sigma_{B2} \\ \rho_{01}\sigma_{B0}\sigma_{B1} & \sigma_{B1}^2 & \rho_{12}\sigma_{B1}\sigma_{B2} \\ \rho_{02}\sigma_{B0}\sigma_{B2} & \rho_{12}\sigma_{B1}\sigma_{B2} & \sigma_{B2}^2 \end{pmatrix}. \\ &\quad i = 1, ..., N; j = 0,\ 1, ..., 4 \end{aligned}$$

However, the number of random effects $\boldsymbol{b}_i$ in this model is 3, which seems to be the maximum number (depending on the models) in the sense that the adaptive Gauss-Hermite quadrature method with a reasonable number of nodes (around 13 or more) can successfully converge to the true value (see Appendix B, Section B.3.3.3). Unfortunately, the above model faced the convergence problem with a reasonable number of nodes 15. So, we shall consider the following three covariance structures less complex than Model VIIQ with "full" covariance structures:

- Model VIIQ-1:

$$\boldsymbol{\Phi} = \begin{pmatrix} \sigma_{B0}^2 & 0 & 0 \\ 0 & \sigma_{B1}^2 & 0 \\ 0 & 0 & 0 \end{pmatrix}$$

- Model VIIQ-2:

$$\boldsymbol{\Phi} = \begin{pmatrix} \sigma_{B0}^2 & \rho_{01}\sigma_{B0}\sigma_{B1} & 0 \\ \rho_{01}\sigma_{B0}\sigma_{B1} & \sigma_{B1}^2 & 0 \\ 0 & 0 & 0 \end{pmatrix}$$

- Model VIIQ-3:

$$\Phi = \begin{pmatrix} \sigma_{B0}^2 & 0 & 0 \\ 0 & \sigma_{B1}^2 & 0 \\ 0 & 0 & \sigma_{B2}^2 \end{pmatrix}$$

Now, let us apply four Models VIQ, VIIQ-1, VIIQ-2, and VIIQ-3 to the *Respiratory Data* using the SAS procedure `PROC GLIMMIX`. The respective sets of SAS programs are shown in Program 8.5. In these programs, we need to create a continuous variable `xvisit2` indicating the quadratic term t_j^2 in the `DATA` step. Then, the `MODEL` statement should be

```
model status (event="1") = centre gender age treatment
xvisit xvisit2 treatment*xvisit treatment*xvisit2/s cl ddfm=sat;
```

and the `RANDOM` statement for Model VIIQ-2, for example, should be

```
random intercept xvisit/ type=un subject= subject g gcorr ;
```

Program 8.5: SAS procedure `PROC GLIMMIX` for Models VIQ, VIQ-1 and VIQ-2

```
<SAS program>
data resplong ;
  infile 'c:\book\RepeatedMeasure\longresp.txt' missover;
  input no centre subject visit treatment status gender age;
  xvisit=visit;
  xvisit2=xvisit*xvisit;

 proc glimmix data=resplong method=quad (qpoints=15);
   class subject centre visit/ref=first  ;
   model status (event="1")  = centre gender age treatment
             xvisit xvisit2 treatment*xvisit treatment*xvisit2
                                       / d=bin link=logit s cl ;
  /* model VIQ    */
  random intercept /  subject= subject g gcorr ;
  /* model VIIQ-1  */
  random intercept xvisit / type=simple subject= subject g gcorr ;
  /* model VIIQ-2  */
  random intercept xvisit / type=un subject= subject g gcorr ;
  /* model VIIQ-3  */
  random intercept xvisit xvisit2 / type=simple subject= subject g gcorr ;
 run ;
```

Output 8.5: SAS procedure `PROC GLIMMIX` for Models VIQ

```
<A part of the results for Model VIQ >
Covariance Parameter Estimates
Cov Parm  Subject Estimate S.E.
Intercept subject 5.8189 1.6200

Fit statistics
-2 Res Log Likelihood 569.29
AIC (smaller is better) 589.29
BIC (smaller is better) 616.38

Solution for Fixed Effects
Effect     centre   Estimate S.E.  DF t Value Pr>|t| Alpha Lower Upper
Intercept             -0.1705 0.8420 106 -0.20 0.8400 0.05 -1.8398  1.4989
centre        2        2.0071 0.5839 440  3.44 0.0006 0.05  0.8595  3.1546
centre        1        0  . . . . . . .
gender                -0.4083 0.7314 440 -0.56 0.5769 0.05 -1.8457  1.0291
age                   -0.0300 0.0217 440 -1.38 0.1674 0.05 -0.07256 0.01262
treatment             -0.1819 0.7090 440 -0.26 0.7977 0.05 -1.5754  1.2117
xvisit                -0.2123 0.4140 440 -0.51 0.6083 0.05 -1.0260  0.6014
xvisit2                0.0393 0.0992 440  0.40 0.6921 0.05 -0.1557  0.2343
treatment*xvisit       2.1757 0.6373 440  3.41 0.0007 0.05  0.9232  3.4283
treatment*xvisit2     -0.4461 0.1516 440 -2.94 0.0034 0.05 -0.7440 -0.1483
```

The results for Model VIQ are shown in Output 8.5, where we have the variance estimates $\hat{\sigma}^2_{B0} = 5.8189$ ($s.e. = 1.620$) and AIC $= 589.29$ and BIC $= 616.38$. In Model VIIQ-1, we have the variance estimates $\hat{\sigma}^2_{B0} = 6.0638$ ($s.e. = 1.8856$), $\hat{\sigma}^2_{B1} = 0.2202$ ($s.e. = 0.1887$), and AIC $= 588.76$ and BIC $= 618.56$. Model VIIQ-2 has the covariance estimates $\hat{\sigma}^2_{B0} = 6.1765$ ($s.e. = 2.9335$), $\hat{\sigma}^2_{B1} = 0.2222$ ($s.e. = 0.1922$), $\hat{\rho}_{01} = -0.02433$, and AIC $= 590.75$ and BIC $= 623.27$. Unfortunately, Model VIIQ-3 did not converge. However, AIC and BIC seem to select Model VIQ with the simplest covariance structure as the best model. Furthermore, Model VIQ seems to fit better than Model VI (AIC $= 599.39$, BIC $= 621.07$), the best model for the treatment by linear time interaction, indicating that Model VIQ is better than Model VI. The estimated mean quadratic trend (via Model VIQ) of the odds ratio by the treatment group is

$$
\begin{aligned}
\hat{\mathrm{OR}}(t) &= \begin{cases} e^{\hat{\beta}_2 t+\hat{\beta}_4 t^2}, & \text{(Placebo)} \\ e^{(\hat{\beta}_2+\hat{\beta}_3)t+(\hat{\beta}_4+\hat{\beta}_5)t^2}, & \text{(New treatment)} \end{cases} \\
&= \begin{cases} e^{-0.2123t+0.03932t^2}, & \text{(Placebo)} \\ e^{(-0.2123+2.1757)t+(0.03932-0.4461)t^2}, & \text{(New treatment).} \end{cases}
\end{aligned}
$$

These two quadratic lines are plotted in Figure 8.4, which seems to be similar to the estimated *subject-specific* odds ratio (via Model I) by treatment group shown in Figure 8.2. In this case, the estimated treatment effect

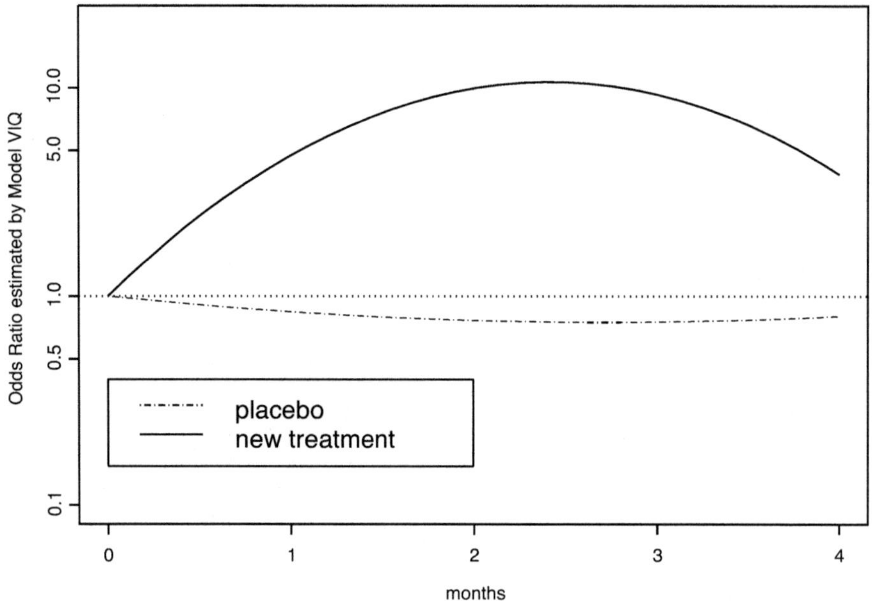

FIGURE 8.4
Estimated changes from baseline by treatment group based on the estimated odds ratios (via Model VIQ) of being "good" at each visit versus at baseline.

$e^{\hat{\beta}_3} = 1.47(95\%CI : 1.04, 2.06)$, assuming the *treatment by linear time interaction* may not be acceptable.

8.7 ANCOVA-type models adjusting for baseline measurement

As described in Chapter 1 and Section 7.7, many RCTs tend to try to narrow the evaluation period down to one time point (ex., the last Tth measurement), leading to the *pre-post* design or the *1:1* design. In these simple *1:1* designs, traditional analysis of covariance (ANCOVA) has been used to analyze data where the baseline measurement is used as a covariate.

So, in this section, we shall apply some ANCOVA-type models to the *Respiratory Data* with *1:4* repeated measures design where the baseline measurement is used as a covariate and compare the results with those of the corresponding repeated measures models.

8.7.1 Model VIII: Random intercept model for the treatment effect at each visit

Let us consider here the following *random intercept model* where the random intercept $b_{i(Ancova)}$ is assumed to be constant during the evaluation period.

$$\text{logit}\Pr(y_{ij}=1\mid b_{i(Ancova)}) = \begin{cases} b_{i(Ancova)}+\beta_0+\beta_{2j}+\theta y_{i0}+\boldsymbol{w}_i^t\boldsymbol{\xi}, & \text{(Placebo)} \\ b_{i(Ancova)}+\beta_0+\beta_1+\beta_{2j}+\beta_{3j}+\theta y_{i0} \\ \quad +\boldsymbol{w}_i^t\boldsymbol{\xi} & \text{(New treatment)} \end{cases}$$
$$j=1,...,4,\quad \beta_{21}=\beta_{31}=0$$

where:

1. β_0 denotes the mean subject-specific log-odds of being "good" in the placebo group at the 1st visit.
2. $e^{b_{i(Anova)}+\beta_0}$ denotes the subject-specific odds of being "good" in the placebo group at the 1st visit.
3. $\beta_0+\beta_1$ denotes the mean subject-specific log-odds of being "good" in the new treatment group at the 1st visit.
4. $e^{b_{i(Anova)}+\beta_0+\beta_1}$ denotes the subject-specific odds of being "good" in the new treatment group at the 1st visit.
5. e^{β_1} denotes the subject-specific odds ratio comparing the odds of being "good" in the new treatment group versus in the placebo group at the 1st visit.
6. θ denotes the coefficient for the baseline measurement y_{i0}.
7. $e^{\beta_0+\beta_{2j}}$ denotes the subject-specific odds of being "good" in the placebo group at the jth visit.
8. $e^{\beta_0+\beta_1+\beta_{2j}+\beta_{3j}}$ denotes the subject-specific odds of being "good" in the new treatment group at the jth visit.
9. $e^{\beta_1+\beta_{3j}}$ denotes the subject-specific odds ratio comparing the odds of being "good" in the new treatment group versus in the placebo group at the jth visit, i.e., the treatment effect of the new treatment compared with placebo at the jth visit in terms of the *odds ratio (OR)*.

This model is re-expressed as

$$\begin{aligned}
\text{logit}\Pr(y_{ij} = 1 \mid b_{i(Ancova)}) &= \beta_0 + b_{i(Ancova)} + \theta y_{i0} + \beta_1 x_{1i} + \beta_{2j} \\
&\quad + \beta_{3j} x_{1i} + \boldsymbol{w}_i^t \boldsymbol{\xi} \qquad (8.32) \\
i &= 1, ..., N; \;\; j = 1, 2, 3, 4; \;\; \beta_{21} = 0, \;\; \beta_{31} = 0 \\
b_{i(Ancova)} &\sim N(0, \sigma^2_{B(Ancova)}).
\end{aligned}$$

In the ANCOVA-type model, the treatment effect at time j can be expressed via some linear contrast. For example, the treatment effect at month 4 ($j = 4$) can be expressed as

$$\beta_1 + \beta_{34} = (1)\beta_1 + (0, 0, 0, 1)(\beta_{31}, \beta_{32}, \beta_{33}, \beta_{34})^t. \qquad (8.33)$$

8.7.2 Model IX: Random intercept model for the average treatment effect

In this section, we shall consider Model IX, in which the treatment effect is assumed to be constant during the evaluation period.

$$\begin{aligned}
\text{logit}\Pr(y_{ij} = 1 \mid b_{i(Ancova)}) &= \beta_0 + b_{i(Ancova)} + \theta y_{i0} + \beta_3 x_{1i} + \boldsymbol{w}_i^t \boldsymbol{\xi} \\
&\qquad (8.34) \\
i &= 1, ..., N; \;\; j = 1, 2, 3, 4; \\
b_{i(Ancova)} &\sim N(0, \sigma^2_{B(Ancova)}),
\end{aligned}$$

where e^{β_3} denotes the subject-specific odds ratio comparing the odds of being "good" in the new treatment group versus in the placebo group during the evaluation period, i.e., the treatment effect of the new treatment assumed to be constant during the evaluation period in terms of the *odds ratio (OR)*.

8.7.3 Analysis using SAS

Now, let us apply two Models VIII and IX to the *Respiratory Data* using the SAS procedure `PROC GLIMMIX`. But the first step for the analysis is to rearrange the data structure from the long format shown in Table 8.1 into another long format shown in Table 8.7, where the baseline records were deleted and the new variable `base` indicating baseline data was created. The respective sets of SAS programs are shown in Program 8.6. Here also, due to the option

TABLE 8.7
A part of the long format *Respiratory Data* set for the ANCOVA-type model. The variable `base` indi cates the baseline measurement. (Data for the first three patients are shown).

No.	centre	subject	visit	treatment	status	gender	age	base
1	1	1	1	placebo	poor	female	46	poor
2	1	1	2	placebo	poor	female	46	poor
3	1	1	3	placebo	poor	female	46	poor
4	1	1	4	placebo	poor	female	46	poor
5	1	2	1	placebo	poor	female	28	poor
6	1	2	2	placebo	poor	female	28	poor
7	1	2	3	placebo	poor	female	28	poor
8	1	2	4	placebo	poor	female	28	poor
9	1	3	1	treatment	good	female	23	good
10	1	3	2	treatment	good	female	23	good
11	1	3	3	treatment	good	female	23	good
12	1	3	4	treatment	good	female	23	good

`/ref=first` used in the `CLASS` statement, the coefficients of the linear contrast for the `treatment*visit` interaction needs the order change (e.g., see Section 7.7.3). For example, according to the equation (8.33), the linear contrast for the treatment effect at month 4 ($j = 4$) can be expressed in SAS as:

```
estimate 'treatment at 4m' treatment 1 treatment*visit  0 0 0 1
```

However, due to the option `/ref=first`, the following change should be made for the `treatment*visit` interaction:

```
estimate 'treatment at 4m' treatment 1 treatment*visit  0 0 1 0
```

Furthermore, the fixed effects β_3 in Model IX can be expressed by the variable `treatment` and the `MODEL` statement and the `RANDOM` statement should be:

```
 model status (event="1")  = centre gender age base treatment
                                             / s cl ddfm=sat ;
 random intercept /  subject= subject g gcorr ;
```

The results of these two programs are shown in Output 8.6.

Program 8.6: SAS procedure `PROC GLIMMIX` for Models VIII and IX

```
 data resplong2 ;
  infile 'c:\book\RepeatedMeasure\longrespbase.txt' missover;
  input no centre subject visit treatment status gender age base;

<Model VIII>
proc glimmix data=resplong2 method=quad (qpoints=15);
 class subject centre visit/ref=first  ;
 model status (event="1")  = centre gender age base
                       treatment visit treatment*visit
                                  / d=bin link=logit s cl ;
 random intercept /  subject= subject g gcorr ;
 estimate 'treatment at 1m'
  treatment 1  treatment*visit 0 0 0 1/divisor=1 cl alpha=0.05;
 estimate 'treatment at 2m'
  treatment 1  treatment*visit 1 0 0 0/divisor=1 cl alpha=0.05;
 estimate 'treatment at 3m'
  treatment 1  treatment*visit 0 1 0 0/divisor=1 cl alpha=0.05;
 estimate 'treatment at 4m'
  treatment 1  treatment*visit 0 0 1 0/divisor=1 cl alpha=0.05;

<Model IX>
proc glimmix data=resplong2 method=quad (qpoints=15);
   class subject centre visit/ref=first  ;
   model status (event="1")  = centre gender age base treatment
                                  / d=bin link=logit s ;
   random intercept /  subject= subject g gcorr ;
```

Output 8.6: SAS procedure `PROC GLIMMIX` for Models VIII and IX

```
/* Model VIII */
Fit statistics 421.12
-2 Res Log Likelihood
AIC (smaller is better)  447.12

Covariance Parameter Estimates
Cov Parm   Subject  Estimate S.E.
Intercept subject 4.3658 1.4458

Estimates
Label          Estimate S.E.   DF t Value Pr>|t| Alpha Lower Upper
treatment at 1m 1.7681 0.7502 327 2.36 0.0190 0.05 0.2923 3.2439
treatment at 2m 2.8309 0.7788 327 3.63 0.0003 0.05 1.2988 4.3630
treatment at 3m 2.4227 0.7716 327 3.14 0.0018 0.05 0.9048 3.9407
treatment at 4m 1.6972 0.7398 327 2.29 0.0224 0.05 0.2418 3.1525

/* Model IX */
Fit statistics
-2 Res Log Likelihood 426.27
AIC (smaller is better)  440.27

Covariance Parameter Estimates
Cov Parm   Subject  Estimate S.E.
Intercept         subject      4.1214 1.3641

Solution for Fixed Effects
Effect    centre  Estimate S.E.    DF   t Value Pr>|t| Alpha Lower Upper
Intercept          -1.6207  0.7975  105 -2.03 0.0447 0.05 -3.2021 -0.03937
centre       2      1.0396  0.5585  333   1.86 0.0635 0.05 -0.05896 2.1381
centre       1      0 . . . . . . .
gender              0.1974  0.6868  333   0.29 0.7739 0.05 -1.1535  1.5484
age                -0.02507 0.02064 333 -1.21 0.2254 0.05 -0.06566 0.01553
base                3.0276  0.5995  333   5.05 <.0001 0.05  1.8483  4.2069
treatment           2.1280  0.5615  333   3.79 0.0002 0.05  1.0235  3.2324
```

For example, the average treatment effect from Model IX is estimated as $e^{2.128} = 8.40$ with 95% confidence interval ($e^{1.0235} = 2.78$, $e^{3.2324} = 25.34$) and two-tailed $p = 0.0002$.

Here also, it will be interesting to compare the estimates of the treatment effect obtained from the ANCOVA-type Models VIII and IX with those from the repeated measures models, Models I and IV, which are shown in Table 8.8. It should be noted that the treatment effect is estimated in terms of the *odds ratio* for the ANOVA-type models, while the treatment effect is estimated in terms of the *odds ratio ratio* for the repeated measures models. In the *Beat the Blues Data*, the repeated measures models tend to give smaller p-values than the ANCOVA-type models, although all the estimates are not statistically significant (see Table 7.8). In the *Respiratory Data*, on the other hand, the ANCOVA-type models tend to give a little bit smaller p-values than repeated measures models, although all the estimates are statistically significant.

TABLE 8.8
Comparison of estimated treatment effects between repeated measurements models (Models I and IV, in terms of the *ORR*) and the ANCOVA-type models (Models VIII, IX, in terms of the *OR*).

Treatment	Repeated measures models Models I, IV		ANCOVA-type models Models VIII, IX	
effect	Estimate (95%CI)	Two-tailed p-value	Estimate (95%CI)	Two-tailed p-value
Model I vs. Model VIII				
$\hat{\beta}_{31}$: month 1	5.57 (1.18, 26.42)	0.0306	5.86 (1.34, 25.63)	0.0190
$\hat{\beta}_{32}$: month 2	15.31 (3.12, 74.95)	0.0008	16.96 (3.66, 78.49)	0.0003
$\hat{\beta}_{33}$: month 3	10.46 (2.13, 51.20)	0.0039	11.28 (2.47, 51.45)	0.0018
$\hat{\beta}_{34}$: month 4	5.16 (1.12, 23.81)	0.0355	5.46 (1.27, 23.39)	0.0224
Model IV vs. Model IX				
$\hat{\beta}_3$: Average	7.94 (2.32, 27.19)	0.0010	8.40 (2.78, 25.34)	0.0002

8.8 Example 2: The daily symptom data with *7:7* design

The second example used in this chapter comes from a randomized, double-blind, placebo-controlled parallel-group clinical trial (two-armed) in an area of gastrointestinal disease where the week before randomization (day: -6, -5, -4, -3, -2, -1, and 0) is defined as the *baseline week* and the 4th week after randomization (day: 22, 23, 24, 25, 26, 27 and 28) is defined as the *evaluation week* (Takada and Tango, 2014). This trial has a 7 : 7 *repeated measures design.* Patients are instructed to keep a daily record of their symptom scores in their diary from the baseline week to the evaluation week. The presence or elimination of symptoms for patient i at day j is denoted by y_{ij} (presence of symptoms $= 0$, elimination of symptoms $= 1$), where the day number in the evaluation week is renumbered as *1,2,3, ... ,7*. The primary endpoint of this trial is to evaluate the average treatment effect of eliminating symptoms based on the patient's daily symptoms.

Table 8.9 shows a set of *hypothetical* daily records of patient symptoms from the baseline week before randomization to the evaluation week after randomization from a gastroenterology clinical trial consisting of $N = 40$ patients. The first $n_1 = 20$ patients are assigned to the placebo group and the last $n_2 = 20$ patients are assigned to the new treatment group. Unfortunately, the real data is not available at present.

Before analyzing these data using the SAS procedure `PROC GLIMMIX`, we have to rearrange the data structure from the wide format (Table 8.9) into the long format structure in which separate repeated measurements and associated covariate values appear as separate rows in the data set. The rearranged data set is omitted here and includes the following five variables:

1. `no`: serial number for each record within the data set.
2. `subject`: categorical variable indicating the subject ID.
3. `visit`: categorical variable indicating the day of visit to the center: -6, -5, ... , 0, 1, 2, ... , 7.
4. `treatment`: binary variable for the treatment group (the new treatment = 1, placebo = 0).
5. `symptom`: binary variable for the respiratory status at each visit (elimination = 1, with symptoms = 0)

8.8.1 Models for the average treatment effect

To this *7:7* repeated measures design, it is quite natural to apply Models IV, Va, and Vb introduced in Section 8.5 to estimate e^{β_3}, the average treatment effect over the evaluation week, in terms of the ratio of odds ratios, i.e., *odds ratio ratio* (ORR). It should be noted that we find it not so simple to apply the ANCOVA-type model introduced in Section 8.7 to these repeated measurements since there is no natural way of dealing with repeated measurements made before randomization.

$$\begin{aligned}\textbf{Model IV}: \text{logit}\Pr(y_{ij}=1\mid b_{0i}) &= \beta_0+b_{0i}+\beta_1x_{1i}+\beta_2x_{2ij}\\ &\quad +\beta_3x_{1i}x_{2ij} \qquad (8.35)\\ b_{0i} &\sim N(0,\sigma^2_{B0})\end{aligned}$$

$$\begin{aligned}\textbf{Model V}: \text{logit}\Pr(y_{ij}=1\mid b_{0i},b_{1i}) &= \beta_0+b_{0i}+\beta_1x_{1i}+(\beta_2+b_{1i})x_{2ij}\\ &\quad +\beta_3x_{1i}x_{2ij} \qquad (8.36)\\ \boldsymbol{b}_i &= (b_{0i},b_{1i})\sim N(0,\Phi)\end{aligned}$$

where $i = 1, ..., 40;\ j = -6, -5, ..., 0,\ 1, ..., 7$ and the interpretations of the fixed-effects parameters are as follows:

1. e^{β_2} denotes the odds ratio comparing the odds of the symptom being "eliminated" at the evaluation week versus at the baseline week in the placebo group.

TABLE 8.9

A *hypothetical* data. Daily record of patient symptom (elimination = 1; with symptoms = 0) during the baseline week (day: -6,-5, ... , 0) before randomization and the evaluation week (day: 22, 23, ... , 28) after randomization in a gastroenterology clinical trial. The placebo group consists of the first 20 patients and the new treatment group has the last 20 patients.

id	-6	-5	-4	-3	-2	-1	0	22	23	24	25	26	27	28	(day)
	-6	-5	-4	-3	-2	-1	0	1	2	3	4	5	6	7	(j)
1	0	0	0	0	0	0	0	0	0	0	0	0	0	0	
2	0	0	0	0	0	0	0	0	0	1	0	1	0	0	
3	0	0	0	0	0	0	0	0	0	0	0	0	0	0	
4	0	0	0	0	0	0	0	0	0	0	1	0	0	1	
5	0	0	0	1	0	0	1	0	0	0	1	0	0	0	
6	0	0	0	0	0	0	0	0	0	0	0	1	1	1	
7	0	0	0	0	0	0	0	0	0	0	0	0	0	0	
8	0	0	0	0	0	0	0	0	0	0	0	0	0	0	
9	0	0	0	0	0	1	0	0	1	0	0	0	0	1	
10	0	0	0	0	0	0	0	0	0	0	1	0	0	1	
11	0	0	0	0	0	0	0	0	0	0	0	0	0	0	
12	0	0	0	0	0	0	0	0	0	0	0	0	0	0	
13	0	0	1	0	1	0	0	0	1	0	1	1	0	0	
14	0	0	0	1	0	0	0	0	1	1	1	1	0	0	
15	0	0	0	0	0	0	0	0	0	0	0	0	0	0	
16	0	0	0	0	0	0	0	1	1	1	1	1	1	1	
17	0	0	0	0	0	0	0	0	0	0	0	0	1	0	
18	0	0	0	0	0	0	0	0	0	0	0	0	0	0	
19	0	0	0	0	0	0	0	0	0	0	0	0	0	0	
20	0	0	0	0	0	0	0	0	0	0	0	1	0	0	
21	0	0	0	0	0	0	0	0	0	0	0	0	0	0	
22	0	0	0	0	0	0	0	0	0	0	1	0	0	0	
23	0	0	0	0	0	0	0	0	1	1	1	1	1	1	
24	0	0	0	0	0	0	0	1	1	1	1	1	1	1	
25	0	0	0	0	0	0	0	1	1	1	1	1	1	1	
26	0	1	0	0	1	0	0	1	0	1	1	0	1	0	
27	0	0	0	1	0	0	0	0	0	0	0	1	0	1	
28	0	0	0	0	0	0	0	0	0	0	0	0	0	0	
29	0	0	0	0	0	0	0	1	1	1	1	1	1	1	
30	0	0	0	0	0	0	0	1	1	0	0	1	0	1	
31	0	0	0	0	0	0	0	1	1	1	1	1	1	1	
32	0	0	0	0	0	0	0	1	1	1	1	1	1	1	
33	0	1	0	0	1	0	0	1	0	1	0	1	0	1	
34	0	1	1	1	0	0	0	0	0	1	0	0	1	0	
35	0	0	0	0	0	1	0	0	1	1	1	1	1	1	
36	0	1	0	0	0	0	0	1	0	1	1	1	1	1	
37	0	0	1	0	0	0	0	1	0	1	1	0	1	0	
38	0	0	0	0	0	0	0	0	0	1	1	1	1	1	
39	0	0	0	0	0	0	0	0	1	0	1	0	0	1	
40	0	0	0	0	0	0	0	1	1	1	1	1	1	1	

2. $e^{\beta_2+\beta_3}$ denotes the same quantity in the new treatment group.
3. e^{β_3} denotes the *ratio* of these two odds ratios. In other words, the ratio means the average treatment effect of the new treatment compared with placebo in terms of the *odds ratio ratio.*

8.8.2 Analysis using SAS

Now, let us apply Models IV, Va, and Vb to the *Respiratory Data* using `PROC GLIMMIX`. The respective sets of SAS programs and the results for Model Va ($\rho_B = 0$) are shown in Program and Output 8.7.

Program and Output 8.7. SAS procedure `PROC GRIMMIX` for Models IV, Va, Vb

```
data resplong ;
  infile 'c:\book\RepeatedMeasure\longgastro.txt' missover;
  input no subject treatment visit status ;
  if visit<=0 then post=0; else post=1;
  run;

proc glimmix data=resplong method=quad (qpoints=15);
   class subject visit  / ref=first  ;
   model status (event="1")  = treatment  post treatment*post
                              /d=bin link=logit s cl ;
/* IV */
   random intercept /  subject= subject g gcorr ;
/* Va */
   random intercept post /subject= subject g gcorr ;
/* Vb */
   random intercept post /type=un  subject= subject g gcorr ;
  run ;

<A part of the results for Model Va >
Fit statistics
-2 Res Log Likelihood 395.33
AIC (smaller is better) 407.33
BIC (smaller is better) 417.46

Covariance Parameter Estimates
Cov Parm   Subject   Estimate S.E.
Intercept subject 0.6456 0.6534
post subject      4.1401 1.9713

Solution for Fixed Effects
Effect            Estimate S.E.  DF t Value Pr>|t| Alpha Lower Upper
Intercept         -3.4085 0.5527  38  -6.17 <.0001 0.05 -4.5275 -2.2895
treatment          0.7045 0.6074 480   1.16 0.2467 0.05 -0.4890  1.8980
post               1.1435 0.7649  38   1.49 0.1432 0.05 -0.4049  2.6919
treatment*post     2.4944 0.9924 480   2.51 0.0123 0.05  0.5445  4.4443
```

TABLE 8.10
Estimated average treatment effect $e^{\hat{\beta}_3}$ for Models, IV, Va, and Vb. The model with the asterisk (*) indicates the best model based on AIC and BIC.

Model	Estimate (95%CI)	Two-tailed p-value	AIC	BIC
IV	4.96 (1.39, 17.7)	0.0138	425.95	434.40
Va* ($\rho_B = 0$)	12.11 (1.72, 85.1)	0.0123	407.33	417.46
Vb ($\rho_B \neq 0$)	11.02 (1.29, 94.0)	0.0283	407.68	419.51

In Model Va, the variances of the random intercept and random slope are estimated as $\hat{\sigma}^2_{B0} = 0.6456$ ($s.e. = 0.6534$) and $\hat{\sigma}^2_{B1} = 4.1401$ ($s.e. = 1.9713$), respectively. The values of AIC and BIC are 407.33 and 417.46, respectively. The average treatment effect is estimated as $\exp(2.4944) = 12.11$ in terms of the *odds ratios ratio* and the 95% confidence interval is $(1.72, 85.1)$. The results of other models are summarized in Table 8.10. Model Va is selected as the best model based on AIC and BIC.

8.9 Sample size

In this chapter, various mixed-effects models were illustrated with the *Respiratory Data*, which has a *1:4* repeated measures design. In this section, we shall consider the sample size determination. The sample size determinations for longitudinal data analysis in the literature (Diggle et al., 2002; Hedeker and Gibbons, 1999 Fitzmaurice, Laird and Ware, 2011) are based on the *basic 1:T design* where the baseline data is usually used as a covariate. In other words, this design is essentially the *0:T design*. In this section, we shall consider the sample size (the number of subjects) needed for the *S:T design* with $S > 0$, which is different from what appears in the literature. For technical details of the derivation of sample size formula, see Appendix A (Tango, 2016a).

8.9.1 Sample size for the average treatment effect

We shall consider here a typical situation where investigators are interested in estimating the average treatment effect during the evaluation period. To do this, let us consider the sample size for Model V, which includes Model IV as a special case within the framework of the *S:T* design, where the sample size formula with closed form is not available but we can easily obtain sample sizes via Monte Carlo simulations.

Model V within the framework of the $S{:}T$ design is expressed as

$$
\begin{aligned}
\text{logit}\Pr(y_{ij} = 1 \mid b_{0i}, b_{1i}) &= \beta_0 + b_{0i} + \beta_1 x_{1i} + (\beta_2 + b_{1i})x_{2ij} \\
&\qquad + \beta_3 x_{1i} x_{2ij} \qquad (8.37) \\
\boldsymbol{b}_i &= (b_{0i}, b_{1i}) \sim N(0, \Phi) \\
i &= 1, ..., n_1 \text{ (control);} \\
&= n_1 + 1, ..., n_1 + n_2 = N \text{ (new treatment)} \\
j &= -(S-1), -(S-2), ..., 0, 1, ..., T,
\end{aligned}
$$

where it is assumed that all observation periods have an equal length and the parameter β_3 denotes the average treatment effect of the new treatment compared with placebo treatment. Therefore, the null and alternative hypotheses of interest will be one of the following three sets of hypotheses as discussed in Section 1.3:

1. Test for superiority: If a negative β_3 indicates benefits, the superiority hypotheses are given by

$$H_0 \ : \ \beta_3 \geq 0, \text{ versus } H_1 : \beta_3 < 0. \qquad (8.38)$$

If a positive β_3 indicates benefits as in the Respiratory example, then they are

$$H_0 \ : \ \beta_3 \leq 0, \text{ versus } H_1 : \beta_3 > 0. \qquad (8.39)$$

2. Test for non-inferiority: If a negative β_3 indicates benefits, the non-inferiority hypotheses are given by

$$H_0 \ : \ e^{\beta_3} \geq 1 + \Delta, \text{ versus } H_1 : e^{\beta_3} < 1 + \Delta. \qquad (8.40)$$

where $\Delta (> 0)$ denotes the non-inferiority margin in terms of the *odds ratio ratio*. If a positive β_3 indicates benefits as in the Respiratory example, then they are

$$H_0 \ : \ e^{\beta_3} \leq 1 - \Delta, \text{ versus } H_1 : e^{\beta_3} > 1 - \Delta. \qquad (8.41)$$

3. Test for *substantial* superiority: If a negative β_3 indicates benefits, the *substantial* superiority hypotheses are given by

$$H_0 \ : \ e^{\beta_3} \geq 1 - \Delta, \text{ versus } H_1 : e^{\beta_3} < 1 - \Delta. \qquad (8.42)$$

where $\Delta (> 0)$ denotes the *substantial* superiority margin in terms of the *odds ratio ratio*. If a positive β_3 indicates benefits as in the Respiratory example, then they are

$$H_0 \ : \ e^{\beta_3} \leq 1 + \Delta, \text{ versus } H_1 : e^{\beta_3} > 1 + \Delta. \qquad (8.43)$$

For the *non-inferiority test* and the *substantial superiority test*, we have to replace β_3 with

$$\beta_3 \Longrightarrow \beta_3 - \log\{1 - \Delta \text{sign}(\beta_3)\} \tag{8.44}$$

in the basic simulation process described below.

The basic process to obtain Monte Carlo simulated sample size $n(= n_1 = n_2)$ for the $S{:}T$ repeated measures design discussed here assumes

1. no difference in the odds of being "good" between two treatment groups at the baseline period due to randomization, i.e., $\beta_1 = 0$ and

2. no change in the odds of being "good" before and after randomization in the placebo group, i.e., $\beta_2 = 0$.

and consists of the following steps:

Step 0 Set the values of (S, T).

Step 1 Set the sample size $n \leftarrow m_1$.

Step 2 Set the number of repetitions N_{rep} (for example, $N_{rep} = 1000, 10000$) of the simulation.

Step 3 Simulate one data set $\{y_{ij} : i = 1, ..., 2n; j = -(S-1), ..., T\}$ independently under the assumed model shown below:

$$\begin{aligned}
y_{ij} \mid b_{0i}, b_{1i} &\sim \text{Bernoulli}(p_{ij}) \\
p_{ij} &= \frac{1}{1 + \exp\{-(\beta_0 + b_{0i} + b_{1i}x_{2ij} + \beta_3 x_{1i} x_{2ij})\}} \\
i &= 1, ..., n \text{ (Control)},\ n+1, ..., 2n \text{ (New treatment)} \\
j &= -(S-1), -(S-2), ..., 0,\ 1, ..., T \\
\boldsymbol{b}_i &= (b_{0i}, b_{1i}) \sim N(\mathbf{0}, \boldsymbol{\Phi}) \\
\boldsymbol{\Phi} &= \begin{pmatrix} \sigma_{B0}^2 & \rho_{01}\sigma_{B0}\sigma_{B1} \\ \rho_{01}\sigma_{B0}\sigma_{B1} & \sigma_{B1}^2 \end{pmatrix}
\end{aligned}$$

where the values of $\beta_0, \beta_3, \sigma_{B0}^2, \sigma_{B1}^2, \rho_{01}$ must be determined based on similar randomized controlled trials done in the past.

Step 4 Repeat Step 3 N_{rep} times.

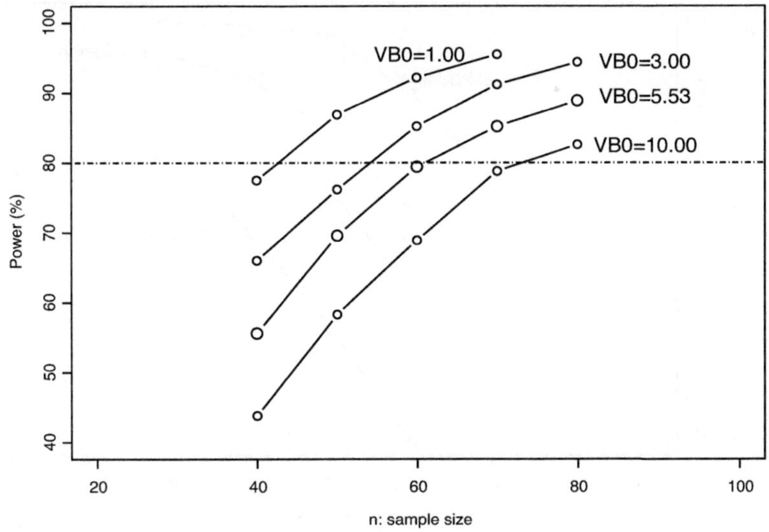

FIGURE 8.5
Simulated power (the effect size $e^{\beta_3} = 8$) for the *1:1 design* of Model IV versus common sample size n for four different values of variance σ^2_{B0} (indicated by "VB0" in the figure).

Step 5 Calculate the Monte Carlo simulated power as the number of results with significant treatment effect at significance level α, k_1, divided by the number of repetitions, i.e., $power_1 = k_1/N_{rep}$.

Step 6 Repeat Step 1 to Step 5 using different sample sizes, $m_2, m_3, \ldots$ and obtain the simulated power, $power_2, power_3, \ldots$. Then, plot the simulated powers against the sample sizes used and obtain a *simulated power curve* by drawing a curve connecting these points. Finally, we can estimate a simulated sample size that attains the pre-specified power $100(1-\phi)\%$ based on the simulated power curve.

Example: *Respiratory Data*

Let us consider here the simulated sample sizes for the *superiority test* based on the estimates from Model IV applied to the *Respiratory Data* shown in Output 8.3 and Table 8.5 where we have

$$\hat{\beta}_3 = 2.07(e^{\hat{\beta}_3 = 7.94}), \quad \hat{\sigma}^2_{B0} = 5.53.$$

Because the observed proportion of respiratory status "good" at baseline was $50/111 = 0.45$, let us set β_0 as $\log(0.45/(1-0.45))$ here. So, based on the results

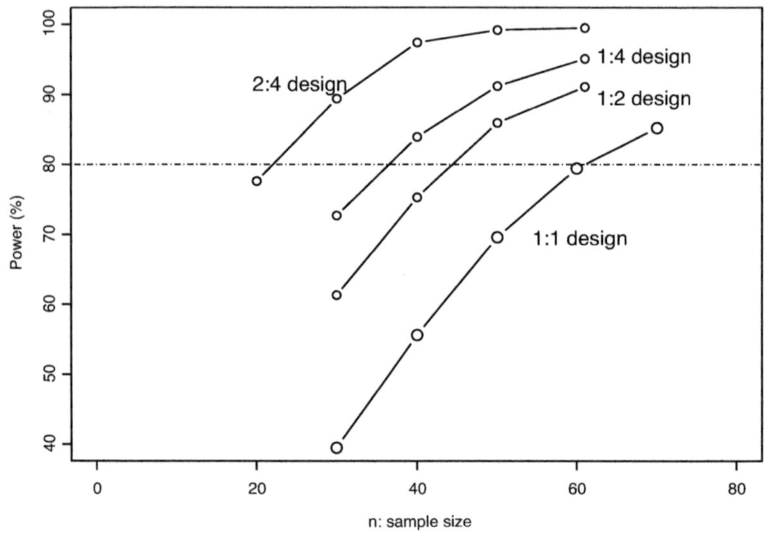

FIGURE 8.6
Simulated power (the effect size $e^{\beta_3} = 8$) of Model IV versus common sample size n for four different repeated measures designs with variance $\sigma^2_{B0} = 5.53$ estimated in the *Respiratory Data* (*1:4 design*).

from the *Respiratory Data*, let us set the values of the necessary parameters as

$$\beta_0 = \log(0.45/(1-0.45)), \beta_3 = 2.08\ (e^{\beta_3} = 8.0),\ \sigma^2_{B0} = 5.50,\ \sigma^2_{B1} = 0$$

and consider the *1:1 design*, *1:4 design*, and *4:4 design*. Figure 8.5 shows the simulated power (N_{rep} = 1000 repetitions) for the *1:1 design* as a function of a common sample size n and the value of intercept variance σ^2_{B0}. Different from normal linear regression models and Poisson regression models described later, the power of the random intercept logistic regression model depends on the value of variance σ^2_{B0} of the *random intercept*. The simulated sample size n with 80% power at $\alpha = 0.05$ is close to 61 for $\sigma^2_{B0} = 5.53$.

Next, we shall conduct a Monte Carlo simulation to compare the sample size (80% power at $\alpha = 0.05$) needed for each of several designs compared with that of the simplest *1:1 design* where the same value of intercept variance $\sigma^2_{B0} = 5.53$ is assumed. Figure 8.6 shows the simulated power of Model IV with $\sigma^2_{B0} = 5.53$ versus common sample size $n(= 20, 30, ..., 70)$ for four different repeated measures designs, *1:1 design*, *1:2 design*, *1:4 design*, and *2,4 design*. The sample sizes needed for each of these designs are 61, 45, 36, and 23, respectively. In other words, compared with the sample size of the *1:1 design*, the *1:2 design* has a 26.2% reduction, the *1:4 design* has a 41.0% reduction, and the *2:2 design* has a 62.3% reduction.

8.9.2 Sample size for the treatment by linear time interaction

In this section, we shall consider the situation where the primary interest is estimating the treatment by *linear* time interaction. In other words, the treatment effect can be expressed in terms of the difference in the slopes of linear trend or rates of improvement. To do this, we shall consider Model VII or the *random intercept plus slope* model within the framework of the *S:T* design. Needless to say, Model VII includes Model VI as a special case. Namely, the model is expressed as

$$\begin{aligned}
\text{logit}\Pr(y_{ij}=1 \mid b_{0i}, b_{1i}) &= b_{0i} + \beta_0 + \beta_1 x_{1i} + (\beta_2 + \beta_3 x_{1i} + b_{1i}) t_j \qquad (8.45)\\
\boldsymbol{b}_i &= (b_{0i}, b_{1i}) \sim N(\mathbf{0}, \boldsymbol{\Phi})\\
\boldsymbol{\Phi} &= \begin{pmatrix} \sigma_{B0}^2 & \rho_{01}\sigma_{B0}\sigma_{B1} \\ \rho_{01}\sigma_{B0}\sigma_{B1} & \sigma_{B1}^2 \end{pmatrix}\\
i &= 1, ..., n_1 \text{ (control)};\\
&= n_1+1, ..., n_1+n_2 \text{ (new treatment)}\\
j &= -(S-1), -(S-2), ..., 0, 1, ..., T,
\end{aligned}$$

where t_j denotes the jth measurement time but all the measurement times during the baseline period are set to be the same time as t_0, which is usually set to be zero, i.e.,

$$t_{-S+1} = t_{-S+2} = \cdots = t_0 = 0. \qquad (8.46)$$

Here also, the parameter β_3 denotes the treatment effect. Then, the null and alternative hypotheses of interest will be one of the three sets of hypotheses described in (8.38)–(8.43). In other words, investigators are interested in establishing whether the new treatment is *superior, non-inferior*, or *substantially superior* to the placebo regarding the rate of improvement.

As in the case of the sample size determination for Model V, the sample size formula with closed form is not available for Model VII. So, let us consider the sample size determination via Monte Carlo simulations. The basic process to obtain Monte Carlo simulated sample size $n(= n_1 = n_2)$ for the *S:T* repeated measures design is exactly the same as that for Model V (Section 8.9.1) and assumes

1. no difference in the odds of being "good" between two treatment groups at baseline period due to randomization, i.e., $\beta_1 = 0$, and

2. no temporal trend in the log odds of being "good" in the placebo group, i.e., $\beta_2 = 0$

and you have only to replace Step 3 in Model V with that arranged for Model VII:

Step 3 Simulate one data set $\{y_{ij} : i = 1, ..., 2n; j = -(S-1), ..., T\}$ independently under the assumed model shown below:

$$
\begin{aligned}
y_{ij} \mid b_{0i} &\sim \text{Bernoulli}(p_{ij}) \\
p_{ij} &= \frac{1}{1 + \exp\{-(\beta_0 + b_{0i} + (\beta_3 x_{1i} + b_{1i}) t_j)\}} \\
i &= 1, ..., n \text{ (Control)}, \ n+1, ..., 2n \text{ (New treatment)} \\
j &= -(S-1), -(S-2), ..., 0, \ 1, ..., T \\
\boldsymbol{b}_i &= (b_{0i}, b_{1i}) \sim N(\mathbf{0}, \boldsymbol{\Phi}) \\
\boldsymbol{\Phi} &= \begin{pmatrix} \sigma_{B0}^2 & \rho_{01}\sigma_{B0}\sigma_{B1} \\ \rho_{01}\sigma_{B0}\sigma_{B1} & \sigma_{B1}^2 \end{pmatrix}
\end{aligned}
$$

where the values of $\beta_0, \beta_3, \sigma_{B0}^2, \sigma_{B1}^2, \rho_{01}$ must be determined based on similar randomized controlled trials done in the past.

Here also, for the *non-inferiority test* and the *substantial superiority test*, we have to replace β_3 with

$$\beta_3 \Longrightarrow \beta_3 - \log\{1 - \Delta \text{sign}(\beta_3)\}$$

in the basic process described above.

8.10 Discussion

In this chapter, several mixed-effects logistic regression models are introduced and are illustrated with real data from a randomized controlled trial, called

Respiratory Data, with the *1:4* design. Needless to say, selection of the appropriate model depends on the purpose of the trial and an appropriate model should be examined cautiously using data from the previous trials.

Especially, we would like to stress that the set of models for the average treatment effect within the framework of $S{:}T$ repeated measures design should be considered as a practical and important trial design that is a better extension of the ordinary *1:1* design combined with an ANCOVA-type logistic regression model in terms of *sample size reduction* and *easier handling of missing data*. Section 8.7.3 compared the estimates of the treatment effect obtained from the ANCOVA-type models VIII and IX with those from the repeated measures models, Models I and IV, which are shown in Table 8.8. In the *Respiratory Data*, the ANCOVA-type models are shown to give a little bit smaller p-values than repeated measures models, although all the estimates are statistically significant.

However, the repeated measures models can be more natural for the $S{:}T$ repeated measures design with $S > 1$ than the ordinary ANCOVA-type logistic regression model because we find it difficult to apply the ANCOVA-type model to these repeated measurements since there is no natural way of dealing with repeated measurements made before randomization, as is shown in the daily symptom data with *7:7* design in Section 8.8.

9

Mixed-effects Poisson regression models

In this chapter, we shall introduce the following three practical and important types of statistical analysis plans or statistical models that you frequently encounter in many randomized controlled trials:

◇ models for the treatment effect at each scheduled visit,
◇ models for the average treatment effect, and
◇ models for the treatment by linear time interaction,

which are illustrated with real data from a randomized controlled trial called *Epilepsy Data*. It should be noted that the problem of *which model should be used in our trial* largely depends on the purpose of the trial. Furthermore, to contrast the traditional ANCOVA-type analysis frequently used in the pre-post design (*1:1* design), where the baseline measurement is used as a covariate, we shall introduce

◇ANCOVA-type models adjusting for baseline measurement

for the *1:T* design. Finally, sample size calculations needed for some models with *S:T* repeated measures design are presented and illustrated with real data.

9.1 Example: The Epilepsy Data with *1:4* design

In this chapter, we shall illustrate the mixed-effects Poisson regression models with data from a clinical trial for patients suffering from epilepsy which was designed to investigate whether an anti-epileptic drug called *progabide* reduces the rate of seizures when compared with placebo (Leppik et al., 1987). This data set, called here the *Epilepsy Data*, is very famous in the sense that it has been analyzed by many authors including Thall and Vail (1990), Diggle et al. (2002), Cook and Wei (2002, 2003), Everitt and Hothorn (2010) and Fitzmaurice et al. (2011). The full data set is provided in Thall and Vail (1990) and Diggle et al. (2002). N = 59 epileptic patients enrolled in this study were randomized to either progabide ($n_2 = 31$) or a placebo ($n_1 = 28$) in addition to a standard anti-epileptic chemotherapy. Prior to randomization, age and the number of epileptic seizures during the baseline period of eight

TABLE 9.1
Epilepsy Data: Data set with long format from a randomized placebo-controlled clinical trial to investigate whether an anti-epileptic drug called *progabide* reduces the rate of seizures when compared with placebo. Data of the first three patients are shown here.

No.	subject	treatment	visit	seizure	age
1	1	placebo	0	11	31
2	1	placebo	1	5	31
3	1	placebo	2	3	31
4	1	placebo	3	3	31
5	1	placebo	4	3	31
6	2	placebo	0	11	30
7	2	placebo	1	3	30
8	2	placebo	2	5	30
9	2	placebo	3	3	30
10	2	placebo	4	3	30
11	3	placebo	0	6	25
12	3	placebo	1	2	25
13	3	placebo	2	4	25
14	3	placebo	3	0	25
15	3	placebo	4	5	25

weeks were recorded. After randomization, patients were assessed biweekly for eight weeks and the number of seizures was recorded in four consecutive two-week intervals. The original trial design seems to be the *4:4 design* with two weeks as a unit interval, but they took the total number of seizures during eight weeks as the baseline count data.[1] Many authors considered the overall or average treatment effect during the eight-week treatment period.

A part of the *Epilepsy Data* in the long format is shown in Table 8.1 which includes the following five variables:

1. `subject`: a numeric factor indicating the subject ID.
2. `treatment`: a binary variable for the treatment group (progabide = 1, placebo = 0).
3. `visit`: a numeric factor indicating the period of observation, 0 = baseline (eight weeks), 1, 2, 3, 4 (for each of four two-week periods).
4. `seizure`: a continuous variable for the number of seizures observed in each of five observation periods.
5. `age`: a continuous variable for age.

[1]This data set is available as the data frame `epilepsy` in the `R` system for statistical computing using the following code: data("epilepsy", package="HSAUR2")

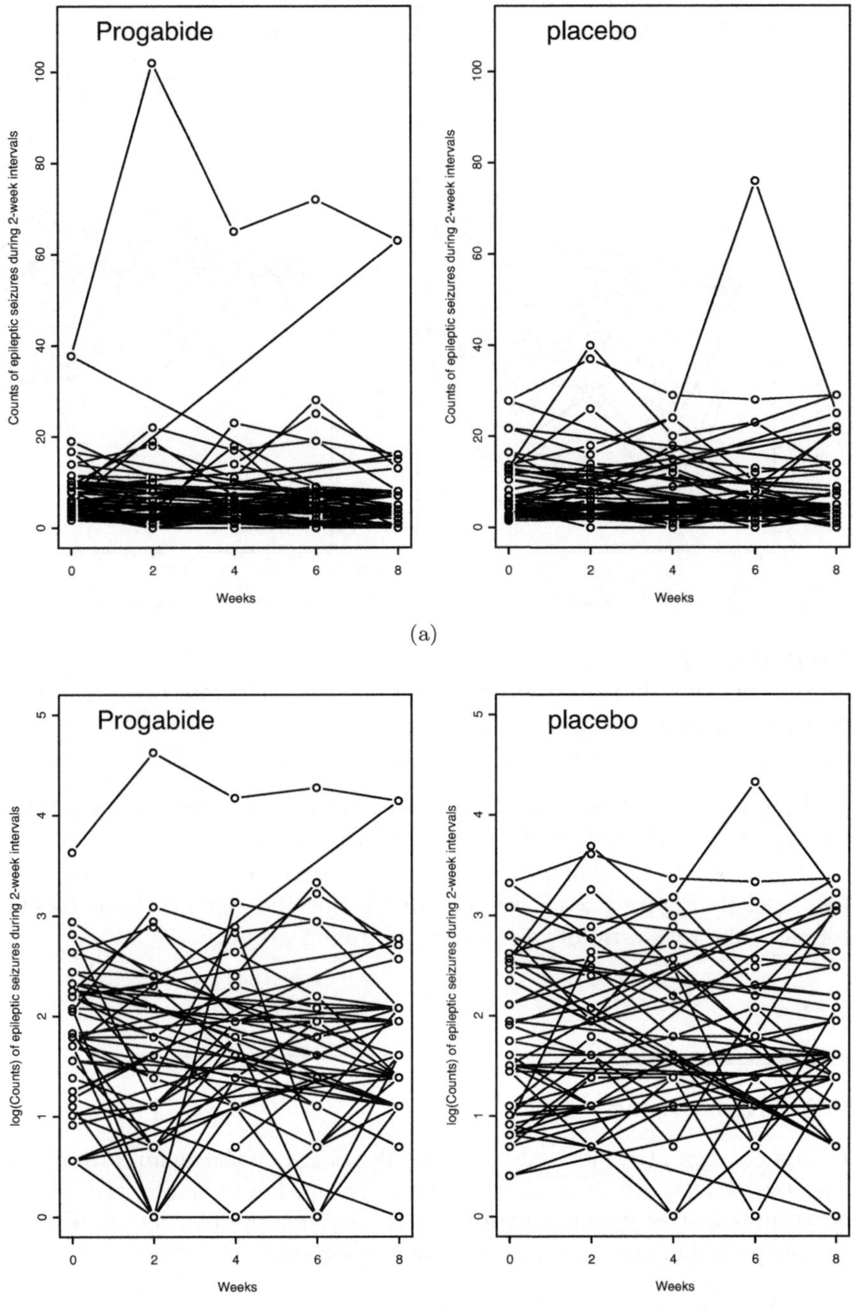

FIGURE 9.1
Subject-specific response profiles by treatment group based on (a) the rate of seizures (per two weeks) and (b) the logarithm of the rate of seizures (per two weeks).

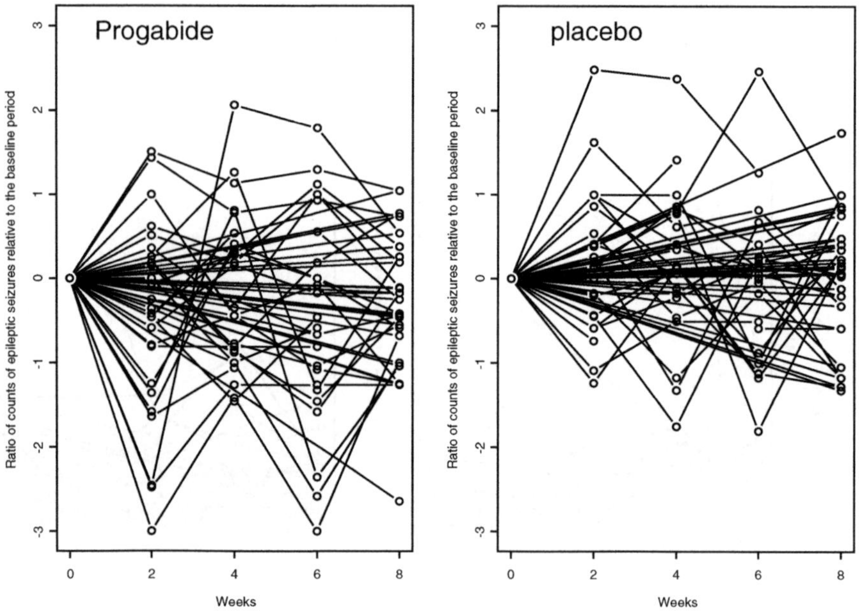

FIGURE 9.2
Subject-specific changes from baseline in terms of the rate ratio of seizures by treatment group.

Figure 9.1(a) shows the subject-specific response profiles over time by treatment group based on the number of seizures (per two weeks) and Figure 9.1(b) shows the similar profiles based on the log of the rate of seizures (per two weeks). Figure 9.2 shows the subject-specific changes from baseline in terms of the rate ratio of seizures by treatment group.

9.2 Rate ratio

In Figure 9.3(a), the mean response profiles based on the mean rates of seizures (per two weeks) are shown by treatment group. For example, the mean rates of seizures at the jth observation period, R_{1j} for the placebo group and R_{2j} for the progabide group, are calculated as follows:

1. At baseline for the placebo group:

$$R_{10} = \frac{1}{4n_1} \sum_{i=1}^{n_1+n_2} y_{i0}(1 - x_{1i}) = 7.70,$$

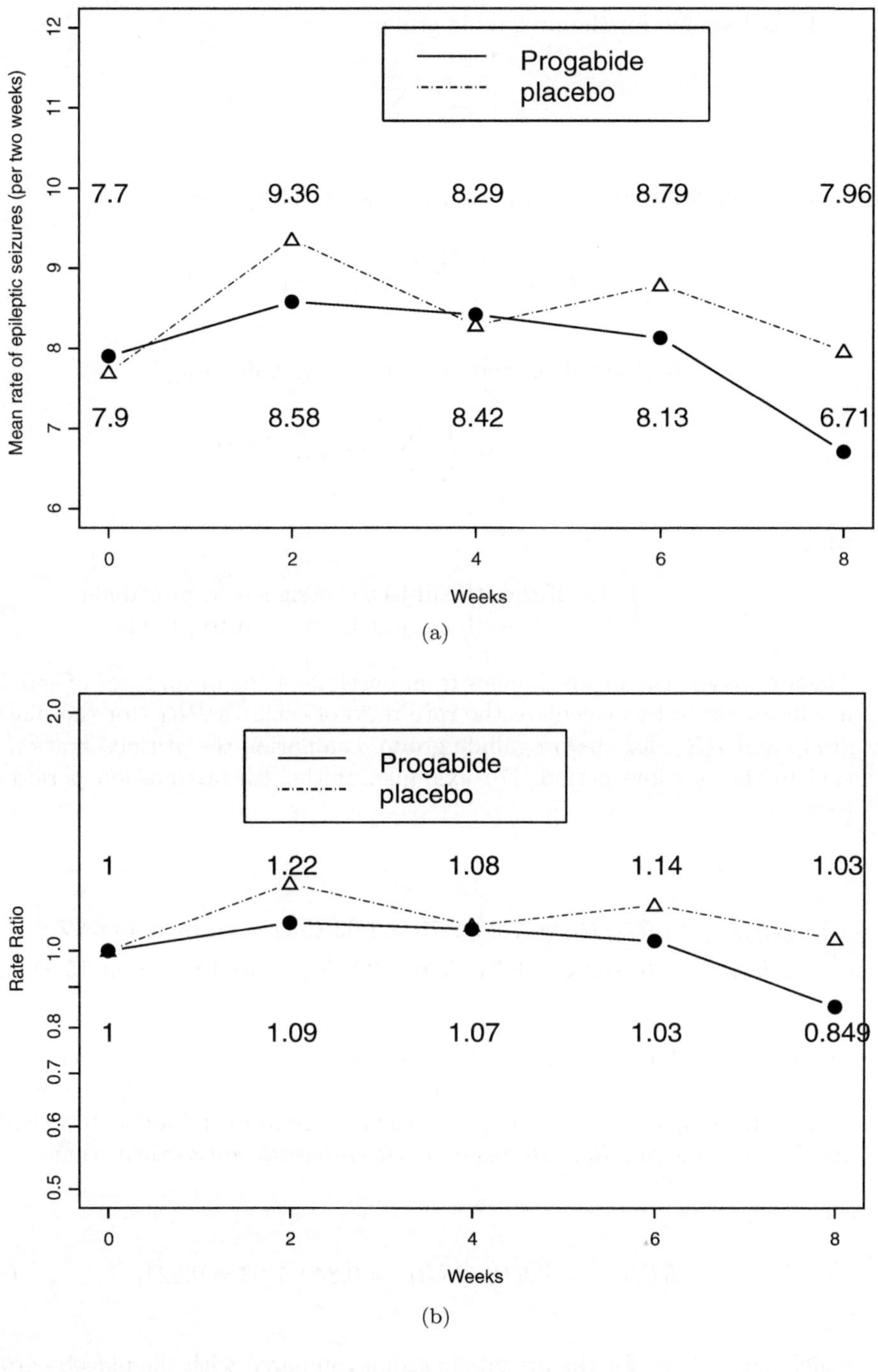

FIGURE 9.3
(a) Mean response profiles by treatment group based on the mean rate of seizures (per two weeks). (b) Mean changes from baseline by treatment group in terms of the rate ratio of seizures.

2. At baseline for the progabide group:

$$R_{20} = \frac{1}{4n_2} \sum_{i=1}^{n_1+n_2} y_{i0} x_{1i} = 7.90.$$

3. At the 4th observation period for the placebo group:

$$R_{14} = \frac{1}{n_1} \sum_{i=1}^{n_1+n_2} y_{i4}(1 - x_{1i}) = 7.96.$$

4. At the 4th observation period for the progabide group:

$$R_{24} = \frac{1}{n_2} \sum_{i=1}^{n_1+n_2} y_{i4} x_{1i} = 6.71.$$

where

$$x_{1i} = \begin{cases} 1, & \text{if the } i\text{th subject is assigned to progabide} \\ 0, & \text{if the } i\text{th subject is assigned to placebo.} \end{cases} \tag{9.1}$$

Then, to assess the mean changes from baseline of the mean rates of seizures, it will be natural to calculate the rate ratio of seizures RR_{1j} for the placebo group and RR_{2j} for the progabide group, comparing the jth observation period to the baseline period. For example, at the 4th observation period, we have

$$RR_{14} = R_{14}/R_{10} = 7.96/7.70 = 1.03 \text{ (increased by about 3\%)} \tag{9.2}$$

$$RR_{24} = R_{24}/R_{20} = 6.71/7.90 = 0.849 \text{ (reduced by about 15\%).} \tag{9.3}$$

Figure 9.3(b) shows the mean changes from baseline in terms of these rate ratios by treatment group. Then, one way to estimate the treatment effect of progabide compared with placebo at each observation period is to calculate the *Ratio of the two Rate Ratios* or *RRR (rate ratio ratio)* such that

$$RRR_4 = RR_{24}/RR_{14} = 0.849/1.03 = 0.824, \tag{9.4}$$

which means that, for the progabide group compared with the placebo group, the rate ratio of seizures is relatively reduced by about 17.6% at the 4th observation period.

9.3 Poisson regression models

The number of epileptic seizures is so-called *count* data. Although we can apply a linear regression approach to the count data, there are two problems. The response variable that is a count can take only positive values and the variable is unlikely to follow a normal distribution symmetric about the mean. Instead, the Poisson distribution has a long history as a model for count data. Let y_{ij} denote the number of seizures of the ith subject at the jth observation period. Then, we can formulate the Poisson model as

$$y_{ij} \sim \text{Poisson}(\lambda_{ij}) = \text{Poisson}(e^{\mu_{ij}}) \tag{9.5}$$

$$p(y_{ij}) = \frac{(e^{\mu_{ij}})^{y_{ij}}}{y_{ij}!} \exp(-e^{\mu_{ij}}), \tag{9.6}$$

where $\lambda_{ij} = e^{\mu_{ij}}(> 0)$ is the expected number of seizures for the ith subject at the jth observation period. Then, a *fixed-effects* Poisson regression model with covariates $(x_1, ..., x_q)$ is defined as

$$\log \lambda = \beta_0 + \beta_1 x_1 + \cdots + \beta_q x_q. \tag{9.7}$$

However, the Poisson distribution has a very strong assumption that the variance is equal to the expected value, i.e.,

$$\text{Var}(y_{ij}) = E(y_{ij}) = \lambda_{ij} = e^{\mu_{ij}}(> 0).$$

In many medical and biological applications, this relationship is rarely satisfied, and usually the variance exceeds the expected value, i.e.,

$$\text{Var}(y_{ij}) = \phi e^{\mu_{ij}} > e^{\mu_{ij}}, \ (\phi > 1). \tag{9.8}$$

This is usually called "over-dispersion" and ϕ is called a over-dispersion parameter. This over-dispersion can be explained by an inter-subject variability of the expected value $\lambda_{ij} = e^{\mu_{ij}}$. Namely, we can deal with this situation by introducing the random-effects b_{0i} reflecting inter-subject variability such that

1. Conditional on the subject-specific expected value $e^{b_{0i}} e^{\mu_{ij}} = e^{b_{0i} + \mu_{ij}}$, the response variable y_{ij} has a Poisson distribution.

2. The random effects b_{0i} are independent realizations from some distribution. We assume here a normal distribution with mean 0 and variance σ^2_{B0}.

In other words, we have

$$E(y_{ij} \mid b_{0i}) = \lambda_{ij} e^{b_{0i}} = e^{b_{0i}+\mu_{ij}} \quad (9.9)$$

$$y_{ij} \mid b_{0i} \sim \text{Poisson}(e^{b_{0i}+\mu_{ij}}) \quad (9.10)$$

$$p(y_{ij} \mid b_{0i}) = \frac{(e^{b_{0i}+\mu_{ij}})^{y_{ij}}}{y_{ij}!} \exp(-e^{b_{0i}+\mu_{ij}}). \quad (9.11)$$

Namely, a mixed-effects Poisson regression model can be expressed as

$$\log E(y_{ij} \mid b_{0i}) = \log e^{b_{0i}+\mu_{ij}} = b_{0i} + \beta_0 + \beta_1 x_{1i} + \cdots + \beta_q x_{qi}. \quad (9.12)$$

9.4 Models for the treatment effect at each scheduled visit

As in the case of the logistic regression model in Section 8.4, we shall apply two types of mixed-effects models: (1) a random intercept model and (2) a random intercept plus slope model with slope constant during the evaluation period.

9.4.1 Model I: Random intercept model

In the Poisson model, it is quite natural to consider the following multiplicative model at first, rather than the usual additive model. The *random intercept model* with random intercept b_{0i} reflecting the inter-subject variability of the rate of seizures at baseline can be given as

$$E(y_{i0} \mid b_{0i}) = \begin{cases} e^{b_{0i}} e^{\beta_0} e^{\boldsymbol{w}_i^t \boldsymbol{\xi}} L_{i0}, & \text{(placebo)} \\ e^{b_{0i}} e^{\beta_0} e^{\beta_1} e^{\boldsymbol{w}_i^t \boldsymbol{\xi}} L_{i0}, & \text{(progabide)} \end{cases}$$

$$E(y_{ij} \mid b_{0i}) = \begin{cases} e^{b_{0i}} e^{\beta_0} e^{\beta_{2j}} e^{\boldsymbol{w}_i^t \boldsymbol{\xi}} L_{ij}, & \text{(placebo)} \\ e^{b_{0i}} e^{\beta_0} e^{\beta_1} e^{\beta_{2j}} e^{\beta_{3j}} e^{\boldsymbol{w}_i^t \boldsymbol{\xi}} L_{ij}, & \text{(progabide)} \end{cases}$$

$$j = 1, ..., 4,$$

where:

1. L_{ij} denotes the length of the observation period (= 4 for $j = 0$; = 1 for $j = 1, 2, 3, 4$) in the unit of "**two weeks.**" In the Poisson regression models described below, the $\log(L_{ij})$ is set as an *offset.*

2. e^{β_0} denotes the mean subject-specific rate of seizures (per two weeks) for the placebo group at baseline.

3. $e^{b_{0i}}e^{\beta_0}$ denotes the subject-specific rate of seizures for the placebo group at baseline.

4. e^{β_1} denotes the subject-specific rate ratio of seizures, comparing the progabide group to the placebo group at baseline.

5. $e^{\beta_{2j}}$ denotes the subject-specific rate ratio of seizures, comparing the jth observation period to the baseline period for the placebo group.

6. $e^{\beta_{2j}}e^{\beta_{3j}}$ denotes the subject-specific rate ratio of seizures, comparing the jth observation period to the baseline period for the progabide group.

7. β_{3j} denotes the effect of the treatment-by-time interaction at the jth visit or $e^{\beta_{3j}}$ denotes the *ratio* of these two rate ratios or the *RRR, rate ratio ratio.* In other words, $e^{\beta_{3j}}$ means the subject-specific treatment effect of the new treatment compared with the control treatment at the jth visit in terms of *RRR.*

8. $\boldsymbol{w}_i^t = (w_{1i}, ..., w_{qi})$ is a vector of covariates.

9. $\boldsymbol{\xi}^t = (\xi_1, ..., \xi_q)$ is a vector of coefficients for covariates.

Needless to say, we should add the phrase "adjusted for covariates" to the interpretations of fixed-effects parameters β, but we omit the phrase in what follows. In terms of the generalized linear model discussed in Chapter 1, the canonical link function for the Poisson model is the log transformation. So the most common Poisson model is the *log-linear* model. Then the above random intercept model is expressed by the following log-linear model:

$$
\begin{aligned}
\log E(y_{i0} \mid b_{0i}) &= \begin{cases} b_{0i} + \beta_0 + \boldsymbol{w}_i^t\boldsymbol{\xi} + \log L_{i0}, & \text{(placebo)} \\ b_{0i} + \beta_0 + \beta_1 + \boldsymbol{w}_i^t\boldsymbol{\xi} + \log L_{i0}, & \text{(progabide)} \end{cases} \\
\log E(y_{ij} \mid b_{0i}) &= \begin{cases} b_{0i} + \beta_0 + \beta_{2j} + \boldsymbol{w}_i^t\boldsymbol{\xi} + \log L_{ij}, & \text{(placebo)} \\ b_{0i} + \beta_0 + \beta_1 + \beta_{2j} + \beta_{3j} + \boldsymbol{w}_i^t\boldsymbol{\xi} + \log L_{ij}, & \text{(progabide)} \end{cases} \\
& \quad j = 1, ..., 4.
\end{aligned}
$$

Then, as in Section 7.4.1, by introducing the two dummy variables x_{1i}, x_{2ij}, the above model can be re-expressed as

$$
\begin{aligned}
\log E(y_{ij} \mid b_{0i}) &= \log L_{ij} + \beta_0 + b_{0i} + \beta_1 x_{1i} + \beta_{2kj} x_{2ij} \\
&\quad + \beta_{3j} x_{1i} x_{2ij} + \boldsymbol{w}_i^t \boldsymbol{\xi} \qquad (9.13) \\
i &= 1, ..., N;\ j = 0, 1, 2, 3, 4;\ \beta_{20} = 0,\ \beta_{30} = 0 \\
b_{0i} &\sim N(0, \sigma_{B0}^2),
\end{aligned}
$$

where

$$
x_{2ij} = \begin{cases} 1, & \text{for } j \geq 1 \text{ (evaluation period)} \\ 0, & \text{for } j \leq 0 \text{ (baseline period).} \end{cases} \qquad (9.14)
$$

It should be noted here also that an important assumption is, given the random intercept b_{0i}, the subject-specific repeated measures $(y_{i0}, ..., y_{i4})$ are *mutually independent.*

9.4.2 Model II: Random intercept plus slope model

As the second model, consider a *random intercept plus slope model* by simply adding the random effects b_{1i} taking account of the inter-subject variability of the response assumed to be constant during the treatment period, which is given by

$$
\begin{aligned}
\log E(y_{i0} \mid b_{0i}) &= \begin{cases} \beta_0 + b_{0i} + \boldsymbol{w}_i^t \boldsymbol{\xi} + \log L_{i0}, & \text{(placebo)} \\ \beta_0 + b_{0i} + \beta_1 + \boldsymbol{w}_i^t \boldsymbol{\xi} + \log L_{i0}, & \text{(progabide)} \end{cases} \\
\log E(y_{ij} \mid b_{0i}, b_{1i}) &= \begin{cases} \beta_0 + b_{0i} + b_{1i} + \beta_{2j} + \boldsymbol{w}_i^t \boldsymbol{\xi} + \log L_{ij}, & \text{(placebo)} \\ \beta_0 + b_{0i} + b_{1i} + \beta_1 + \beta_{2j} + \beta_{3j} + \boldsymbol{w}_i^t \boldsymbol{\xi} + \log L_{ij}, & \\ \qquad\qquad\qquad\qquad \text{(progabide)} \end{cases} \\
& j = 1, ..., 4,
\end{aligned}
$$

which is re-expressed as

$$
\begin{aligned}
\log E(y_{ij} \mid b_{0i}, b_{1i}) &= \log L_{ij} + \beta_0 + b_{0i} + b_{1i} x_{2ij} + \beta_1 x_{1i} + \beta_{2j} x_{2ij} \\
&\quad + \beta_{3j} x_{1i} x_{2ij} + \boldsymbol{w}_i^t \boldsymbol{\xi} \qquad (9.15) \\
i &= 1, ..., N;\ j = 0, 1, 2, 3, 4;\ \beta_{20} = 0,\ \beta_{30} = 0 \\
\boldsymbol{b}_i &= (b_{0i}, b_{1i}) \sim N(0, \Phi) \\
\boldsymbol{\Phi} &= \begin{pmatrix} \sigma_{B0}^2 & \rho_B \sigma_{B0} \sigma_{B1} \\ \rho_B \sigma_{B0} \sigma_{B1} & \sigma_{B1}^2 \end{pmatrix}.
\end{aligned}
$$

We shall call Model II with $\rho_B = 0$, Model IIa, and the one with $\rho_B \neq 0$, Model IIb. It should be noted that the *random slope* introduced in the above model does not mean the *slope* on the time or a linear time trend, which will be considered in Section 9.6.

9.4.3 Analysis using SAS

Now, let us apply these three models to the *Epilepsy Data* using the SAS procedure `PROC GRIMMIX`. The respective sets of SAS programs are shown in Program 9.1. The following considerations are required for coding the SAS programs (some of them have already been described in Sections 3.5, 7.4.4 and 8.4.3):

1. A binary variable `treatment` indicates x_{1i}.

2. Create a new binary variable `post` indicating x_{2ij} in the `DATA` step as

   ```
   if visit=0 then post=0; else post=1;
   ```

3. The fixed effects β_{2j} can be expressed via the variable `visit` (main factor), which must be specified as a numeric factor by the `CLASS` statement.

4. The fixed effects β_{3j} can be expressed via the `treatment * visit` interaction.

5. As already explained in Section 3.5, the `CLASS` statement needs the option `/ref=first` to specify the first category be the reference category.

6. The option `method=quad` specifies the adaptive Gauss-Hermite quadrature method for evaluating integrals involved in the calculation of the log-likelihood. For details, see Section B.3 in Appendix B.

7. The option `(qpoints=7)` specifies the number of nodes used for evaluating integrals. For the details to select the number of nodes, see Section B.3.3.2 in Appendix B.

8. The Poisson regression model specifies the `MODEL` statement with option

   ```
   / d=poi link=log offset=logt s cl ;
   ```

   where the *offset* variable `logt` indicating $\log(L_{ij})$ must be created as follows:

   ```
   if visit=0 then logt=log(4); else logt=log(1);
   ```

9. When you want to fit the *random intercept and slope model* with $\rho_B = 0$, you have to use the following `RANDOM` statement:

```
random intercept post /type=simple subject=id g gcorr ;
```

When you want to fit the model with $\rho_B \neq 0$, then

```
random intercept post /type=un subject=id g gcorr ;
```

10. In this example, we want to obtain the confidence interval of the estimate $\beta_{24} + \beta_{34}$, which denotes the log of rate ratio of seizures, comparing the 4th observation period to the baseline period for the progabide group. To do this, we use the following linear contrast

$$\begin{aligned}\beta_{24} + \beta_{34} &= (\beta_{24} - \beta_{20}) + (\beta_{34} - \beta_{30}) \\ &= (-1, 0, 0, 0, 1)(\beta_{20}, \beta_{21}, \beta_{22}, \beta_{23}, \beta_{24})^t \\ &\qquad + (-1, 0, 0, 0, 1)(\beta_{30}, \beta_{31}, \beta_{32}, \beta_{33}, \beta_{34})^t.\end{aligned}$$

However, due to the option `/ref=first` used, the coefficients of the linear contrast in SAS programs needs the following change (for example, see Section 3.5)

$$(-1, 0, 0, 0, 1) \rightarrow (0, 0, 0, 1, -1),$$

and then the `ESTIMATE` statement should be:

```
estimate 'progabide at 8w ' visit 0 0 0 1 -1
 treatment*visit 0 0 0 1 -1 /divisor=1  cl  alpha=0.05;
```

11. As in the case of the normal linear regression models, let us perform the same diagnostic based on *studentized conditional residuals*, which is useful to examine whether the subject-specific model is adequate, although `PROC GLIMMIX` provides several kinds of panels of residual diagnostics. Each panel consists of a plot of residuals versus predicted values, a histogram with normal density overlaid, a Q-Q plot, and the box plots of residuals. We can do this in the same manner as explained in Section 7.4.4.

Program 9.1. SAS procedure PROC GLIMMIX for Models I, IIa, IIb

```
data epilong ;
  infile 'c:\book\RepeatedMeasure\epilepsy_long.txt' missover;
  input no  subject treatment  visit seizure age;
  if visit=0 then post=0; else post=1;
  if visit=0 then logt=log(4); else logt=log(1);

  ods graphics on;
  proc glimmix data=epilong method=quad (qpoints=7)
   plots=studentpanel( conditional blup) ;
   class subject visit/ref=first  ;
   model seizure  =  age treatment  visit treatment*visit
                                   / d=poi link=log offset=logt s cl ;
 /* Model I  */
  random intercept  / subject= subject g gcorr ;
 /* Model IIa */
   random intercept post / subject= subject g gcorr ;
 /* Model IIb*/
   random intercept post / type=un subject= subject g gcorr ;
   estimate 'progabide at 8w' visit 0 0 0 1 -1
                         treatment*visit 0 0 0 1 -1
                                  /divisor=1  cl  alpha=0.05;
run;
```

The results of Model I are shown in Output 9.1. The estimated variance of the random intercept is $\hat{\sigma}^2_{B0} = 0.5999$ ($s.e. = 0.1153$) and $e^{\hat{\beta}_{2j}}$, the rate ratio of seizures comparing the jth observation period to baseline period for the placebo group, is estimated as

1. visit 1: $e^{0.1954} = 1.21$
2. visit 2: $e^{0.07378} = 1.08$
3. visit 3: $e^{0.1324} = 1.14$
4. visit 4: $e^{0.0342} = 1.03$

which are exactly the same as RR_{1j} shown in Figure 9.3(b). As a matter of fact, in Model I we have

$$e^{\hat{\beta}_{2j}} = RR_{1j} \quad (9.16)$$
$$e^{\hat{\beta}_{2j}+\hat{\beta}_{3j}} = RR_{2j} \quad (9.17)$$
$$e^{\hat{\beta}_{3j}} = RR_{2j}/RR_{1j} = RRR_j. \quad (9.18)$$

Output 9.1. SAS procedure PROC GLIMMIX for Model I

```
Fit statistics
-2 Res Log Likelihood 2007.88
AIC (smaller is better) 2031.88
BIC (smaller is better) 2056.81

Covariance Parameter Estimates
Cov Parm    Subject   Estimate S.E.
Intercept subject 0.5999 0.1153

Solution for Fixed Effects
Effect        visit Estimate S.E. DF t Value Pr>|t| Alpha Lower Upper
Intercept         2.1735  0.5045   56  4.31 <.0001 0.05  1.1629  3.1840
age              -0.01543 0.01659 228 -0.93 0.3534 0.05 -0.04812 0.01726
treatment        -0.04395 0.2103  228 -0.21 0.8347 0.05 -0.4584  0.3705
visit          1  0.1954  0.07055 228  2.77 0.0061 0.05  0.05637 0.3344
visit          2  0.07378 0.07396 228  1.00 0.3195 0.05 -0.07195 0.2195
visit          3  0.1324  0.07228 228  1.83 0.0684 0.05 -0.01005 0.2748
visit          4  0.03420 0.07513 228  0.46 0.6494 0.05 -0.1138  0.1822
visit          0  0 . . . . . . .
treatment*visit 1 -0.1131  0.09878 228 -1.15 0.2533 0.05 -0.3078  0.08149
treatment*visit 2 -0.01053 0.1016  228 -0.10 0.9176 0.05 -0.2107  0.1897
treatment*visit 3 -0.1042  0.1011  228 -1.03 0.3036 0.05 -0.3034  0.09492
treatment*visit 4 -0.1979  0.1071  228 -1.85 0.0659 0.05 -0.4090  0.01313
treatment*visit 0 0 . . . . . . .

Estimate
Label            Estimate  S.E.   DF  t Value Pr>|t| Alpha Lower Upper
progabide at 8w  -0.1637  0.07634 228 -2.14 0.0331 0.05 -0.3141 -0.01329
```

The results of Model IIa are shown in Output 9.2. The results of Model IIb are omitted here. The values of the AIC for Models I, IIa, and IIb are 2031.88, 1861.92, and 1862.45, respectively. The values of the BIC for these three models are 2056.81, 1888.93, and 1891.54, respectively. Therefore, based on the AIC and BIC, Model IIa is selected as the best model.

Output 9.2. SAS procedure PROC GLIMMIX for Model IIa

```
Fit statistics
-2 Res Log Likelihood 1835.92
AIC (smaller is better) 1861.92
BIC (smaller is better) 1888.93

Covariance Parameter Estimates
Cov Parm   Subject   Estimate S.E.
Intercept subject 0.5004 0.09985
post       subject 0.2415 0.06191

Solution for Fixed Effects
Effect           visit Estimate S.E.   DF t Value Pr>|t| Alpha Lower Upper
Intercept              2.3739  0.4709  56   5.04 <.0001 0.05 1.4305    3.3172
age                  -0.02144 0.0154 171 -1.39 0.1663 0.05 -0.05188 0.009005
treatment             0.02059 0.1942 171   0.11 0.9157 0.05 -0.3628  0.4039
visit            1  0.1028   0.1220 171   0.84 0.4006 0.05 -0.1381  0.3438
visit            2 -0.02078 0.1241 171 -0.17 0.8672 0.05 -0.2657  0.2242
visit            3  0.04036 0.1230 171   0.33 0.7433 0.05 -0.2025  0.2832
visit            4 -0.05572 0.1247 171 -0.45 0.6556 0.05 -0.3019  0.1904
visit            0  0 . . . . . . .
treatment*visit 1 -0.3278   0.1705 171 -1.92 0.0562 0.05 -0.6644  0.008796
treatment*visit 2 -0.2216   0.1722 171 -1.29 0.1999 0.05 -0.5614  0.1183
treatment*visit 3 -0.3198   0.1719 171 -1.86 0.0645 0.05 -0.6590  0.01947
treatment*visit 4 -0.4168   0.1755 171 -2.38 0.0186 0.05 -0.7631 -0.07040
treatment*visit 0 0 . . . . . . .

Estimate
Label              Estimate  S.E.  DF t Value Pr>|t| Alpha Lower Upper
progabide at 8w   -0.4725   0.1241 171 -3.81 0.0002 0.05 -0.7174  -0.2276
```

From the estimates of Model IIa ($\rho_B = 0$), we have the following information:

1. Estimates of the variance of random effects are

$$\hat{\sigma}^2_{B0} = 0.5004 \ (s.e. = 0.09985), \ \hat{\sigma}^2_{B1} = 0.2415 \ (s.e. = 0.0619).$$

2. The rate ratio of seizures comparing the 4th observation period (7–8 weeks after randomization) to the baseline period for the placebo group is estimated as $e^{\hat{\beta}_{24}} = e^{-0.05572} = 0.946$, and its 95% confidence interval is $(e^{-0.3019}, e^{0.1904}) = (0.739, 1.209)$.

3. On the other hand, the rate ratio for the progabide group is estimated as $e^{\hat{\beta}_{24}+\hat{\beta}_{34}} = e^{-0.4725} = 0.623$ and its 95% confidence interval is $(e^{-0.7174}, e^{-0.2276}) = (0.488, 0.796)$ by reading the results of ESTIMATE statement. These results indicate a reduction of 37.7%.

4. The treatment effect of progabide compared with placebo at the 4th observation period is estimated as $e^{\hat{\beta}_{34}} = e^{-0.4168}$ $(95\%CI : e^{-0.7631}, e^{-0.07040}) = 0.66$ $(95\%CI : 0.47, 0.93)$, indicating a relative reduction of 34%.

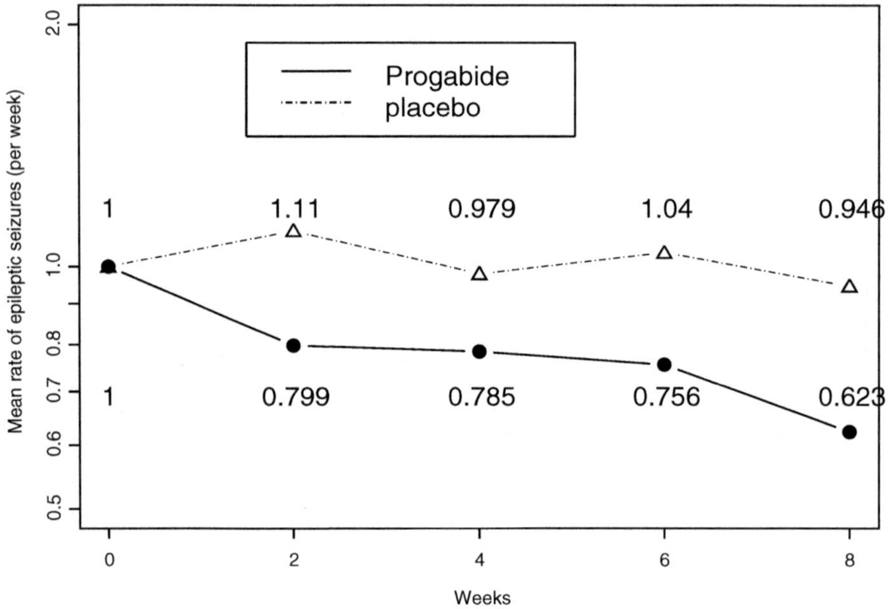

FIGURE 9.4
The changes from baseline by treatment group in terms of the estimated rate ratios of seizures ($e^{\hat{\beta}_{2j}}$ for the placebo group and $e^{\hat{\beta}_{2j}+\hat{\beta}_{3j}}$ for the progabide group) via Model IIa.

5. Figure 9.4 shows the changes from baseline by treatment group based on the estimated rate ratio of seizures, comparing the jth observation period to the baseline period.

6. The panel of graphics of the studentized conditional residuals of Model IIa is shown in Figure 9.5. There is one outlying point having studentized residuals larger than 7.5, but there seems to be no systematic alarming patterns in these plots.

Table 9.2 shows the estimated treatment effect $e^{\hat{\beta}_{3j}}$ (rate ratio ratio) at each of four observation periods for Model I and Model IIa ($\rho_B = 0$).

9.5 Models for the average treatment effect

In Chapter 1 we introduced a new *S:T* repeated measures design both as an extension of the *1:1* design or pre-post design and as a formal confirmatory trial design for randomized controlled trials. The primary interest in this de-

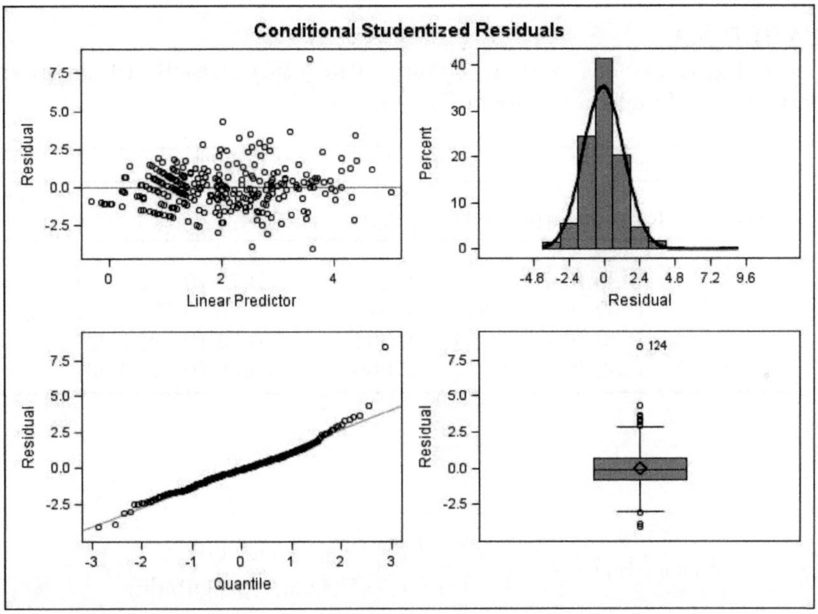

FIGURE 9.5
The panel of graphics of studentized conditional residuals of Model IIa consisting of a plot of residuals versus predicted values, a histogram with normal density overlaid, a Q-Q plot, and a box plot.

sign is to estimate the overall or average treatment effect during the evaluation period. So, in the trial protocol, it is important to select the evaluation period during which the treatment effect could be expected to be stable to a certain extent. So, in this section, let us assume that **the primary interest of the *Epilepsy Trial* with the *1:4* design is to estimate the average treatment effect over eight weeks after randomization (evaluation period)**, although many readers may not think it reasonable for the real situation of the *Epilepsy Trial*. In this case, as already described in Sections 1.2.2, 7.5 and 8.5, we can introduce two models, a *random intercept* model and a *random intercept plus slope* model.

9.5.1 Model IV: Random intercept model

The *random intercept model* with random intercept b_{0i} is expressed as

TABLE 9.2
Estimated treatment effect $e^{\hat{\beta}_{3j}}$ (rate ratio ratio) at each of four observation periods for Model I and Model IIa ($\rho_B = 0$).

	Model I (AIC = 2031.88)		Model IIa (AIC = 1861.92)	
Weeks	Estimate (95%CI)	Two-tailed p	Estimate (95%CI)	Two-tailed p
2	0.89 (0.74, 1.08)	0.253	0.72 (0.51, 1.01)	0.056
4	0.99 (0.81, 1.21)	0.918	0.80 (0.57, 1.13)	0.200
6	0.90 (0.74, 1.10)	0.304	0.73 (0.52, 1.02)	0.065
8	0.82 (0.66, 1.01)	0.066	0.66 (0.47, 0.93)	0.019

$$
\begin{aligned}
E(y_{i0} \mid b_{0i}) &= \begin{cases} e^{b_{0i}} e^{\beta_0} e^{\boldsymbol{w}_i^t \boldsymbol{\xi}} L_{i0}, & \text{(placebo)} \\ e^{b_{0i}} e^{\beta_0} e^{\beta_1} e^{\boldsymbol{w}_i^t \boldsymbol{\xi}} L_{i0}, & \text{(progabide)} \end{cases} \\
E(y_{ij} \mid b_{0i}) &= \begin{cases} e^{b_{0i}} e^{\beta_0} e^{\beta_2} e^{\boldsymbol{w}_i^t \boldsymbol{\xi}} L_{ij}, & \text{(placebo)} \\ e^{b_{0i}} e^{\beta_0} e^{\beta_1} e^{\beta_2} e^{\beta_3} e^{\boldsymbol{w}_i^t \boldsymbol{\xi}} L_{ij}, & \text{(progabide)} \end{cases} \\
& \quad j = 1, ..., 4,
\end{aligned}
$$

which can be re-expressed as

$$
\begin{aligned}
\log E(y_{ij} \mid b_{0i}) &= \log L_{ij} + \beta_0 + b_{0i} + \beta_1 x_{1i} + \beta_2 x_{2ij} \\
& \qquad + \beta_3 x_{1i} x_{2ij} + \boldsymbol{w}_i^t \boldsymbol{\xi} \qquad (9.19) \\
i &= 1, ..., N; \ j = 0, 1, 2, 3, 4 \\
b_{0i} &\sim N(0, \sigma_{B0}^2),
\end{aligned}
$$

where the interpretations of the parameters different from Model I are as follows:

1. $e^{\beta_0 + b_{i0}}$ denotes the subject-specific rate of seizures for the placebo group at baseline.

2. $e^{\beta_0 + b_{i0} + \beta_1}$ denotes the subject-specific rate of seizures for the new treatment group at baseline.

3. $e^{\beta_0 + b_{i0} + \beta_2}$ denotes the subject-specific rate of seizures for the placebo group in the evaluation period.

4. $e^{\beta_0+b_{i0}+\beta_1+\beta_2+\beta_3}$ denotes the subject-specific rate of seizures for the new treatment group in the evaluation period.

5. e^{β_2} denotes the subject-specific rate ratio of seizures, comparing the treatment period to the baseline period for the placebo group.

6. $e^{\beta_2+\beta_3}$ denotes the same quantity for the progabide group.

7. e^{β_3} denotes the *ratio* of these two rate ratios or the subject-specific average treatment effect of progabide compared with placebo in terms of the *RRR*, *rate ratio ratio.*

9.5.2 Model V: Random intercept plus slope model

The random intercept plus slope model with random slope b_{1i} is expressed as

$$
\begin{aligned}
E(y_{i0} \mid b_{0i}) &= \begin{cases} e^{b_{0i}} e^{\beta_0} e^{\boldsymbol{w}_i^t \boldsymbol{\xi}} L_{i0}, & \text{(placebo)} \\ e^{b_{0i}} e^{\beta_0} e^{\beta_1} e^{\boldsymbol{w}_i^t \boldsymbol{\xi}} L_{i0}, & \text{(progabide)} \end{cases} \\
E(y_{ij} \mid b_{0i}, b_{1i}) &= \begin{cases} e^{b_{0i}} e^{b_{1i}} e^{\beta_0} e^{\beta_2} e^{\boldsymbol{w}_i^t \boldsymbol{\xi}} L_{ij}, & \text{(placebo)} \\ e^{b_{0i}} e^{b_{1i}} e^{\beta_0} e^{\beta_1} e^{\beta_2} e^{\beta_3} e^{\boldsymbol{w}_i^t \boldsymbol{\xi}} L_{ij}, & \text{(progabide)} \end{cases} \\
& \quad j = 1, ..., 4,
\end{aligned}
$$

which can be re-expressed as

$$
\begin{aligned}
\log E(y_{ij} \mid b_{0i}) &= \log L_{ij} + \beta_0 + b_{0i} + \beta_1 x_{1i} + (\beta_2 + b_{1i}) x_{2ij} \\
& \qquad + \beta_3 x_{1i} x_{2ij} + \boldsymbol{w}_i^t \boldsymbol{\xi} \qquad (9.20) \\
i &= 1, ..., N; \; j = 0, 1, 2, 3, 4 \\
\boldsymbol{b}_i &= (b_{0i}, b_{1i}) \sim N(0, \Phi).
\end{aligned}
$$

We shall call Model V with $\rho_B = 0$, Model Va, and the one with $\rho_B \neq 0$, Model Vb.

9.5.3 Analysis using SAS

Now, let us apply Models IV, Va, and Vb to the *Epilepsy Data* using the SAS procedure `PROC GLIMMIX`. The respective sets of SAS programs are shown in Program 9.3.

Program 9.3. SAS procedure PROC GRIMMIX for Models IV, Va, Vb

```
<Model IV>
proc glimmix data=epilong method=quad (qpoints=7);
   class subject visit/ref=first  ;
   model seizure  =  age treatment  post treatment*post
                                  / d=poi link=log offset=logt s cl ;
   random intercept / subject= subject g gcorr ;
<Model V>
proc glimmix data=epilong method=quad (qpoints=7);
   class subject visit/ref=first  ;
   model seizure  =  age treatment  post treatment*post
                                 /  d=poi link=log offset=logt s cl ;
 /* Va */
   random intercept post / type=un subject= subject g gcorr ;
 /* Vb */
   random intercept post / type=simple subject= subject g gcorr ;
run ;
```

The results of Models IV and Va are shown in Output 9.3. In Model IV, the variance of the random intercept is estimated as $\hat{\sigma}^2_{B0} = 0.5999$ ($s.e. = 0.1153$), which is exactly the same as the variance estimate of Model I. Furthermore, the estimated variances of the random intercept and random slope are $\hat{\sigma}^2_{B0} = 0.5014$ ($s.e. = 0.1002$) and $\hat{\sigma}^2_{B1} = 0.2415$ ($s.e. = 0.06192$), respectively, which are also quite similar to those of Model IIa. The values of the AIC and BIC are 2032.29 and 2044.76, respectively, for Model IV and 1862.31 and 1876.85, respectively, for Model Va. Although the results of Model Vb are omitted here, the values of the AIC and BIC are 1862.85 and 1879.47, respectively. Therefore, the best model is selected as Model Va based on these information criteria. The average treatment effect of Model Va is estimated in terms of the *rate ratio ratio*, i.e., $RRR = e^{-0.3087} = 0.73$ and the 95% confidence interval is $(e^{-0.6113}, e^{-0.00620}) = (0.54, 0.99)$. Namely, progabide reduced the rate ratio of seizures (comparing the treatment period to the baseline period) by about 27% compared with placebo. The estimated average treatment effects $RRR = e^{\hat{\beta}_3}$ for Models IV, Va, and Vb are shown in Table 9.3.

TABLE 9.3
The estimated average treatment effects $e^{\hat{\beta}_3}$ (rate ratio ratios) for Models IV, Va, and Vb. The model with the asterisk (*) indicates the best model based on the AIC and BIC.

Model	Estimate (95%CI)	Two-tailed p	AIC	BIC
IV	0.90 (0.79, 1.02)	0.1123	2032.29	2044.76
Va* ($\rho_B = 0$)	0.73 (0.54, 0.99)	0.0455	1862.31	1876.85
Vb ($\rho_B \neq 0$)	0.74 (0.55, 0.99)	0.0461	1862.85	1879.47

Output 9.3. SAS procedure `PROC GRIMMIX` for Models IV and Va

```
<Model IV>
Fit statistics
-2 Res Log Likelihood  2020.29
AIC (smaller is better) 2032.29
BIC (smaller is better) 2044.76

Covariance Parameter Estimates
Cov Parm   Subject   Estimate S.E.
Intercept subject 0.5999 0.1153

Solution for Fixed Effects
Effect          Estimate   S.E.    DF t Value Pr>|t| Alpha Lower Upper
Intercept        2.1735  0.5045   56   4.31 <.0001 0.05  1.1629  3.1840
age             -0.01543 0.01659 234 -0.93 0.3533 0.05 -0.04811 0.01726
treatment       -0.04394 0.2103  234 -0.21 0.8347 0.05 -0.4583  0.3704
post             0.1108  0.04689 234  2.36 0.0189 0.05  0.01842 0.2032
treatment*post  -0.1037  0.06505 234 -1.59 0.1123 0.05 -0.2318  0.02449

<Model Va>
Fit statistics
-2 Res Log Likelihood 1848.31
AIC (smaller is better) 1862.31
BIC (smaller is better) 1876.85

Covariance Parameter Estimates
Cov Parm   Subject   Estimate S.E.
Intercept   subject 0.5014 0.1002
post        subject 0.2415 0.06192

Solution for Fixed Effects
Effect          Estimate S.E.    DF t Value Pr>|t| Alpha Lower Upper
Intercept       2.3228  0.4691   56  4.95 <.0001 0.05  1.3830  3.2625
age            -0.01953 0.01543 177 -1.27 0.2075 0.05 -0.04998 0.01093
treatment       0.02713 0.1944  177  0.14 0.8892 0.05 -0.3565  0.4108
post            0.01198 0.1101  177  0.11 0.9135 0.05 -0.2053  0.2293
treatment*post -0.3087  0.1533  177 -2.01 0.0455 0.05 -0.6113 -0.00620
```

9.6 Models for the treatment by linear time interaction

In the previous section, we focused on the mixed-effects models where we are primarily interested in comparing the average treatment effect during the evaluation period. In this section, we shall consider the situation where the primary interest is testing the treatment by *linear* time interaction (Hedeker and Gibbons, 2006; Bhumik et al., 2008). So, let us assume here that **the primary interest of the *Epilepsy Trial* with the *1:4* design is to estimate the difference in average rates of change or improvement of the seizure rate over time.** To do this, we shall consider the *random intercept* model and the *random intercept plus slope* model.

9.6.1 Model VI: Random intercept model

The *random intercept model* with random intercept b_{0i} is expressed as

$$
\begin{aligned}
E(y_{i0} \mid b_{0i}) &= \begin{cases} e^{b_{0i}} e^{\beta_0} e^{\boldsymbol{w}_i^t \boldsymbol{\xi}} L_{i0}, & \text{(placebo)} \\ e^{b_{0i}} e^{\beta_0} e^{\beta_1} e^{\boldsymbol{w}_i^t \boldsymbol{\xi}} L_{i0}, & \text{(progabide)} \end{cases} \\
E(y_{ij} \mid b_{0i}) &= \begin{cases} e^{b_{0i}} e^{\beta_0} e^{\beta_2 t_j} e^{\boldsymbol{w}_i^t \boldsymbol{\xi}} L_{ij}, & \text{(placebo)} \\ e^{b_{0i}} e^{\beta_0} e^{\beta_1} e^{(\beta_2+\beta_3) t_j} e^{\boldsymbol{w}_i^t \boldsymbol{\xi}} L_{ij}, & \text{(progabide)} \end{cases} \\
& \quad j = 1, ..., 4,
\end{aligned}
$$

where:

1. t_j denotes the jth measurement time in the unit of "**two weeks,**" i.e., $t_0 = 0, t_1 = 1, t_2 = 2, t_3 = 3$ and $t_4 = 4$.
2. Interpretations on β_0 and β_1 are the same as those of Models I–V.
3. β_2 denotes the subject-specific change of the log rate of seizures for an increase of one unit in t_j in the placebo group, in other words, *the subject-specific rate of change of the log rate of seizures per two weeks* in the placebo group. Therefore, e^{β_2} denotes the subject-specific rate ratio of seizures per two weeks in the placebo group.
4. $e^{\beta_2+\beta_3}$ denotes the subject-specific rate ratio of seizures per two weeks in the progabide group.
5. e^{β_3} denotes the subject-specific ratio of these two rate ratios per two weeks, i.e., the subject-specific effect size of the treatment by linear time interaction in terms of the *RRR, rate ratio ratio.*

The above model can be re-expressed as

$$\begin{aligned} \log E(y_{ij} \mid b_{0i}) &= \log L_{ij} + \beta_0 + b_{0i} + \beta_1 x_{1i} \\ &\qquad +(\beta_2 + \beta_3 x_{1i})t_j + \boldsymbol{w}_i^t \boldsymbol{\xi} \qquad (9.21) \\ i &= 1, ..., N;\ j = 0, 1, 2, 3, 4 \\ b_{0i} &\sim N(0, \sigma_{B0}^2). \end{aligned}$$

9.6.2 Model VII: Random intercept plus slope model

The *random intercept plus slope* model with random intercept b_{1i} is expressed as

$$\begin{aligned} E(y_{i0} \mid b_{0i}) &= \begin{cases} e^{b_{0i}} e^{\beta_0} e^{\boldsymbol{w}_i^t \boldsymbol{\xi}} L_{i0}, & \text{(placebo)} \\ e^{b_{0i}} e^{\beta_0} e^{\beta_1} e^{\boldsymbol{w}_i^t \boldsymbol{\xi}} L_{i0}, & \text{(progabide)} \end{cases} \\ E(y_{ij} \mid b_{0i}, b_{1i}) &= \begin{cases} e^{b_{0i}} e^{\beta_0} e^{(b_{1i}+\beta_2)t_j} e^{\boldsymbol{w}_i^t \boldsymbol{\xi}} L_{ij}, & \text{(placebo)} \\ e^{b_{0i}} e^{\beta_0} e^{\beta_1} e^{(b_{1i}+\beta_2+\beta_3)t_j} e^{\boldsymbol{w}_i^t \boldsymbol{\xi}} L_{ij}, & \text{(progabide)} \end{cases} \\ & j = 1, ..., 4, \end{aligned}$$

which can be re-expressed as

$$\begin{aligned} \log E(y_{ij} \mid b_{0i}, b_{1i}) &= \log L_{ij} + \beta_0 + b_{0i} + \beta_1 x_{1i} \\ &\qquad +(b_{1i} + \beta_2 + \beta_3 x_{1i})t_j + \boldsymbol{w}_i^t \boldsymbol{\xi} \qquad (9.22) \\ i &= 1, ..., N;\ j = 0, 1, 2, 3, 4 \\ \boldsymbol{b}_i &= (b_{0i}, b_{1i}) \sim N(\boldsymbol{0}, \boldsymbol{\Phi}) \\ \boldsymbol{\Phi} &= \begin{pmatrix} \sigma_{B0}^2 & \rho_B \sigma_{B0} \sigma_{B1} \\ \rho_B \sigma_{B0} \sigma_{B1} & \sigma_{B1}^2 \end{pmatrix}. \end{aligned}$$

We shall call Model VII with $\rho_B = 0$, Model VIIa, and the one with $\rho_B \neq 0$, Model VIIb.

9.6.3 Analysis using SAS

Now, let us apply Models VI, VIIa, and VIIb to the *Epilepsy Data* using the SAS procedure `PROC GLIMMIX`. The respective sets of SAS programs and part of the results for Model VIIa are shown in Program and Output 9.4. In this program, we need to create the continuous variable `xvisit` indicating t_j in the `DATA` step as follows:

```
xvisit = visit;
```

and the `MODEL` statement should be

```
model seizure = age treatment xvisit treatment*xvisit
              /d=poisson link=log offset=logt s cl ;
```

Program and Output 9.4: SAS procedure `PROC GLIMMIX` for Models VI, VIIa, VIIb

```
<SAS program>
data epilong ;
  infile 'c:\book\RepeatedMeasure\epilepsy_long.txt' missover;
  input no  subject treatment  visit seizure age;
  if visit=0 then post=0; else post=1;
  if visit=0 then logt=log(4); else logt=log(4);
  xvisit=visit;
  run;

proc glimmix data=epilong method=quad (qpoints=7);
   class subject visit/ref=first  ;
   model seizure  =  age treatment  xvisit treatment*xvisit
               /d=poisson link=log offset=logt s cl ;
 /* model VI */
   random intercept /  subject= subject g gcorr ;
 /* model VIIa */
   random intercept xvisit/  subject= subject g gcorr ;
 /* model VIIb */
   random intercept xvisit/ type=un subject= subject g gcorr ;
run;

 <A part of the results for Model VIIa>
Covariance Parameter Estimates
Cov Parm   Subject  Estimate S.E.
Intercept  subject   0.5348  0.1052
xvisit     subject   0.02096 0.005939

Fit statistics
-2 Res Log Likelihood 1909.06
AIC (smaller is better) 1923.06
BIC (smaller is better) 1937.61

Solution for Fixed Effects
Effect                Estimate  S.E.    DF t Value Pr>|t| Alpha Lower Upper
Intercept              2.2681  0.4810   56  4.72 <.0001 0.05  1.3045  3.2317
age                  -0.01653 0.01583 177 -1.04 0.2975 0.05 -0.04777 0.01470
treatment            -0.00178 0.1991  177 -0.01 0.9929 0.05 -0.3946  0.3911
xvisit               -0.01697 0.03384  57 -0.50 0.6179 0.05 -0.08473 0.05079
treatment*xvisit     -0.09448 0.04760 177 -1.98 0.0487 0.05 -0.1884 -0.00054
```

In Model VIIa, the variances of the random-effects parameters are estimated as

$$\hat{\sigma}^2_{B0} = 0.5348 \ (s.e. = 0.1052), \ \hat{\sigma}^2_{B0} = 0.02096 \ (s.e. = 0.005939).$$

The subject-specific rate of change of the log rate of seizures (per two weeks) is estimated as $\hat{\beta}_2 = -0.01697$ in the placebo group and $\hat{\beta}_2 + \hat{\beta}_3 = -0.01697 - 0.09448 = -0.11145$ in the progabide group, respectively. The estimated lines by treatment group are plotted in Figure 9.6 together with the estimates shown in Figure 9.4 by Model VIIa. Both models seem to give similar estimates or time trends of each other. The difference in average changes is estimated as $\hat{\beta}_3 = -0.09448$ $(s.e. = 0.0476), p = 0.0487$. Namely, the estimated rate ratio of seizures per two weeks is $e^{-0.01697} = 0.9832$ in the placebo group and $e^{-0.11145} = 0.8945$ in the progabide group, respectively. These results indicate that for every increase of 2 weeks, the rate of seizures reduces $100(1 - 0.9832) = 1.68\%$ in the placebo group and $100(1 - 0.8945) = 10.55\%$ in the progabide group in terms of the rate ratio, respectively. Therefore, the treatment effect of progabide compared with placebo is expressed as the relative reduction of the rate ratio of seizures, i.e,

$$100(1 - e^{-0.09448}) = 100(1 - 0.8945/0.9832) = 100(1 - 0.9098) = 9.02\%.$$

Namely, the speed of improvement of the seizure rate is more rapid for the progabide group compared with the placebo group. Table 9.4 shows the treatment effect with 95% confidence interval for each of the three models.

9.6.4 Checking the goodness-of-fit of linearity

However, as discussed and illustrated in Sections 7.6.4 and 8.6.4, we should be cautious about the goodness-of-fit of the models for the treatment by *linear* time interaction because the *linear trend model* has very strong assumptions on the linearity. Although Figure 9.6 shows that the trend could be linear, let us check here also the goodness-of-fit of the linear model. To do this, we can apply the following *random intercept* model and the *random intercept plus slope* model including the treatment by quadratic time interaction.

1. Model VIQ: Random intercept model

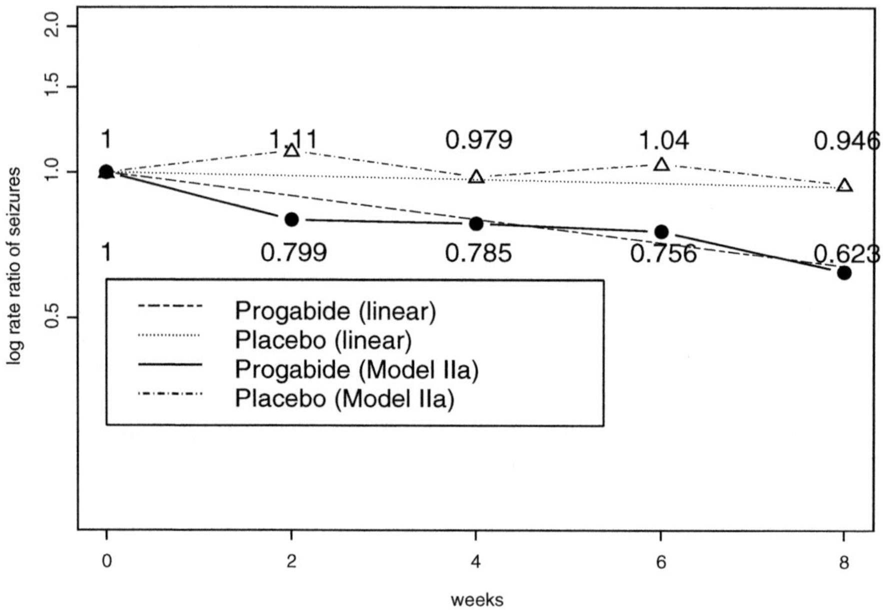

FIGURE 9.6
The changes from baseline by treatment group based on the estimated rate ratios via Model VIIa (linear) and those via Model IIa of seizures at each visit versus the baseline.

$$\begin{aligned}\log E(y_{ij} \mid b_{0i}) &= \log L_{ij} + \beta_0 + b_{0i} + \beta_1 x_{1i} + (\beta_2 + \beta_3 x_{1i})t_j + \\ &\quad (\beta_4 + \beta_5 x_{1i})t_j^2 + \boldsymbol{w}_i^t \boldsymbol{\xi} \\ b_{0i} &\sim N(\mathbf{0}, \sigma_{B0}^2) \\ i &= 1, ..., N;\ j = 0, 1, 2, 3, 4.\end{aligned} \tag{9.23}$$

2. Model VIIQ: Random intercept plus slope model

The random intercept plus slope model with a random intercept b_{0i}, random slopes b_{1i} on the linear term, and b_{2i} on the quadratic term is expressed by:

TABLE 9.4
Estimated treatment effect $e^{\hat{\beta}_3}$ (rate ratio ratio) and variance components for Models, VI, VIIa and VIIb. The model with the asterisk (*) indicates the best model.

Model	$e^{\hat{\beta}_3}$ (95%CI)	Two-tailed p-value	$\hat{\sigma}^2_{B0}$	$\hat{\sigma}^2_{B1}$
VI	0.962 (0.922, 1.005)	0.0853	0.599 (0.115)	
VIIa*	0.910 (0.828, 0.999)	0.0487	0.535 (0.105)	0.0210 (0.0059)
VIIb	0.911 (0.931, 0.999)	0.0492	0.515 (0.102)	0.0201 (0.0058)

Model	$\hat{\rho}_B$	AIC	BIC
VI		2034.92	2047.38
VIIa*		1923.06	1937.61
VIIb	0.2442	1923.04	1939.66

$$
\begin{aligned}
\log E(y_{ij} \mid b_{0i}, b_{1i}, b_{2i}) &= \log L_{ij} + \beta_0 + b_{0i} + \beta_1 x_{1i} + (\beta_2 + \beta_3 x_{1i} + b_{1i})t_j + \\
& \quad (\beta_4 + \beta_5 x_{1i} + b_{2i})t_j^2 + \boldsymbol{w}_i^t \boldsymbol{\xi} \qquad (9.24) \\
\boldsymbol{b}_i &= (b_{0i}, b_{1i}, b_{2i}) \sim N(\mathbf{0}, \boldsymbol{\Phi}) \\
\boldsymbol{\Phi} &= \begin{pmatrix} \sigma^2_{B0} & \rho_{B01}\sigma_{B0}\sigma_{B1} & \rho_{B02}\sigma_{B0}\sigma_{B2} \\ \rho_{B01}\sigma_{B0}\sigma_{B1} & \sigma^2_{B1} & \rho_{B12}\sigma_{B1}\sigma_{B2} \\ \rho_{B02}\sigma_{B0}\sigma_{B2} & \rho_{B12}\sigma_{B1}\sigma_{B2} & \sigma^2_{B2} \end{pmatrix} \\
i &= 1, ..., N; \; j = 0, 1, 2, 3, 4.
\end{aligned}
$$

Now, let us apply Models VIQ and VIIQ to the *Epilepsy Data* using the SAS procedure `PROC GLIMMIX`. The respective sets of SAS programs and a part of the results for Model VIIQ are shown in Program and Output 9.5. In this program, we need to create the continuous variable `xvisit2` indicating that the quadratic term in the `DATA` step and the `MODEL` statement should be

```
model seizure = age treatment xvisit xvisit2 treatment*xvisit
      treatment*xvisit2 / d=poisson link=log offset=logt s cl ;
```

and the `RANDOM` statement for Model VIIQ should be

```
random intercept xvisit xvist2/type=un subject= subject g gcorr;
```

Program and Output 9.5: SAS procedure PROC GLIMMIX for Models VIQ, VIIQ

```
<SAS program>
data epilong ;
  infile 'c:\book\RepeatedMeasure\epilepsy_long.txt' missover;
  input no  subject treatment  visit seizure age;
  if visit=0 then post=0; else post=1;
  if visit=0 then logt=log(4); else logt=log(1);
  xvisit=visit;
  xvisit2=xvisit * xvisit;
  run;

proc glimmix data=epilong method=quad (qpoints=7);
   class subject visit/ref=first  ;
   model seizure  =  age treatment  xvisit xvisit2 treatment*xvisit
              treatment*xvisit2 / d=poisson link=log offset=logt s cl ;

/* model VIQ  */
  random intercept / subject= subject g gcorr ;
/* model VIIQ  */
  random intercept xvisit xvisit2/ type=un subject= subject g gcorr ;
run ;

<A part of the results for Model VIIQd >
Covariance Parameter Estimates
Cov Parm  Subject Estimate S.E.
UN(1,1) subject  0.5063  0.1042
UN(2,1) subject  0.05625 0.06004
UN(2,2) subject  0.2334  0.06828
UN(3,1) subject -0.01135 0.01388
UN(3,2) subject -0.04842 0.01565
UN(3,3) subject  0.01043 0.003716

Fit statistics
-2 Res Log Likelihood 1830.67
AIC (smaller is better) 1856.67
BIC (smaller is better) 1883.68

Solution for Fixed Effects
Effect             Estimate   S.E.   DF t Value  Pr>|t| Alpha Lower Upper
Intercept           2.5869  0.4786   56   5.40 <.0001 0.05   1.6281 3.5457
age                -0.02759 0.01578 118 -1.75 0.0830 0.05 -0.0588 0.003658
treatment          -0.01002 0.1949  118 -0.05 0.9591 0.05 -0.3960 0.3760
xvisit             -0.00959 0.1173   57 -0.08 0.9352 0.05 -0.2445 0.2253
xvisit2            -0.00377 0.02750  57 -0.14 0.8914 0.05 -0.0588 0.05130
treatment*xvisit   -0.1468  0.1601  118 -0.92 0.3608 0.05 -0.4638 0.1701
treatment*xvisit2   0.01744 0.03722 118   0.47 0.6403 0.05 -0.0562 0.09114
```

TABLE 9.5
The estimated coefficients (s.e.) of fixed effects $\beta_2, \beta_3, \beta_4, \beta_5$ and covariance structure Φ for Models VIQ and VIIQ.

Model	$\hat{\beta}_2$	$\hat{\beta}_3$	$\hat{\beta}_4$	$\hat{\beta}_5$
VIQ	0.135 (0.057)	-0.015 (0.079)	-0.0327 (0.015)	-0.0070 (0.021)
VIIQ	-0.0096 (0.12)	-0.147 (0.160)	-0.0038 (0.028)	0.0174 (0.037)

Model	$\hat{\sigma}^2_{B0}$	$\hat{\sigma}^2_{B1}$	$\hat{\sigma}^2_{B2}$	AIC	BIC
VIQ	0.599 (0.115)			2027.4	2044.0
VIIQ	0.506 (0.104)	0.233 (0.0683)	0.0104 (0.00372)	1856.7	1883.7

$\hat{\rho}_{B01} = 0.1636, \hat{\rho}_{B02} = -0.1561, \hat{\rho}_{B12} = -0.9814$ for Model VIIQ.

The results are summarized in Table 9.5. Based on the values of the AIC and BIC, Model VIIQ is the best model among Models VI, VIIa, VIIb, VIQ, and VIIQ. The estimated mean quadratic trend of the rate ratio of seizures by treatment group is

$$\begin{aligned}\hat{\text{RR}}(t) &= \begin{cases} e^{\hat{\beta}_2 t + \hat{\beta}_4 t^2}, & \text{(placebo)} \\ e^{(\hat{\beta}_2+\hat{\beta}_3)t + (\hat{\beta}_4+\hat{\beta}_5)t^2}, & \text{(progabide)} \end{cases} \\ &= \begin{cases} e^{-0.00959t - 0.00377t^2}, & \text{(placebo)} \\ e^{(-0.00959-0.1468)t + (-0.00377+0.01744)t^2}, & \text{(progabide)}. \end{cases}\end{aligned}$$

These two quadratic lines are plotted in Figure 9.7 together with the estimated linear trends by Model VIIa. Both models estimated quite similar time trends, which also seems to be similar to the changes from baseline in terms of the estimated rate ratio of seizures via Model IIa by treatment group shown in Figure 9.4. However, the estimated covariance structures are different between the two models and, consequently, the treatment effects are statistically non-significant at the 5% significance level, i.e., $\hat{\beta}_3 = -0.1468(0.1601), p = 0.36$ for the linear trend and $\hat{\beta}_5 = 0.01744(0.03722), p = 0.64$ for the quadratic trend. These results suggest that the results derived by Model VIIa, the best model for the treatment by linear time interaction, is not acceptable.

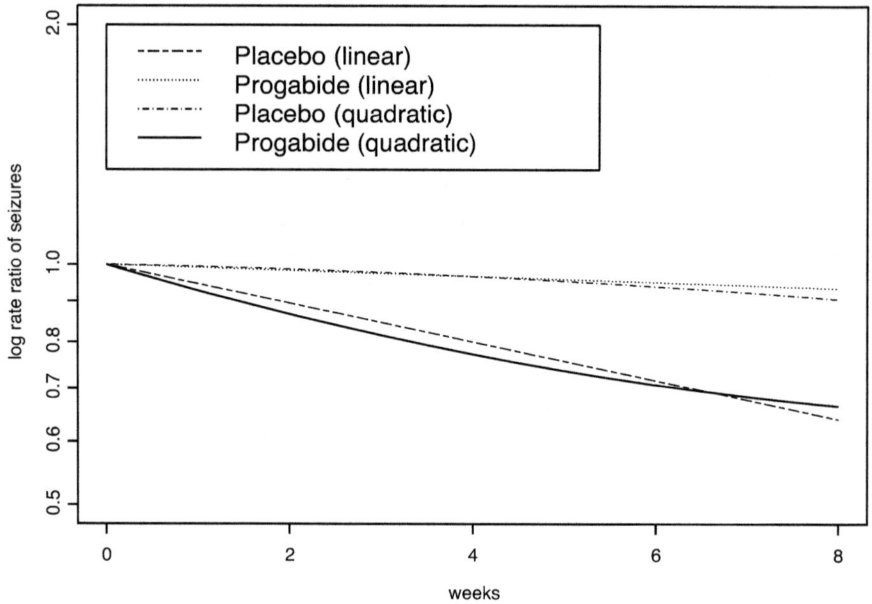

FIGURE 9.7
The changes from baseline by treatment group based on the estimated rate ratio via Model VIIa (linear) and Model VIIQ (quadratic) of seizures at each visit versus the baseline.

9.7 ANCOVA-type models adjusting for baseline measurement

As described in Chapter 1 and Sections 7.7 and 8.7, many RCTs tend to try to narrow the evaluation period down to one time point (ex., the last Tth measurement), leading to the so-called the *pre-post* design or the *1:1* design. In these simple *1:1* designs, traditional analysis of covariance (ANCOVA) has been used to analyze data where the baseline measurement is used as a covariate.

So, in this section, we shall apply some of the ANCOVA-type models to the *Epilepsy Data* with a *1:4* repeated measures design where the baseline measurement is used as a covariate, and compare the results with those of the corresponding repeated measures models.

9.7.1 Model VIII: Random intercept model for the treatment effect at each visit

Let us consider the following *random intercept model* where the random intercept $b_{i(Ancova)}$ is assumed to be constant during the evaluation period.

$$\log E(y_{ij} \mid b_{i(Ancova)}) = \begin{cases} b_{i(Ancova)} + \beta_0 + \beta_{2j} + \theta y_{i0} + \boldsymbol{w}_i^t \boldsymbol{\xi}, & \text{(placebo)} \\ b_{i(Ancova)} + \beta_0 + \beta_1 + \beta_{2j} + \beta_{3j} + \theta y_{i0} + \boldsymbol{w}_i^t \boldsymbol{\xi} & \text{(progabide)} \end{cases}$$
$$j = 1, ..., 4;\ \beta_{21} = \beta_{31} = 0,$$

where:

1. β_0 denotes the mean subject-specific log rate of seizures in the placebo group at the 1st visit.
2. $e^{b_{i(Anova)}+\beta_0}$ denotes the subject-specific rate of seizures in the placebo group at the 1st visit.
3. $\beta_0 + \beta_1$ denotes the mean subject-specific log rate of seizures in the new treatment group at the 1st visit.
4. $e^{b_{i(Anova)}+\beta_0+\beta_1}$ denotes the subject-specific log rate of seizures in the new treatment group at the 1st visit.
5. e^{β_1} denotes the subject-specific rate ratio comparing the rate of seizures in the new treatment group versus in the placebo group at the 1st visit.
6. θ denotes the coefficient for the baseline measurement y_{i0}.
7. $e^{\beta_0+\beta_{2j}}$ denotes the subject-specific rate of seizures in the placebo group at the jth visit.
8. $e^{\beta_0+\beta_1+\beta_{2j}+\beta_{3j}}$ denotes the subject-specific rate of seizures in the new treatment group at the jth visit.
9. $e^{\beta_1+\beta_{3j}}$ denotes the subject-specific rate ratio comparing the rate of seizures in the new treatment group versus in the placebo group at the jth visit, i.e., the treatment effect of the new treatment compared with placebo at the jth visit in terms of the *rate ratio (RR)*.

This model is re-expressed as

$$
\begin{aligned}
\log E(y_{ij} \mid b_{i(Ancova)}) &= \beta_0 + b_{i(Ancova)} + \theta y_{i0} + \beta_1 x_{1i} + \sum_{k=2}^{4} \beta_{2k} z_{kij} \\
&\quad + \sum_{k=2}^{4} \beta_{3k} x_{1i} z_{kij} + \boldsymbol{w}_i^t \boldsymbol{\xi} \qquad (9.25) \\
i &= 1, ..., N; \ j = 1, 2, 3, 4; \ \beta_{21} = 0, \ \beta_{31} = 0 \\
b_{i(Ancova)} &\sim N(0, \sigma^2_{B(Ancova)}).
\end{aligned}
$$

In the ANOVA-type model, the treatment effect at time j can be expressed via some linear contrast. For example, the treatment effect at weeks 7–8 ($j = 4$) can be expressed as

$$
\begin{aligned}
\tau_{21}^{(4)} &= \beta_1 + \beta_{34} \\
&= (1)\beta_1 + (0, 0, 0, 1)(\beta_{31}, \beta_{32}, \beta_{33}, \beta_{34})^t. \qquad (9.26)
\end{aligned}
$$

9.7.2 Model IX: Random intercept model for the average treatment effect

In this section, we shall consider Model IX in which the treatment effect is assumed to be constant during the evaluation period:

$$
\begin{aligned}
\log E(y_{ij} \mid b_{i(Ancova)}) &= \beta_0 + b_{i(Ancova)} + \theta y_{i0} + \beta_3 x_{1i} + \boldsymbol{w}_i^t \boldsymbol{\xi} \qquad (9.27) \\
i &= 1, ..., N; \ j = 1, 2, 3, 4; \\
b_{i(Ancova)} &\sim N(0, \sigma^2_{B(Ancova)}),
\end{aligned}
$$

where the parameter e^{β_3} is the treatment effect of progabide compared with placebo in terms of the rate ratio.

9.7.3 Analysis using SAS

Now, let us apply Models VIII and IX to the *Epilepsy Data* using the SAS procedure `PROC GLIMMIX`. The first step for the analysis is to rearrange the data structure from the long format shown in Table 9.1 into another long format shown in Table 9.6 where the baseline records were deleted and the new variable `base`, indicating baseline seizure counts, was created.

The respective sets of SAS programs are shown in Program 9.6. Here also, due to the option `/ref=first` used in the `CLASS` statement, the coefficients of the linear contrast for the `treatment*visit` interaction needs the order change (e.g., see Section 7.7.3). For example, according to Equation (9.26), the linear contrast for the treatment effect at week 8 ($j = 4$) can be expressed in SAS as

```
estimate 'treatment at 8w' treatment 1 treatment*visit  0 0 0 1
```

However, due to the option `/ref=first`, the following change should be made for the `treatment*visit` interaction:

```
estimate 'treatment at 8w' treatment 1 treatment*visit  0 0 1 0
```

Furthermore, the fixed effects β_3 in Model IX can be expressed by the variable `treatment` and the `MODEL` statement and the `RANDOM` statement should be

```
model seizure  =  logbase age  treatment
                / d=poisson link=log s cl ;
random intercept /  subject= subject g gcorr ;
```

where `logbase` denotes the log count of seizures during the baseline per two weeks and was created in the `DATA` step as

```
logbase=log(base/4);
```

The results of these two programs are shown in Output 9.6.

TABLE 9.6
A part of the long format *Epilepsy Data* set for the ANCOVA-type model rearranged from the data file shown in Table 9.1. The newly created variable base indicates the baseline measurement. (Data for the first four patients are shown.)

No.	subject	treatment	visit	seizure	age	base
1	1	0	1	5	31	11
2	1	0	2	3	31	11
3	1	0	3	3	31	11
4	1	0	4	3	31	11
5	2	0	1	3	30	11
6	2	0	2	5	30	11
7	2	0	3	3	30	11
8	2	0	4	3	30	11
9	3	0	1	2	25	6
10	3	0	2	4	25	6
11	3	0	3	0	25	6
12	3	0	4	5	25	6
13	4	0	1	4	36	8
14	4	0	2	4	36	8
15	4	0	3	1	36	8
16	4	0	4	4	36	8

Program 9.6: SAS procedure PROC GLIMMIX for Models VIII, IX

```
data epilongB ;
  infile 'c:\book\RepeatedMeasure\epilepsyB_long.txt' missover;
  input no  subject treatment  visit seizure age base;
  logbase=log(base/4);

<Model VIII>
proc glimmix data=epilongB method=quad (qpoints=7);
   class subject visit/ref=first  ;
   model seizure  =  logbase  age treatment  visit treatment*visit
                                / d=poisson link=log s cl ;
   random intercept /  subject= subject g gcorr ;
   estimate 'treatment at 2w'
      treatment 1  treatment*visit  0 0 0 1 /divisor=1 cl alpha=0.05;
   estimate 'treatment at 4w'
      treatment 1  treatment*visit  1 0 0 0 /divisor=1 cl alpha=0.05;
   estimate 'treatment at 6w'
      treatment 1  treatment*visit  0 1 0 0 /divisor=1 cl alpha=0.05;
   estimate 'treatment at 8w'
      treatment 1  treatment*visit  0 0 1 0 /divisor=1 cl alpha=0.05;
run ;
<Model IX>
proc glimmix data=epilongB method=quad (qpoints=7);
   class subject visit  ;
   model seizure  =  logbase age  treatment
                  / d=poisson link=log offset=logt s cl ;
   random intercept /  subject= subject g gcorr ;
run ;
```

Output 9.6: SAS procedure `PROC GLIMMIX` for Models VIII and IX

```
/* Model VIII */
Fit statistics
-2 Res Log Likelihood 1330.02
AIC (smaller is better) 1352.02
BIC (smaller is better) 1374.88

Covariance Parameter Estimates
Cov Parm   Subject  Estimate S.E.
Intercept subject  0.2694 0.06202

Estimates
Label          Estimate S.E.   DF t Value Pr>|t| Alpha  Lower    Upper
treatment at 2w -0.3297 0.1685 170 -1.96 0.0520 0.05 -0.6623  0.002955
treatment at 4w -0.2271 0.1702 170 -1.33 0.1839 0.05 -0.5630  0.1089
treatment at 6w -0.3207 0.1699 170 -1.89 0.0607 0.05 -0.6560  0.01458
treatment at 8w -0.4145 0.1735 170 -2.39 0.0180 0.05 -0.7570 -0.07193

/* Model IX */
Fit statistics
-2 Res Log Likelihood 1342.44
AIC (smaller is better) 1352.44
BIC (smaller is better) 1362.83

Covariance Parameter Estimates
Cov Parm   Subject  Estimate S.E.
Intercept subject  0.2694 0.06202

Solution for Fixed Effects
Effect         Estimate S.E.  DF t Value Pr>|t| Alpha Lower    Upper
Intercept      -0.3024 0.4035  56 -0.75 0.4567 0.05 -1.1107  0.5059
logbase         1.0253 0.1016 176 10.09 <.0001 0.05  0.8249  1.2258
age             0.0107 0.0122 176  0.88 0.3815 0.05 -0.01339 0.03483
treatment      -0.3202 0.1512 176 -2.12 0.0356 0.05 -0.6187 -0.02176
```

For example, the average treatment effect from Model IX is estimated as $e^{-0.3202} = 0.73$ with 95% confidence interval ($e^{-0.6187} = 0.54, e^{-0.02176} = 0.98$) and two-tailed $p = 0.0356$.

Here also, it will be interesting to compare the estimates of treatment effect obtained from the ANCOVA-type Models VIII and IX with those from Models IIa and Va, which are shown in Table 9.7. It should be noted that the treatment effect is estimated in terms of *rate ratio* for the ANOVA-type models, while the treatment effect is in terms of the *rate ratio ratio* for the latter models. In the *Epilepsy Data* also, the ANCOVA-type Models VIII (and IX) tend to give just a little smaller p-values than Models IIa (and Va).

TABLE 9.7
Comparison of the estimated treatment effect at each observation period between Models IIa and Va (in terms of *RRR*) and the ANCOVA-type Models VIII and IX (in terms of *RR*).

Treatment effect	Models IIa, Va		ANCOVA-type model Models VIII, IX	
	Estimate (95%CI)	Two-tailed p-value	Estimate (95%CI)	Two-tailed p-value
Model IIa vs. Model VIII				
$\hat{\beta}_{31}$: week 1-2	0.72 (0.51, 1.01)	0.056	0.72 (0.52, 1.00)	0.052
$\hat{\beta}_{32}$: week 3-4	0.80 (0.57, 1.13)	0.200	0.80 (0.57, 1.01)	0.184
$\hat{\beta}_{33}$: week 5-6	0.73 (0.52, 1.02)	0.065	0.73 (0.52, 1.01)	0.061
$\hat{\beta}_{34}$: week 7-8	0.66 (0.47, 0.93)	0.019	0.66 (0.47, 0.93)	0.018
Model Va vs. Model IX				
$\hat{\beta}_3$: Average	0.73 (0.54, 0.99)	0.046	0.73 (0.54, 0.98)	0.036

9.8 Sample size

In this chapter, various mixed-effects models were illustrated with the *Epilepsy Data*, which has a *1:4* repeated measures design with unequal length of observation periods. In this section, we shall consider the sample size determination. The sample size determinations for longitudinal data analysis in the literature (Diggle et al., 2002; Hedeker and Gibbons 2006; Fitzmaurice, Laird and Ware, 2011) are based on the *basic 1:T design* where the baseline data is used as a covariate. In other words, this design is essentially the *0:T design*. In this section, we shall consider the sample size (the number of subjects) needed for the *S:T design* with $S > 0$, which is different from what appears in the literature. For technical details of the derivation of the sample size formula, see Appendix A (Tango, 2016a).

9.8.1 Sample size for the average treatment effect

We shall consider here a typical situation where investigators are interested in estimating the average treatment effect during the evaluation period. To do this, let us first consider the sample size for Model IV or the *random intercept* model within the framework of the *S:T* design, where the sample size formula with closed form is available. Secondly, we shall consider the sample size for Model V, where the sample size formula with closed form is not available, but we can easily obtain sample sizes via Monte Carlo simulations.

9.8.1.1 Sample size for Model IV

Model IV within the framework of the *S:T* design is generally expressed as

$$\begin{aligned}
\log E(y_{ij} \mid b_{0i}) &= \beta_0 + b_{0i} + \beta_1 x_{1i} + \beta_2 x_{2ij} + \beta_3 x_{1i} x_{2ij} \qquad (9.28)\\
b_{0i} &\sim N(0, \sigma_{B0}^2)\\
i &= 1, ..., n_1 \text{ (control treatment);}\\
&= n_1 + 1, ..., n_1 + n_2 = N \text{ (new treatment)}\\
j &= -(S-1), -(S-2), ..., 0, 1, ..., T,
\end{aligned}$$

where it is assumed that all the observation periods have an equal length and that we need no so-called *offset* variable such as $\log L_{ij}$ used in the analysis of the *Epilepsy Data*.. The maximum likelihood estimator $\hat{\beta}_3$ is given by

$$e^{\hat{\beta}_3} = \frac{y_{+1}^{(2)} y_{+0}^{(1)}}{y_{+0}^{(2)} y_{+1}^{(1)}}, \qquad (9.29)$$

where

$$\begin{aligned}
y_{+0}^{(1)} &= \sum_{i=1}^{n_1} \sum_{j(\leq 0)} y_{ij}, \; y_{+1}^{(1)} = \sum_{i=1}^{n_1} \sum_{j(>0)} y_{ij},\\
y_{+0}^{(2)} &= \sum_{i=n_1+1}^{n_1+n_2} \sum_{j(\leq 0)} y_{ij}, \; y_{+1}^{(2)} = \sum_{i=n_1+1}^{n_1+n_2} \sum_{j(>0)} y_{ij}
\end{aligned}$$

and its standard error is approximated by

$$S.E.(e^{\hat{\beta}_3}) = \sqrt{\frac{1}{y_{+0}^{(2)}} + \frac{1}{y_{+1}^{(2)}} + \frac{1}{y_{+0}^{(1)}} + \frac{1}{y_{+1}^{(1)}}}. \qquad (9.30)$$

As explained in Chapters 7 and 8, the parameter β_3 denotes the treatment effect (*average* here) of the new treatment compared with the control treatment. Therefore, the null and alternative hypotheses of interest will be one of the following three sets of hypotheses as discussed in Section 1.3:

1. Test for superiority: If a negative β_3 indicates benefits as in the Epilepsy example, the superiority hypotheses are given by

$$H_0 \quad : \quad \beta_3 \geq 0, \text{ versus } \; H_1 : \beta_3 < 0. \tag{9.31}$$

If a positive β_3 indicates benefits, then they are

$$H_0 \quad : \quad \beta_3 \leq 0, \text{ versus } \; H_1 : \beta_3 > 0. \tag{9.32}$$

2. Test for non-inferiority: If a negative β_3 indicates benefits as in the Epilepsy example, the non-inferiority hypotheses are given by

$$H_0 \quad : \quad e^{\beta_3} \geq 1 + \Delta, \text{ versus } \; H_1 : e^{\beta_3} < 1 + \Delta. \tag{9.33}$$

where $\Delta(> 0)$ denotes the non-inferiority margin in terms of the rate ratio ratio (RRR). If a positive β_3 indicates benefits, then they are

$$H_0 \quad : \quad e^{\beta_3} \leq 1 - \Delta, \text{ versus } \; H_1 : e^{\beta_3} > 1 - \Delta. \tag{9.34}$$

3. Test for *substantial* superiority: If a negative β_3 indicates benefits as in the Epilepsy example, the *substantial* superiority hypotheses are given by

$$H_0 \quad : \quad e^{\beta_3} \geq 1 - \Delta, \text{ versus } \; H_1 : e^{\beta_3} < 1 - \Delta. \tag{9.35}$$

where $\Delta(> 0)$ denotes the *substantial* superiority margin in terms of the ratio of the rate ratio ratio. If a positive β_3 indicates benefits, then they are

$$H_0 \quad : \quad e^{\beta_3} \leq 1 + \Delta, \text{ versus } \; H_1 : e^{\beta_3} > 1 + \Delta. \tag{9.36}$$

In other words, investigators are interested in establishing whether the new treatment is *superior, non-inferior*, or *substantially superior* to the control treatment on the average.

Then, the sample size formula for the *superiority test* with two equally sized groups ($n_1 = n_2 = n$) to detect an effect size e^{β_3} with power $100(1-\phi)\%$ at the two-tailed significance level α assuming *no period effect*, $\beta_2 = 0$, is given by

$$\begin{aligned} n_{S,T} \quad = \quad & \frac{1}{\mu_b(e^{\beta_3}-1)^2}\left(z_{\alpha/2}\sqrt{\frac{2(S+T)(e^{\beta_3}+1)(S+Te^{\beta_3})}{ST\{2S+T(e^{\beta_3}+1)\}}} + \right. \\ & \left. z_{\phi}\sqrt{\frac{(S+T)^3 e^{\beta_3} + (S+Te^{\beta_3})^3}{ST(S+T)(S+Te^{\beta_3})}}\right)^2, \end{aligned} \tag{9.37}$$

where μ_b denotes the expected number of counts in each unit baseline period ($j = -S+1, -S+2, ..., 0$) and Z_α denotes the upper $100\alpha\%$ percentile of the standard normal distribution. For details of the derivation, see Appendix A, which is an extension of Tango's sample size formula (Tango, 2009). From this formula, we can find the following relationship, i.e., sample size reduction to a considerable extent,

$$n_{T,T} = \frac{1}{T} n_{S=1,T=1}, \tag{9.38}$$

where

$$n_{S=1,T=1} = \frac{1}{\mu_b(e^{\beta_3}-1)^2}\left(z_{\alpha/2}\sqrt{\frac{4(e^{\beta_3}+1)^2}{(e^{\beta_3}+3)}} + z_\phi\sqrt{\frac{8e^{\beta_3}+(1+e^{\beta_3})^3}{2(1+e^{\beta_3})}}\right)^2. \tag{9.39}$$

For reference, the common sample size $n_{S=1,T=1}$ for each group required for $1-\phi = 80\%$ power of the two-tailed score test at $\alpha = 0.05$ level for various values of e^{β_3} and μ_b under the assumption of *no period effect*, $\beta_2 = 0$, are shown in Table 9.8.

The corresponding sample size formula $n_{S,T}^{(NI)}$ for the *non-inferiority test* (9.33), (9.34) is given by

$$n_{S,T}^{(NI)} = \frac{1}{\mu_b(e^{\beta_3^*}-1)^2}\left(z_{\alpha/2}\sqrt{\frac{2(S+T)(e^{\beta_3^*}+1)(S+Te^{\beta_3^*})}{ST\{2S+T(e^{\beta_3^*}+1)\}}} + z_\phi\sqrt{\frac{(S+T)^3e^{\beta_3^*}+(S+Te^{\beta_3^*})^3}{ST(S+T)(S+Te^{\beta_3^*})}}\right)^2, \tag{9.40}$$

where

$$\beta_3^* = \beta_3 - \log\{1 - \Delta\text{sign}(\beta_3)\}. \tag{9.41}$$

The corresponding sample size formula $n_{S,T}^{(SS)}$ for the *substantial superiority test* (9.35), (9.36), on the other hand, is given by the same formula (9.40), but β_3^* is given by

TABLE 9.8
Common sample size $n_{S=1,T=1}$ for each group required for $1-\phi = 80\%$ power of the two-tailed score test at the $\alpha = 0.05$ level for various values of e^{β_3} and μ_b under the *random intercept* Poisson regression model with *no period effect*, $\beta_2 = 0$.

e^{β_3}	μ_b					
	5	10	15	20	25	30
0.90	581	291	194	146	117	97
0.88	397	199	133	100	80	67
0.86	287	144	96	72	58	48
0.84	216	108	73	54	44	36
0.82	168	84	56	42	34	28
0.80	134	67	46	34	27	23
0.78	109	55	37	28	22	19
0.76	90	45	30	23	18	15
0.74	75	38	25	19	15	13
0.72	64	32	22	16	13	11
0.70	55	28	19	14	11	10

$$\beta_3^* = \beta_3 + \log\{1 - \Delta\text{sign}(\beta_3)\}. \tag{9.42}$$

Example: *Epilepsy Data*

This data set appears to contain an outlier. A patient numbered 207 (assigned to the progabide group) had extremely high seizure counts, 151 at baseline and 302 in the treatment period. For the purpose of calculating sample size, let us delete the outlier with extremely high seizure counts. For the sample without patient number 207, the maximum likelihood estimate of treatment effect using the SAS procedure `PROC GLIMMIX` is estimated as $e^{\hat{\beta}_3} = 0.74$ (95%CI: $0.65 - 0.85$). The value of the AIC of the *random intercept* model was 1908.61, whereas the value of the AIC for Model Va applied to the data without the patient 207 was 1899.23, which is a little bit better fit and gave similar results:

$$e^{\hat{\beta}_3} = 0.73 \text{ (95\%CI: } 0.54 - 0.99), \ \hat{\sigma}^2_{B0} = 0.4495, \ \hat{\sigma}^2_{B1} = 0.2190.$$

Furthermore, the result of Model Va applied to the full data shown in Output 9.3 and Table 9.3 had a similar estimate

$$e^{\hat{\beta}_3} = 0.73(95\%\text{CI} : 0.54 - 0.99),\ \hat{\sigma}^2_{B0} = 0.5014,\ \hat{\sigma}^2_{B1} = 0.2415.$$

In this trial, the average number of epileptic seizures at baseline is $\hat{\mu_b} = 31.2$ per eight weeks. So, let us consider here the sample size to detect an effect size $e^{\beta_3} = 0.8$ with power 80% at $\alpha = 0.05$ under Model IV. If we consider the simplest *1:1 design* with an 8-week period each and $\mu_b = 32$, then $n_{S=1,T=1} = 20.88$ from (9.39). However, if we consider the *4:4 design* with eight 2-week observation periods and $\mu_b = 32/4 = 8.0$, then, from (9.38) and (9.39),

$$n_{4,4} = \frac{1}{4} n_{S=1,T=1} = \frac{1}{4} 83.52 = 20.88,$$

which is the same sample size as the *1:1 design* with $\mu_b = 32$, but the former is better in the sense that the former can deal with missing data without any imputations. Then the total sample size is $21 \times 2 = 42$, indicating that the actual sample size 59 is quite sufficient if we can successfully expect $e^{\beta_3} = 0.8$ under the random intercept model. If we adopt the *1:4 design* with $\mu_b = 8.0$, then from (9.37) we have $n_{1,4} = 51$, indicating about $51/21 = 2.5$ times the sample size of the *4:4 design*.

9.8.1.2 Sample size for Model V

Let us consider here Model V or the *random intercept plus slope* model within the framework of the *S:T* design, where the sample size formula with closed form is not available, but we can easily obtain sample sizes via Monte Carlo simulations. Model V within the framework of the *S:T* design is expressed as

$$\begin{aligned}
\log E(y_{ij} \mid b_{0i}, b_{1i}) &= \beta_0 + b_{0i} + \beta_1 x_{1i} + (\beta_2 + b_{1i}) x_{2ij} \\
&\qquad + \beta_3 x_{1i} x_{2ij} + \epsilon_{ij} \qquad (9.43) \\
\boldsymbol{b}_i &= (b_{0i}, b_{1i}) \sim N(0, \Phi) \\
i &= 1, ..., n_1 \text{ (control treatment);} \\
&= n_1 + 1, ..., n_1 + n_2 = N \text{ (new treatment)} \\
j &= -(S-1), -(S-2), ..., 0, 1, ..., T,
\end{aligned}$$

where it is assumed that all the observation periods have an equal length and that we need no so-called *offset* variable such as $\log L_{ij}$ used in the analysis of the *Epilepsy Data*. Here also, the parameter β_3 denotes the treatment effect. Then, the null and alternative hypotheses of interest will be one of the three sets of hypotheses described in (9.31)–(9.36). In other words, investigators are interested in establishing whether the new treatment is *superior, non-inferior*, or *substantially superior* to the control treatment regarding the rate of improvement. For the *non-inferiority test* and the *substantial superiority test*, we have to replace β_3 with

$$\beta_3 \Longrightarrow \beta_3 - \log\{1 - \Delta \text{sign}(\beta_3)\}$$

in the basic process described below.

The basic process to obtain the Monte Carlo simulated sample size $n (= n_1 = n_2)$ for the $S{:}T$ repeated measures design discussed here assumes

1. no difference in expected count between two treatment groups at the baseline period due to randomization, i.e., $\beta_1 = 0$, and

2. no period effects or no change in the log rate of seizures between before and after randomization in the control group, i.e., $\beta_2 = 0$,

and consists of the following steps:

Step 0 Set the values of (S, T).

Step 1 Set the sample size $n \leftarrow m_1$.

Step 2 Set the number of repetitions N_{rep} (for example, $N_{rep} = 1000, 10000$) of the simulation.

Step 3 Simulate one data set $\{y_{ij} : i = 1, ..., 2n; j = -(S-1), ..., T\}$ independently under the assumed model shown below:

$$\begin{aligned}
y_{ij} \mid b_{0i}, b_{1i} &\sim \text{Poisson}(\mu_{ij}) \\
\mu_{ij} &= \exp\{\beta_0 + b_{0i} + b_{1i}x_{2ij} + \beta_3 x_{1i} x_{2ij}\} \\
i &= 1, ..., n \text{ (Control)}, \; n+1, ..., 2n \text{ (New treatment)} \\
j &= -(S-1), -(S-2), ..., 0, \; 1, ..., T \\
\boldsymbol{b}_i &= (b_{0i}, b_{1i}) \sim N(\mathbf{0}, \boldsymbol{\Phi}) \\
\boldsymbol{\Phi} &= \begin{pmatrix} \sigma_{B0}^2 & \rho_B \sigma_{B0} \sigma_{B1} \\ \rho_B \sigma_{B0} \sigma_{B1} & \sigma_{B1}^2 \end{pmatrix}
\end{aligned}$$

where the values of $\beta_0, \beta_3, \sigma_{B0}^2, \sigma_{B1}^2, \rho_B$ must be determined based on similar randomized controlled trials done in the past.

Step 4 Repeat Step 3 N_{rep} times.

Step 5 Calculate the Monte Carlo simulated power as the number of results with significant treatment effect at significance level α, k_1, divided by the number of repetitions, i.e., $power_1 = k_1/N_{rep}$.

Step 6 Repeat Step 1 to Step 5 using different sample sizes, $m_2, m_3, ...$ and obtain the simulated power, $power_2, power_3, ...$ Then, plot the simulated powers against the sample sizes used and obtain a *simulated power curve* by drawing a curve connecting these points. Finally, we can estimate a simulated sample size that attains the pre-specified power $100(1-\phi)\%$ based on the simulated power curve.

Example: *Epilepsy Data*

First of all, let us consider the simulated sample sizes for the *superiority test* using the estimates with some modifications from Model Va applied to the data without patient 207. Based on this result, let us assume here that

$$\beta_0 = \log(\mu_b) = \log(8.0),\ \beta_3 = \log(0.8),\ \sigma_{B0}^2 = 0.45,\ \rho_B = 0.$$

Using four values of variance of b_{1i}, i.e., $\sigma_{B1}^2 = 0.22$ (the estimates in this example), $0.10, 0.05$, and 0 (= Model IV), the corresponding simulated power with $N_{rep} = 1000$ repetitions at $\alpha = 0.05$ is plotted against a common sample size $n(= 20, 40, 60, 80, 100)$ for the *4:4 design* with $\mu_b = 8$ in Figure 9.8. The simulated sample size n that attains 80% power at $\alpha = 0.05$ is close to 80, 52, 35, 20, for $\sigma_{B1}^2 = 0.22,\ 0.10,\ 0.05,\ 0.0$, respectively. It should be noted that the last simulated sample size 20 is close to the sample size 20.88 calculated by the formula (9.37) under Model IV. These simulation results indicate that the actual total sample size 59 in this example is quite insufficient (160 is needed) if we expect $e^{\beta_3} = 0.8$ under Model Va. Furthermore, if we adopt the *1:4 design* with $\mu_b = 8$ and two weeks as a unit interval, then the simulated sample size goes up to 120, indicating about $120/80 = 1.5$ times that of the *4:4 design*.

Secondly, let us consider the simulated sample sizes based on the estimates from Model Va applied to the full data shown in Output 9.3 and Table 9.3. So, let us set the values of necessary parameters as

$$\beta_0 = \log(8),\ \beta_3 = -0.30,\ \sigma_{B0}^2 = 0.50,\ \sigma_{B1}^2 = 0.25,\ \rho_B = 0$$

and consider the *1:1 design*, *1:4 design*, and *4:4 design*. Figure 9.9 shows the simulated power versus common sample size $n(= 15, 20, 25, 30, 40, ..., 70)$ for three different repeated measures designs, the *1:1 design*, *1:4 design*, and *4:4 design*. The sample size needed for each of these designs is close to $n_{1,1} = 54, n_{1,4} = 38, n_{4,4} = 20$, respectively. In other words, compared with the sample size of the *1:1 design*, the *1:4 design* has a 30% reduction, the *1:4*

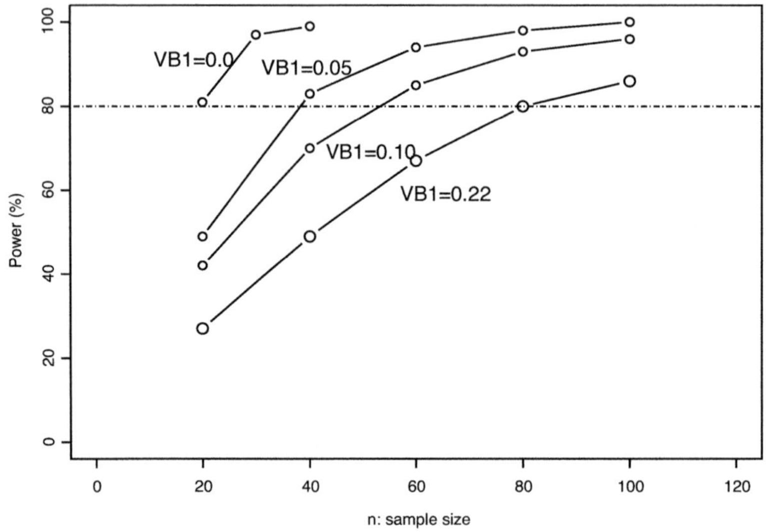

FIGURE 9.8
Simulated power (the effect size $e^{\beta_3} = 0.8$) of Model Va versus common sample size n for four different values of slope variance σ^2_{B1} (indicated by "VB1" in the figure) of the *4:4 design* with $\mu_b = 8$.

design has a 41.0% reduction, and the *4:4 design* has a 63% reduction.

9.8.2 Sample size for the treatment by linear time interaction

In this section, we shall consider the situation where the primary interest is estimating the treatment by *linear* time interaction. In other words, the treatment effect can be expressed in terms of the difference in slopes of linear trend or rates of improvement. To do this, we shall consider Model VII or the *random intercept plus slope* model within the framework of the *S:T* design. Needless to say, Model VII includes Model VI as a special case. Namely, the model is expressed as

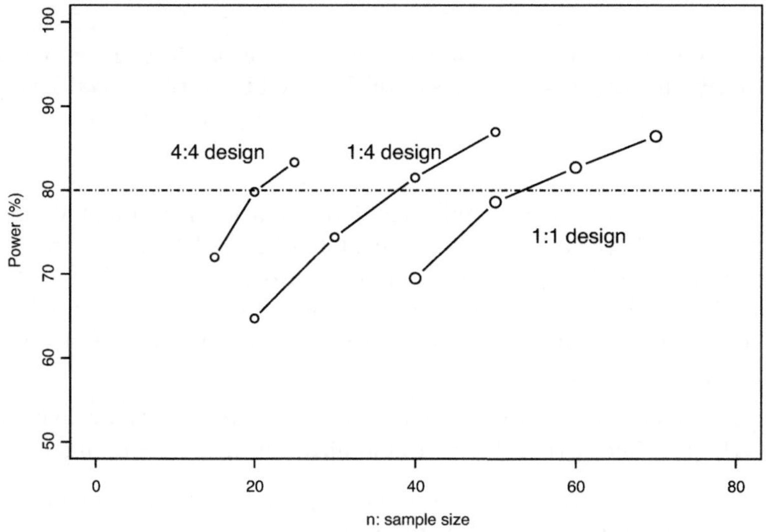

FIGURE 9.9
Simulated power (the effect size $\beta_3 = -0.30, e^{\beta_3} = 0.74$) of Model Va versus common sample size n for three different repeated measures designs, *1:1 design*, *1:4 design* and *4:4 design*, where it is assumed that $\beta_0 = \log(8)$, $\sigma^2_{B0} = 0.50$, $\sigma^2_{B1} = 0.25$, $\rho_B = 0$ based on the the results of Model Va applied to the *Epilepsy Data.*

$$\begin{aligned}
\log E(y_{ij} \mid b_{0i}, b_{1i}) &= \log L_{ij} + b_{0i} + \beta_0 + \beta_1 x_{1i} + (\beta_2 + \beta_3 x_{1i} + b_{1i})t_j \qquad (9.44)\\
\boldsymbol{b}_i &= (b_{0i}, b_{1i}) \sim N(\mathbf{0}, \boldsymbol{\Phi})\\
\boldsymbol{\Phi} &= \begin{pmatrix} \sigma^2_{B0} & \rho_B\sigma_{B0}\sigma_{B1} \\ \rho_B\sigma_{B0}\sigma_{B1} & \sigma^2_{B1} \end{pmatrix}\\
i &= 1, ..., n_1 \text{ (control);}\\
&= n_1 + 1, ..., n_1 + n_2 \text{ (new treatment)}\\
j &= -(S-1), -(S-2), ..., 0, 1, ..., T,
\end{aligned}$$

where t_j denotes the jth measurement time but all the measurement times during the baseline period are set to be the same time as t_0, which is usually set to zero, i.e.,

$$t_{-S+1} = t_{-S+2} = \cdots = t_0 = 0. \qquad (9.45)$$

Here also, the parameter β_3 denotes the treatment effect. Then, the null and alternative hypotheses of interest will be one of the three sets of hypotheses described in (9.31)–(9.36). In other words, investigators are interested in establishing whether the new treatment is *superior, non-inferior*, or *substantially superior* to the control treatment regarding the rate of improvement.

As in the case of the sample size determination for Model V, the sample size formula with closed form is not available for Model VII. So, let us consider the sample size determination via Monte Carlo simulations. The basic process to obtain the Monte Carlo simulated sample size $n(= n_1 = n_2)$ for the $S{:}T$ repeated measures design is exactly the same as that for Model V (Section 9.8.1.2) and assumes

1. no difference in expected count between the two treatment groups at the baseline period due to randomization, i.e., $\beta_1 = 0$, and
2. no temporal trend between the log rate of seizures before and after randomization in the control group, i.e., $\beta_2 = 0$,

and you have only to replace Step 3 for Model V with that arranged for Model VII:

Step 3 Simulate one data set $\{y_{ij} : i = 1, ..., 2n; j = -(S-1), ..., T\}$ independently under the assumed model shown below:

$$
\begin{aligned}
y_{ij} \mid b_{0i}, b_{1i} &\sim \text{Poisson}(\mu_{ij}) \\
\mu_{ij} &= \exp\{\beta_0 + b_{0i} + (\beta_3 x_{1i} + b_{1i}) t_j\} \\
i &= 1, ..., n \text{ (Control)}, \; n+1, ..., 2n \text{ (New treatment)} \\
j &= -(S-1), -(S-2), ..., 0, \; 1, ..., T \\
\boldsymbol{b}_i &= (b_{0i}, b_{1i}) \sim N(\mathbf{0}, \boldsymbol{\Phi}) \\
\boldsymbol{\Phi} &= \begin{pmatrix} \sigma_{B0}^2 & \rho_B \sigma_{B0} \sigma_{B1} \\ \rho_B \sigma_{B0} \sigma_{B1} & \sigma_{B1}^2 \end{pmatrix}
\end{aligned}
$$

where the values of $\beta_0, \beta_3, \sigma_{B0}^2, \sigma_{B1}^2, \rho_B$ must be determined based on similar randomized controlled trials done in the past.

Here also, for the *non-inferiority test* and the *substantial superiority test*, we have to replace β_3 with

$$\beta_3 \Longrightarrow \beta_3 - \log\{1 - \Delta \text{sign}(\beta_3)\}$$

in the basic process described above.

9.9 Discussion

In this chapter, several mixed-effects Poisson regression models are introduced and are illustrated with real data from a randomized controlled trial, called *Epilepsy Data*, with the *1:4* design. Needless to say, selection of the appropriate model depends on the purpose of the trial and an appropriate model should be examined cautiously using data from the previous trials.

Especially, we would like to stress that the set of models for the average treatment effect within the framework of the *S:T* repeated measures design should be considered as a practical and important trial design that is a better extension of the ordinary *1:1* design combined with an ANCOVA-type Poisson regression model in terms of *sample size reduction* and *easier handling of missing data*. Section 9.7.3 compared the estimates of the treatment effect obtained from the ANCOVA-type Models VIII and IX with those from the repeated measures models, Models IIa and Va, which are shown in Table 9.7. In the *Epilepsy Data*, the ANCOVA-type models are shown to give a little bit smaller p-values than repeated measures models, although all the estimates are statistically significant.

However, the repeated measures models can be more natural for the *S:T* repeated measures design with $S > 1$ than the ordinary ANCOVA-type Poisson regression model because we find it difficult to apply the ANCOVA-type model to these repeated measurements because the latter model must additionally consider how to deal with repeated measurements made before randomization.

10

Bayesian approach to generalized linear mixed models

In this chapter, we shall introduce Bayesian models with a non-informative prior for some of the generalized linear mixed-effects models described in previous chapters and show the similarity of the estimates. Bayesian alternatives are presented here in preparation for the situation where frequentist approaches including the generalized linear mixed models face difficulty in estimation. Bayesian models are especially useful for complex models such as generalized linear mixed-effects models with hierarchical random effects, latent class (profile) models, and handling measurement error and missing data.

10.1 Introduction

The generalized linear mixed-effects models discussed so far assumed a probability distribution $p(y \mid \theta)$ for the *frequency distribution* of data y, which includes a parameter of interest θ that is constant (frequentist approach). Statistical inference is essentially an inversion problem. Given a pdf $p(y|\theta)$ and a parameter θ, we can simulate or predict data y. However, we usually observe data y and wish to make inferences about parameter values θ. There are various ways to do this; one is the classical likelihood-based method, and another is the Bayesian method.

In classical inference, we invert our pdf from a function of y given θ to a function of θ given y. This function is called the *likelihood*, $L(\theta|y) = p(y|\theta)$. The value of θ that gives the highest value of the likelihood is the maximum likelihood estimate. On the other hand, the Bayesian approach also assumes the probability distribution $p(\theta)$ for the parameter of interest θ, reflecting the uncertainty about the parameter of interest. When we apply Bayes' theorem to parameters, it becomes Bayesian inference.

$$p(\theta|y) = \frac{p(y|\theta)}{p(y)} p(\theta) \tag{10.1}$$

Taking a pragmatic approach, we may view Bayes' theorem as a formalization of learning from experience. In other words, we update our current view (prior $p(\theta)$) with data obtained (likelihood $p(y|\theta)$) to give our new opinion (posterior $p(\theta|y)$). In general, we wish to obtain a point estimate of θ and some measure of uncertainty in that estimate. In classical analyses, we typically use the maximum likelihood estimate and a 95% confidence interval. In Bayesian analyses, we use the posterior mean, median, or mode as a point estimate and the posterior variance as a basis for an interval. Note that the likelihood is a *function* of θ, whereas the posterior is a *distribution* for θ.

Suppose we wish to estimate the treatment effect of a new therapy versus a standard one. When we carry out a clinical trial, a standard statistical analysis would produce a p-value, a point estimate, and a confidence interval. Bayesian analysis can add to this by focusing on how the trial changes our opinion about the treatment effect. In a Bayesian approach to clinical trials, the analyst needs to explicitly state:

1. an opinion about the value of the treatment effect excluding evidence from the trial (prior) $p(\theta)$,
2. support for different values of treatment effect based only on the data (likelihood) $p(y \mid \theta)$, and
3. a final opinion about the treatment effect (posterior) $p(\theta \mid y)$.

10.2 Non-informative prior and credible interval

So-called "non-informative" priors are those that lead to a posterior distribution which has the same shape as the likelihood, therefore Bayesian estimates will match classical estimates. More appropriate names are reference, default, uniform, or flat priors, as all priors give some information, even if it is that all parameter values are equally likely.

For location parameters, such as regression coefficients, common choices for a prior are a uniform distribution on a wide interval, e.g., U(-100,100), or a normal distribution with a large variance, e.g., N(0,100000). In many cases, the likelihood for a treatment effect can be assumed approximately normal, so it is convenient to use a normal prior provided it summarizes the external evidence. Namely, if the parameter θ satisfies the condition $-\infty \leq \theta \leq \infty$, then we can set

$$p(\theta) = N(0, \sigma^2), \quad \sigma = 100, 1000. \tag{10.2}$$

Sometimes invariance arguments are used to construct priors. A non-informative prior that is uniform in one parameterization will not necessarily be uniform in another. For example, if a prior is uniform for an odds ratio,

OR, then it will not be uniform for 1/OR. If one wishes the prior on an odds ratio to be the same as that on 1/OR, then the prior should be uniform on the log(OR) scale.

For scale parameters, such as sample variance, we may also use similar arguments. A uniform prior on σ, a uniform prior on σ^2 or a uniform prior on the precision $1/\sigma^2$ may be used. A prior which is uniform on $\log(\sigma)$, will also be uniform on $\log(\sigma^2)$ and $\log(1/\sigma^2)$. This can be achieved by directly placing a uniform prior on $\log(\sigma)$. Alternatively,

$$p(1/\sigma^2) = \text{Gamma}(a, a), \quad a = 0.001 \tag{10.3}$$

is commonly used since this is approximately uniform on $\log(\sigma)$. This has mean 1, variance 1000, and favors values of precision near 0, but is almost flat away from 0. Another commonly used prior for the sample variance is a uniform distribution on σ. Again, this can be done by directly placing a uniform prior on σ. Alternatively, a Gamma(1, 0.001) prior on the precision is approximately uniform over σ. This has mean 1000, variance 1,000,000.

As mentioned earlier, an attractive property of Bayesian analysis is that it considers the parameter of interest as uncertain, so we obtain a probability distribution for it, the posterior distribution. In practice, we will need to summarize this distribution using for example the mean, median, or mode as a point estimate. If the posterior is symmetric and unimodal, then these will coincide. If the posterior is skewed, we generally prefer to quote the median as it is less sensitive to the tails of the distribution.

For an interval estimate, any interval containing 95% of the posterior probability is called a 95% credible interval for θ, or more simply a posterior interval. We usually use the following two types of intervals:

- one-tailed interval: For example a one-tailed upper 95% interval would be (θ_L, ∞) where $p(\theta < \theta_L|y) = 0.05$).
- two-tailed equi-tail-area interval: A two-tailed 95% interval with equal probability in each tail area would be (θ_L, θ_U), where $p(\theta < \theta_L|y) = 0.025$) and $p(\theta > \theta_U|y) = 0.025$).

A 95% **credible interval** is an interval within which θ lies with probability 0.95. In contrast, the frequentist 95% **confidence interval** is constructed such that in a long series of 95% confidence intervals, 95% of them should contain the true θ. The width of the confidence interval depends on the standard error of the estimator, whereas the width of the credible interval depends on the posterior standard deviation. If we use a "reference" prior, i.e., one that leads to the posterior distribution being the same shape as the likelihood, then the posterior mode will be equal to the maximum likelihood estimate. In general, in large samples, Bayesian procedures give similar answers to classical ones because the data dominates information from the prior. However, in small samples, they can lead to different answers.

10.3 Markov Chain Monte Carlo methods

For a long time, Bayesian analysis was hampered by the inability to evaluate complex integrals to obtain the posterior distribution. Therefore, analysis was restricted to conjugate analyses, in which the posterior takes the same form as the prior and thus the mean, median, and other summary measures are known without having to do complicated integration. However, with the advent of modern computational power, we now have the ability to calculate complex integrals using simulations, known as Markov Chain Monte Carlo methods. This has led to the growth of Bayesian ideas.

Markov Chain Monte Carlo is Monte Carlo integration using Markov chains. Monte Carlo integration involves sampling from a probability distribution and forming sample averages. Markov chain Monte Carlo does this by running a cleverly constructed Markov chain. Markov Chain Monte Carlo (MCMC) methods are a class of algorithms for sampling from probability distributions based on constructing a Markov chain that has the desired distribution as the equilibrium distribution. Monte Carlo methods are techniques that aim to evaluate integrals by simulation, rather than by exact or approximate algebraic analysis. The essential components of MCMC methods include:

- *Replacing analytic methods by simulation:* Sample from the joint posterior distribution $p(\theta|y)$ and save a large number of plausible values for θ. We then use, e.g., the sample mean of the sampled values as an estimate of the posterior mean $E(\theta|y)$.

- *Sampling from the posterior distribution:* Methods of sampling from a joint posterior distribution that is known to be proportional to a likelihood times a prior focus on producing a Markov chain, in which the distribution for the next simulated value depends only on the current value. The theory of Markov chains states that under broad conditions, the samples will eventually converge to an "equilibrium distribution." A set of algorithms that use the specified form of $p(y|\theta) \times p(\theta)$ to ensure the equilibrium distribution is the posterior distribution of interest are available. Popular techniques include Gibbs sampling and the Metropolis algorithm.

- *Starting the simulation:* The Markov chain must be started somewhere, and initial values are selected for unknown parameters. In theory, the choice of initial values will not have a bearing on the eventual samples, but in practice they make a difference to the rate of convergence.

- *Checking convergence:* Checking whether a Markov chain has converged is a difficult problem. Lack of convergence can be diagnosed by observing the erratic behavior of sampled values, but it is particularly difficult to diagnose convergence. One idea is to run several chains from a diverse set of initial values and check whether they come from the same posterior distribution.

In Bayesian modeling, the *deviance information criterion* (DIC) has been proposed by Spiegelhalter et al. (2002) and is widely used as a criterion of model choice. DIC is intended as a generalization of AIC, Akaike's Information Criterion (3.25) and is defined as

$$DIC = Dhat + 2pD, \tag{10.4}$$

where *Dhat* is a point estimate of the *deviance* (-2 * log(likelihood)) obtained by substituting in the posterior means $\hat{\theta}$, thus

$$Dhat = -2 * \log(p(y \mid \hat{\theta}))$$

and *pD* is the effective number of parameters. Like AIC and BIC, the model with the smallest DIC is estimated to be the model that would best predict a replicate dataset of the same structure. It should be noted that *DIC assumes the posterior mean to be a good estimate of the parameters of interest. If this is not so, say because of extreme skewness or even bimodality, then DIC may not be appropriate. Mixture models discussed in Chapter 12 are one such example in which WinBUGS or OpenBUGS will not permit the calculation of DIC.*

10.4 WinBUGS and OpenBUGS

WinBUGS is statistical software that carries out Bayesian analysis using MCMC methods. BUGS stands for **B**ayesian Inference **U**sing **G**ibbs **S**ampling and runs in Windows. It assumes a Bayesian or full probability model, in which all quantities are treated as random variables. The model consists of a defined joint distribution over all unobserved (parameters and missing data) and observed quantities (the data). We then need to condition the data in order to obtain a posterior distribution over the parameters and unobserved data. Marginalizing over this posterior distribution to obtain inferences on the main quantities of interest is carried out using a Monte Carlo approach to integration (Gibbs sampling). Having specified a full probability model on all the quantities, we wish to sample unknown parameters from their conditional distribution given observed data. The Gibbs sampling algorithm successively samples from the conditional distribution of each node given all the others. Under broad conditions, this process eventually provides a sample from the posterior distribution of the unknown quantities. Inferences can then be drawn about their true values using empirical summary statistics.

WinBUGS is a stand-alone package and the latest version 1.4.x is the last update made, there are many add-on packages such as pkbugs and geobugs. OpenBUGS is open source and runs on Windows and Linux as well as from inside R.

10.5 Getting started

- Download and install WinBUGS 1.4.x from `http://www.mrc-bsu.cam.ac.uk/software/bugs/the-bugs-project-winbugs`
- Download and install the latest patch (if version 1.4.3 were downloaded).
- Download the key for unrestricted use.

The key and the patch are installed by opening the file in WinBUGS (or copying and pasting the code to a new file); go to Tools → Decode → Decode All. (Click yes, if asked to create a new folder.)

The following are suggestions from the WinBUGS manual for new users:

1. Work through the tutorial at the end of the WinBUGS manual.
2. Try some examples in the Help → Examples sections.
3. Find an example similar to the model you'd like to fit and edit the BUGS language according to your problem.

or

- Download and install OpenBUGS from `http://openbugs.net/w/Downloads`

The suggestions from the OpenBUGS manual for new users are the same as those from WinBUGS.

10.6 Bayesian model for the mixed-effects normal linear regression Model V

In this section, let us apply a Bayesian model for the mixed-effects normal linear regression Model Va ($\rho_B = 0$) to the *Beat the Blues Data* (Table 7.2). A frequentist model and the corresponding Bayesian model can be expressed as follows:

A frequentist's model:

$$
\begin{aligned}
y_{ij} &\sim N(\mu_{ij}, \sigma_E^2) \\
\mu_{ij} &= \beta_0 + b_{0i} + \beta_1 x_{1i} + (\beta_2 + b_{1i}) x_{2ij} + \beta_3 x_{1i} x_{2ij} + w_1 \text{drug} + w_2 \text{length} \\
b_{0i} &\sim N(0, \sigma_{B0}^2) \\
b_{1i} &\sim N(0, \sigma_{B1}^2)
\end{aligned}
$$

A Bayesian model:

$$
\begin{aligned}
y_{ij} &\sim N(\mu_{ij}, \sigma_E^2) \\
\mu_{ij} &= \beta_0 + b_{0i} + \beta_1 x_{1i} + (\beta_2 + b_{1i}) x_{2ij} + \beta_3 x_{1i} x_{2ij} + w_1 \text{drug} + w_2 \text{length} \\
\beta_k &\sim N(0, 10^4),\ k = 0, ..., 3 \\
w_k &\sim N(0, 10^4),\ k = 1, 2 \\
b_{0i} &\sim N(0, \sigma_{b0}^2),\ i = 1, ..., N \\
b_{1i} &\sim N(0, \sigma_{b1}^2),\ i = 1, .., N \\
\tau_{b0} &= 1/\sigma_{b0}^2 \sim \text{Gamma}(0.001, 0.001) \\
\tau_{b1} &= 1/\sigma_{b1}^2 \sim \text{Gamma}(0.001, 0.001) \\
\tau &= 1/\sigma_E^2 \sim \text{Gamma}(0.001, 0.001)
\end{aligned}
$$

The OpenBUGS code is shown in Program 10.1 and the corresponding `Initial values` and `Data` are shown in Program 10.2.

Program 10.1. **OpenBUGS code (1) for the Normal Model Va**

```
model {
  for(i in 1:N){
      for(j in 1:5){
          bdi[ 5*(i-1) + j] ~ dnorm(mu[subject[ 5*(i-1) + j], j], tau)
          mu[subject[ 5*(i-1) + j], j] <- a0
               + b0[subject[ 5*(i-1) + j]]
               + b1[subject[ 5*(i-1) + j]] * post[j]
               + beta1*treatment[ 5*(i-1) + j]
               + beta2*post[j]
               + beta3*treatment[ 5*(i-1) + j]*post[j]
               + beta.drug * (drug[ 5*(i-1) + j]    - drug.bar)
               + beta.length*(length[ 5*(i-1) + j] - length.bar)
       }
   }
   for (i in 1:N){
        b0[i] ~ dnorm(0.0, tau.b0)
        b1[i] ~ dnorm(0.0, tau.b1)
   }
   drug.bar <- mean(drug[])
   length.bar<-mean(length[])
# priors:
a0 ~     dnorm(0.0,1.0E-4)
beta1 ~ dnorm(0.0,1.0E-4)
beta2 ~ dnorm(0.0,1.0E-4)
beta3 ~ dnorm(0.0,1.0E-4)
beta.drug ~ dnorm(0.0,1.0E-4)
beta.length ~ dnorm(0.0,1.0E-4)
tau.b0 ~ dgamma(1.0E-3,1.0E-3)
sigma2.b0  <- 1.0/  tau.b0
tau.b1 ~ dgamma(1.0E-3,1.0E-3)
sigma2.b1  <- 1.0/  tau.b1
tau ~ dgamma(1.0E-3,1.0E-3)
sigma2  <- 1.0/  tau
beta0<- a0 - drug.bar*beta.drug - beta.length*length.bar
   }
```

Program 10.2. **OpenBUGS code (2) for the Normal Model Va**

```
# Initial values
list(tau.b0 =1, tau.b1=1, a0=0, beta1=0, beta2=0, beta3=0,
     beta.drug=0, beta.length=0,tau=1)
list(tau.b0 =2, tau.b1=2,  a0=1, beta1=1, beta2=2, beta3=1,
     beta.drug=-1, beta.length= -1,tau=2)

# Data (shown are for the first two patients)
list(N=100,  post=c(0,1,1,1,1))
no[] subject[] drug[] length[] treatment[] visit[] bdi[]
 1          1  0  1     0     0  29
 2          1  0  1     0     2   2
 3          1  0  1     0     3   2
 4          1  0  1     0     5  NA
 5          1  0  1     0     8  NA
 6          2  1  1     1     0  32
 7          2  1  1     1     2  16
 8          2  1  1     1     3  24
 9          2  1  1     1     5  17
10          2  1  1     1     8  20
.....
```

It should be noted that two covariates, `drug` and `length`, had *centering*, i.e., $(x - \bar{x})$. Often, centering a covariate will improve model convergence. In this analysis, we used two chains (i.e., sets of samples to simulate) since running multiple chains is one way to check the convergence. So, we gave two sets of initial values because we need a different set of initial values for each chain. Furthermore, we obtained the results after running the model on 2 chains for 50,000 iterations with a burn-in of 5,000 iterations. Before going on to the results, let us examine whether convergence has been reached. Checking convergence in general requires considerable care. It is very difficult to say conclusively that a chain (simulation) has converged, only to diagnose when it definitely hasn't!

For checking the convergence, the `history` plots for several parameters are shown in Figure 10.1. In this case, we can be reasonably confident that convergence has been achieved because the two chains appear to be overlapping one another. We may also look at the auto-correlation of each chain, which is the cross-correlation of the chain with itself. Informally, it measures the similarity between the values iterated as a function of time separation between them. Figure 10.2 shows auto-correlations for all monitored parameters, where we can see that for all the parameters monitored, the auto-correlation reduces with the lag between iterations as expected.

For a more formal approach to convergence diagnosis, the software also provides an implementation of the techniques described in Brooks and Gelman (1998). When we plot the trace or time series of a chain, it should remain steady around one value. One approach is to run two or more chains from dif-

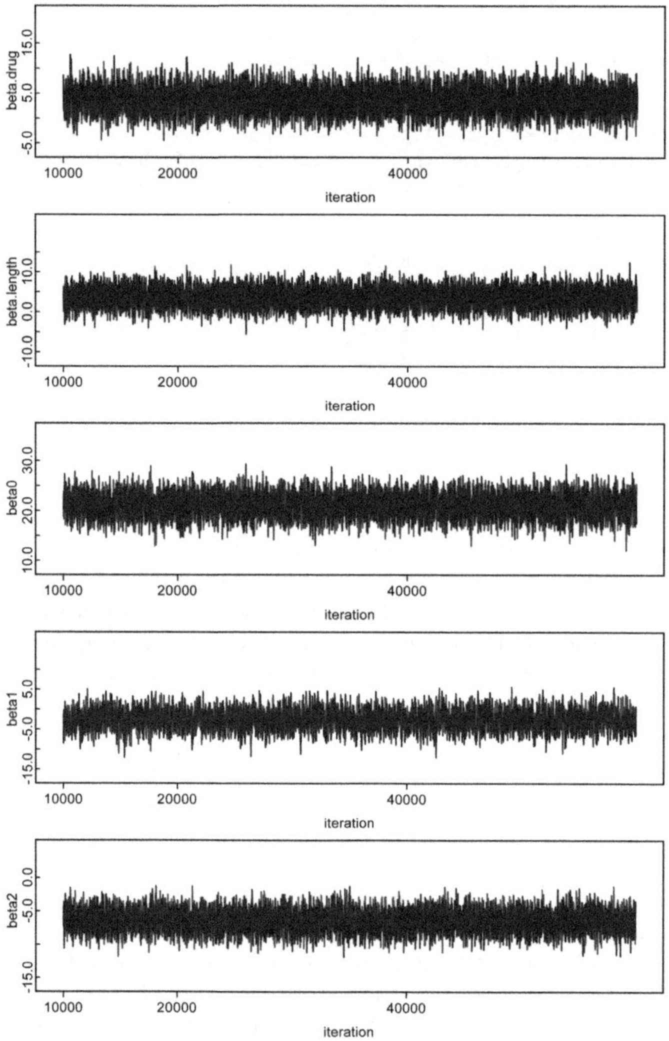

FIGURE 10.1
Beat the Blues Data: History for some parameters of the Bayesian normal linear regression Model Va (2 chains are run for 50,000 iterations with a burn-in of 5,000 iterations).

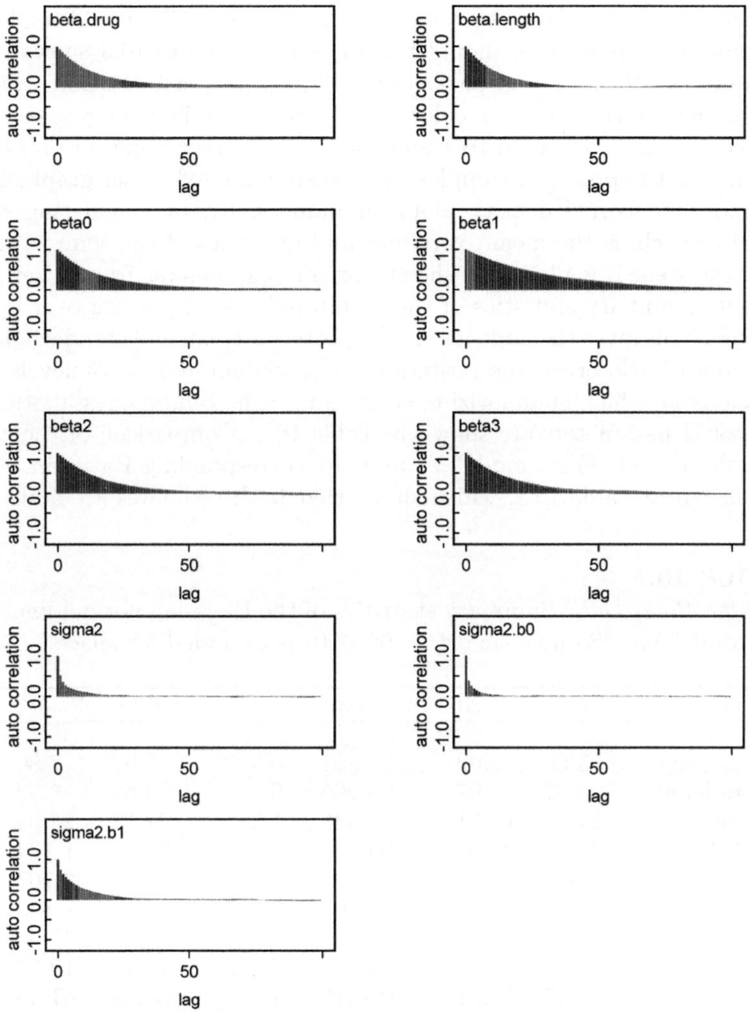

FIGURE 10.2
Beat the Blues Data: Auto-correlation for all monitored parameters of the Bayesian normal linear regression Model Va.

ferent initial values for a long time and see whether they converge to the same distribution. In order to do this, the BGR diagnostic compares the within-chain variance and the between-chain variance. The width of the central 80% interval of the pooled runs is represented by a green line, the average width of the 80% intervals within the individual runs is represented by a blue line, and their ratio R is given by a red line. The red line, R, should tend to 1 and the blue and green lines should become stable. Figure 10.3 shows the BGR diagram for all monitored parameters. Since this is a black and white book, you cannot see three lines in color. If the figure were in color, you can see that the red line has converged to 1 and the blue (= green) lines are both stable.

Finally, the posterior samples may be summarized either graphically, e.g., by smoothed kernel density plots, or numerically, by calculating summary statistics such as the mean, variance, and quantiles of the sample. In Figure 10.4, the `density` plots are shown for all parameters, from where we can estimate summary statistics of the monitored nodes, pooling over the chains selected. This gives the node name, the posterior mean and standard deviation, the Monte Carlo error, the posterior 2.5%, median and 97.5% levels, and the iterations at which summarizing starts and ends. Summary statistics for the monitored parameters are shown in Table 10.1. Comparison of the estimates from the mixed-effects model Va and the corresponding Bayesian model are also shown in Table 10.2, which shows that both estimates are quite similar.

TABLE 10.1
Beat the Blues Data: Summary statistics of the Bayesian normal linear regression Model Va. "Sample size" (= 100,000) is excluded for space.

Node	Mean	sd	MC error	2.5%	Median	97.5%	Start
beta.drug	3.69	2.09	0.0351	-0.373	3.67	7.86	10001
beta.length	3.67	1.97	0.0296	-0.187	3.68	7.52	10001
beta0	21.12	1.951	0.0349	17.28	21.12	24.94	10001
beta1	-2.513	2.159	0.0489	-6.749	-2.513	1.774	10001
beta2	-6.385	1.340	0.0227	-9.018	-6.377	-3.767	10001
beta3	-2.496	1.839	0.0307	-6.106	-2.512	1.155	10001
sigma2	29.04	3.031	0.0251	23.65	28.84	35.53	10001
sigma2.b0	76.44	14.17	0.0971	52.49	75.13	107.7	10001
sigma2.b1	37.37	11.01	0.1316	18.46	36.49	61.48	10001

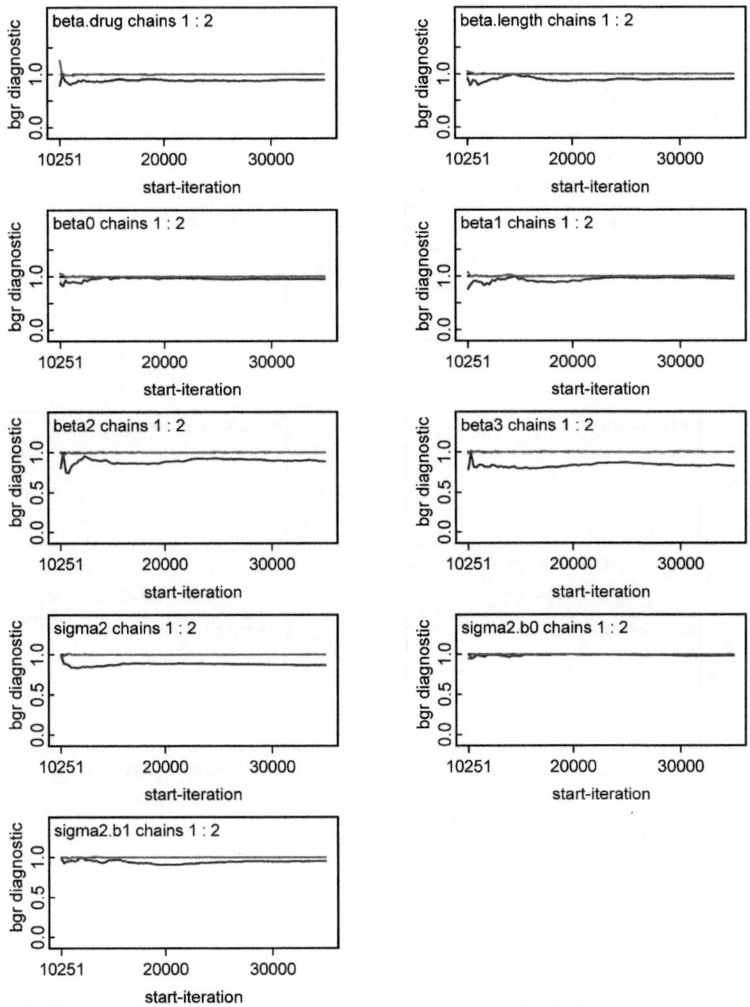

FIGURE 10.3
Beat the Blues Data: BGR diagram for all monitored parameters of the Bayesian normal linear regression Model Va.

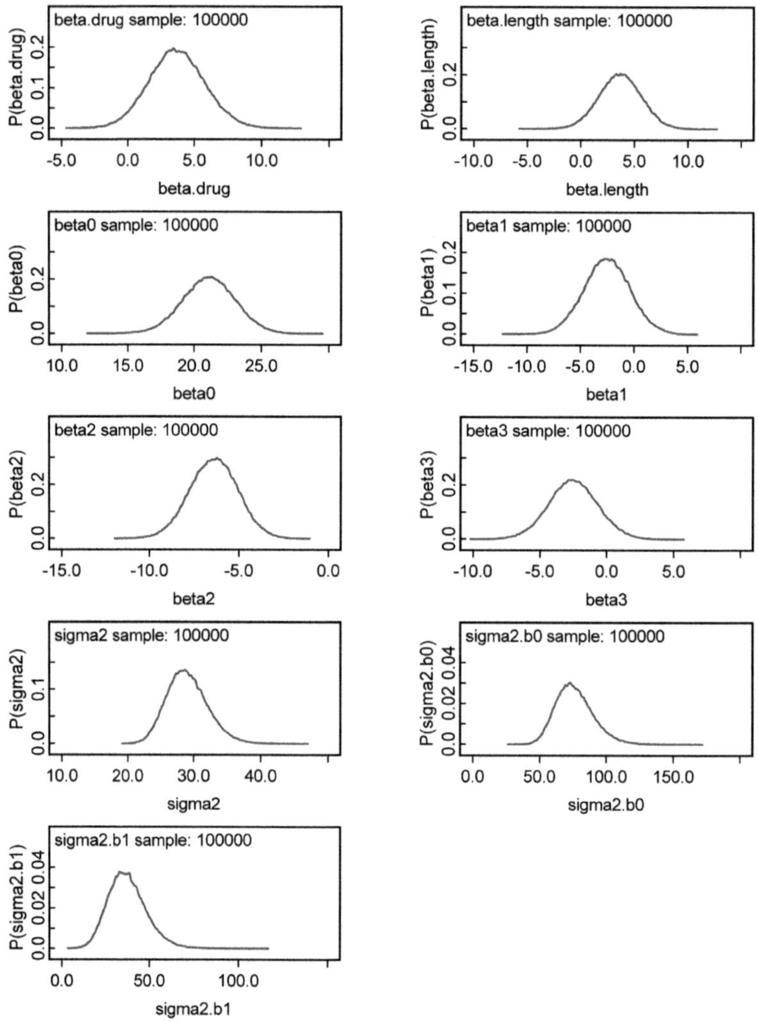

FIGURE 10.4
Beat the Blues Data: Posterior densities for all parameters of the Bayesian normal linear regression Model Va.

TABLE 10.2
Beat the Blues Data: Comparison of the mixed-effects normal linear regression Model Va and the corresponding Bayesian model.

Model	Frequentist			Bayesian		
		95% CI			95% CI	
Parameter	Estimate	Lower	Upper	Estimate	Lower	Upper
Intercept ($\hat{\beta}_0$)	21.186	17.368	25.004	21.12	17.28	24.94
drug	3.805	-0.269	7.879	3.692	-0.3729	7.862
length	3.632	-0.242	7.506	3.674	-0.187	7.52
treatment ($\hat{\beta}_1$)	-2.659	-6.850	1.533	-2.513	-6.749	1.774
post ($\hat{\beta}_2$)	-6.374	-8.972	-3.776	-6.385	-9.018	-3.767
treatment*post ($\hat{\beta}_3$)	-2.514	-6.082	1.055	-2.496	-6.106	1.155
$\hat{\sigma}^2_{B0}$	74.83	(s.e. = 13.63)		75.13	52.49	107.7
$\hat{\sigma}^2_{B1}$	37.48	(s.e. = 10.56)		36.49	18.49	61.48
$\hat{\sigma}^2_{E}$	28.50	(s.e. = 2.92)		28.84	23.65	35.53

10.7 Bayesian model for the mixed-effects logistic regression Model IV

In this section, let us apply a Bayesian model for the mixed-effects logistic regression Model IV to the *Respiratory Data* (Table 8.1). A frequentist model and the corresponding Bayesian model can be expressed as follows:

A frequentist's model:

$$\begin{aligned} y_{ij} &\sim \text{Bernoulli}(p_{ij}) \\ \text{logit } p_{ij} &= \beta_0 + b_{0i} + \beta_1 x_{1i} + \beta_2 x_{2ij} + \beta_3 x_{1i} x_{2ij} \\ &\quad + w_1 \text{age} + w_2 \text{centre} + w_3 \text{gender} \\ b_{0i} &\sim N(0, \sigma^2_{B0}) \end{aligned}$$

A Bayesian model:

$$
\begin{aligned}
y_{ij} &\sim \text{Bernoulli}(p_{ij}) \\
\text{logit } p_{ij} &= \beta_0 + b_{0i} + \beta_1 x_{1i} + \beta_2 x_{2ij} + \beta_3 x_{1i} x_{2ij} \\
&\quad + w_1 \text{age} + w_2 \text{centre} + w_3 \text{gender} \\
\beta_k &\sim N(0, 10^4), \ k = 0, ..., 3 \\
w_k &\sim N(0, 10^4), \ k = 1, 2, 3 \\
b_{0i} &\sim N(0, \sigma_{b0}^2), \ i = 1, ..., N \\
\tau_{b0} &= 1/\sigma_{b0}^2 \sim \text{Gamma}(0.001, 0.001)
\end{aligned}
$$

The OpenBUGS code is shown in Program 10.3 and the corresponding `Initial values` and `Data` are shown in Program 10.4.

Program 10.3. **OpenBUGS code (1) for the logistic Model IV**

```
model {
   for(i in 1:N){
     for(j in 1:5){
status[ 5*(i-1) + j] ~ dbern(p[subject[ 5*(i-1) + j ], j])
#
logit( p[subject[ 5*(i-1) + j], j] ) <- a0
+ b0[subject[ 5*(i-1) +j]
+ beta1*treatment[ 5*(i-1) + j]
+ beta2*post[j]
+ beta3*treatment[ 5*(i-1) + j]*post[j]
+ beta.centre * centre[ 5*(i-1) + j ]
+ beta.gender * gender[ 5*(i-1) + j]
+ beta.age*(age[ 5*(i-1) + j] - age.bar)
  }
   }
#
  for (i in 1:N){
       b0[i] ~ dnorm(0.0, tau.b0)
  }
age.bar <- mean(age[])
# priors:
a0 ~ dnorm(0.0,1.0E-4)
beta1 ~ dnorm(0.0,1.0E-4)
beta2 ~ dnorm(0.0,1.0E-4)
beta3 ~ dnorm(0.0,1.0E-4)
beta.centre ~ dnorm(0.0,1.0E-4)
beta.gender ~ dnorm(0.0,1.0E-4)
beta.age ~ dnorm(0.0,1.0E-4)
tau.b0 ~ dgamma(1.0E-3,1.0E-3)
sigma2.b0  <- 1.0/ tau.b0
#
beta0<- a0 - age.bar*beta.age
}
```

Program 10.4. **OpenBUGS code (2) for the logistic Model IV**

```
# Initial values
list(tau.b0 =1, a0=0, beta1=0, beta2=0, beta3=0, beta.centre=0,
beta.gender=0, beta.age=0)

list(tau.b0 =2,  a0=1, beta1=1, beta2=2, beta3=1, beta.centre=-1,
beta.gender= -1, beta.age=1)

# Data
list(N=111,  post=c(0,1,1,1,1))
no[] centre[] subject[] visit[] treatment[] status[] gender[] age[]
1          1         1       0        0         0         0    46
2          1         1       1        0         0         0    46
3          1         1       2        0         0         0    46
4          1         1       3        0         0         0    46
5          1         1       4        0         0         0    46
6          1         2       0        0         0         0    28
7          1         2       1        0         0         0    28
8          1         2       2        0         0         0    28
9          1         2       3        0         0         0    28
10         1         2       4        0         0         0    28
.....
```

Here also, the variable `age` had *centering*, i.e., $(x-\bar{x})$. In this analysis also, we used two chains and so we gave two sets of initial values. Furthermore, we obtained the results after running the model on 2 chains for 50,000 iterations with a burn-in of 5,000 iterations. For checking the convergence, the `history` plots for several parameters are shown in Figure 10.5, where we can be reasonably confident that convergence has been achieved because the two chains appear to be overlapping one another.

Figure 10.6 shows auto-correlations for all monitored parameters, where we can see that for all the parameters monitored the auto-correlation reduces with the lag between iterations as expected. For a more formal approach to convergence diagnosis, the BGR diagram for all monitored parameters are shown in Figure 10.7. Since this is a black and white book, you cannot see three lines in color. If the figure were in color, you can see that the red line has converged to 1 and the blue (= green) lines are both stable.

In Figure 10.8, the `density` plots are shown for all parameters, from which we can estimate summary statistics of the monitored nodes, pooling over the chains selected. Summary statistics for the monitored parameters are shown in Table 10.3. Comparison of the estimates from the mixed-effects model IV and the corresponding Bayesian model are also shown in Table 10.4, which also shows that both estimates are quite similar.

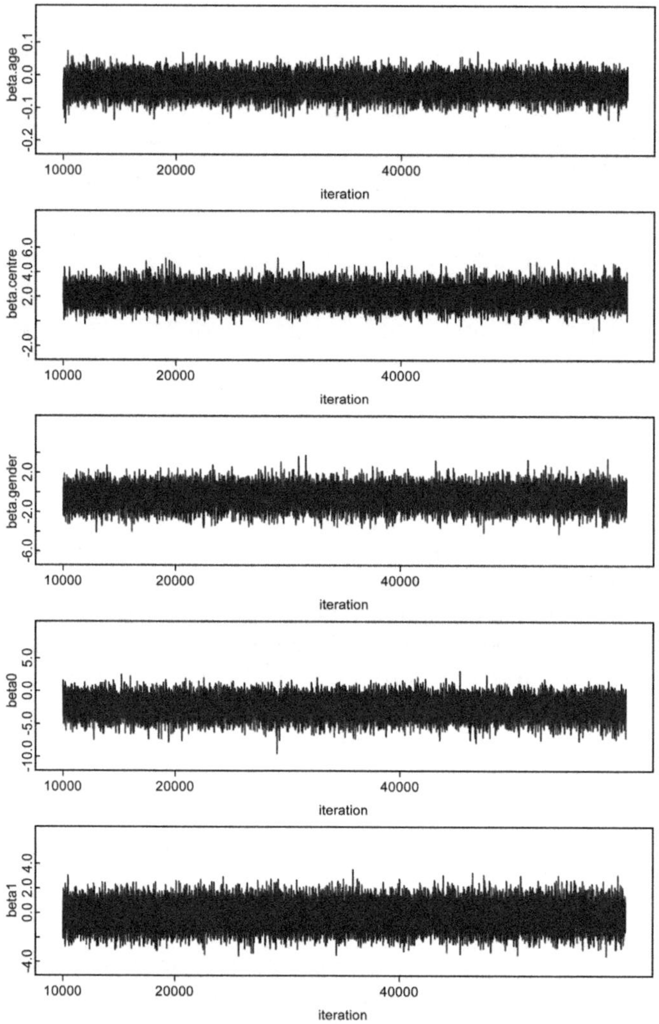

FIGURE 10.5
Respiratory Data: History for some parameters of the Bayesian logistic regression Model IV (2 chains are run for 50,000 iterations with a burn-in of 5,000 iterations).

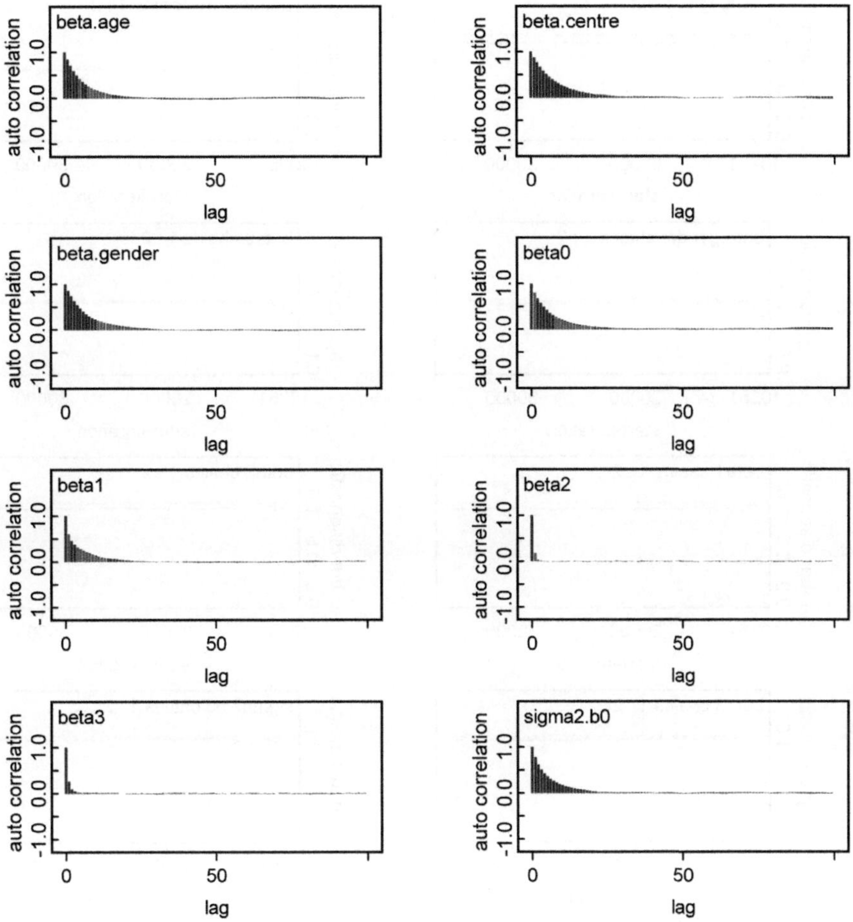

FIGURE 10.6
Respiratory Data: Auto-correlation for all monitored parameters of the Bayesian logistic regression Model IV.

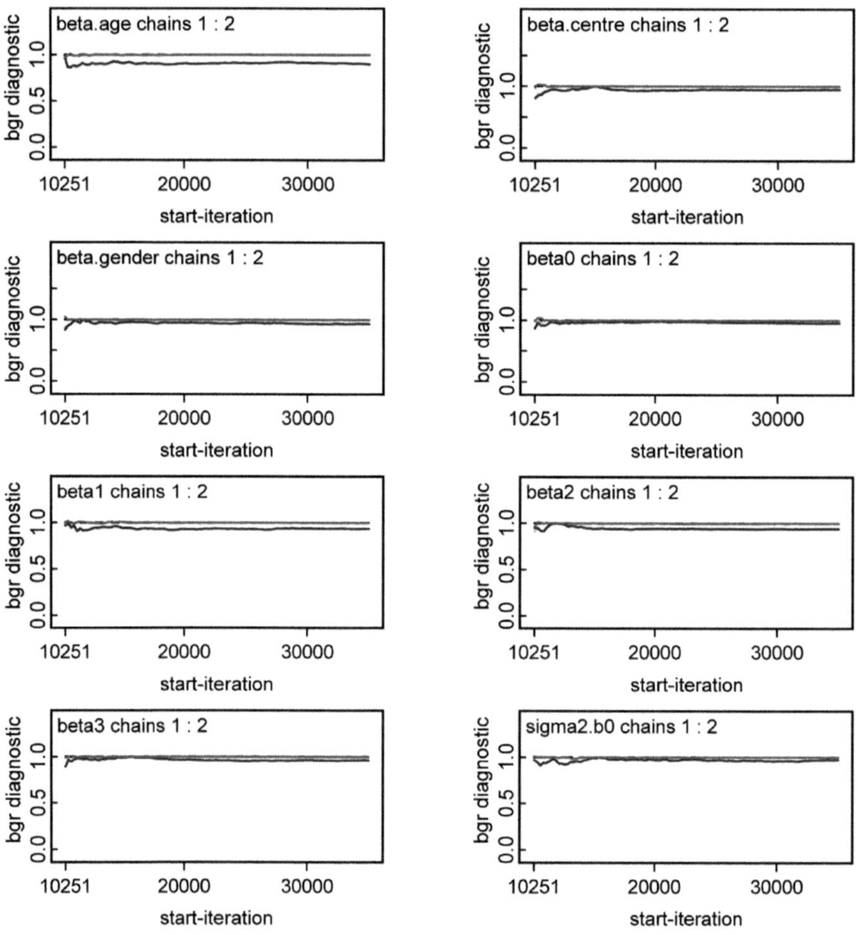

FIGURE 10.7
Respiratory Data: BGR diagram for all monitored parameters of the Bayesian logistic regression Model IV.

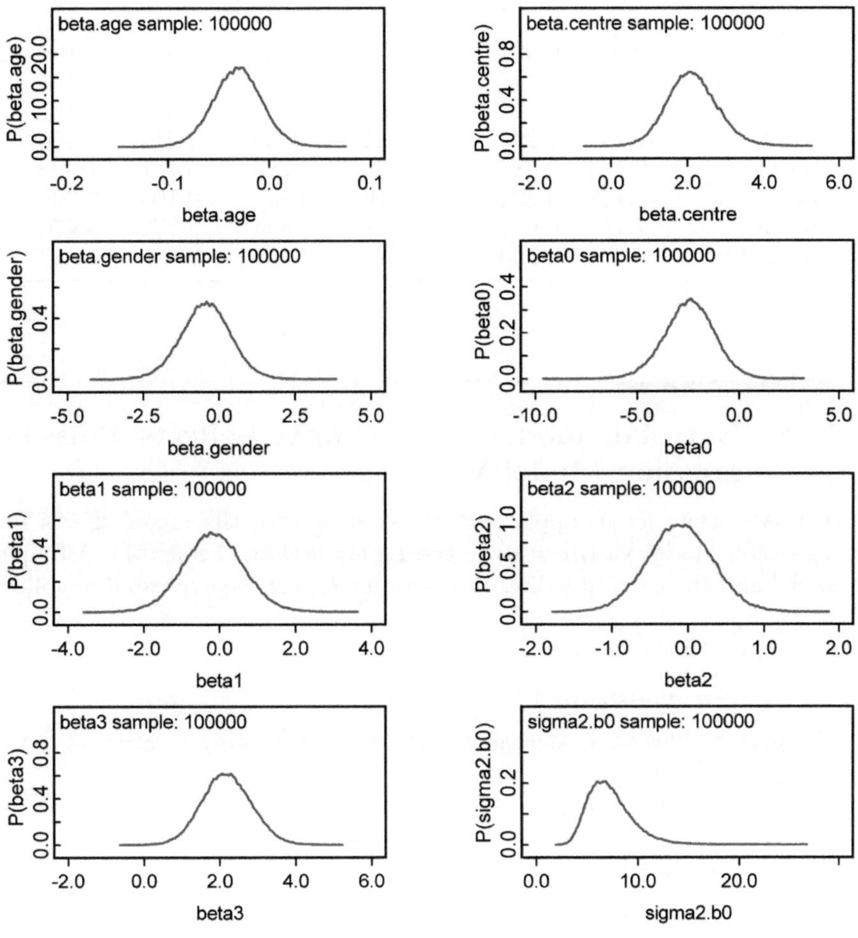

FIGURE 10.8
Respiratory Data: Posterior densities for all parameters of the Bayesian logistic regression Model IV.

TABLE 10.3
Respiratory Data: Summary statistics of the Bayesian Model IV. 'Sample size" (= 100, 000) is excluded for space.

Node	Mean	sd	MC error	2.5%	Median	97.5%	Start
beta.age	-0.031	0.024	2.6E-4	-0.0790	-0.031	0.0154	10001
beta.centre	2.124	0.647	0.0077	0.910	2.103	3.454	10001
beta.gender	-0.434	0.822	0.0095	-2.08	-0.424	1.171	10001
beta0	-2.441	1.207	0.0141	-4.896	-2.412	-0.120	10001
beta1	-0.164	0.788	0.0073	-1.713	-0.167	1.389	10001
beta2	-0.109	0.424	0.0016	-0.942	-0.109	0.723	10001
beta3	2.182	0.647	0.0031	0.934	2.172	3.470	10001
sigma2.b0	7.301	2.165	0.0221	4.001	6.995	12.43	10001

10.8 Bayesian model for the mixed-effects Poisson regression Model V

In this section, let us apply a Bayesian model for the mixed-effects Poisson regression Model Va ($\rho_B = 0$) to the *Epilepsy Data* (Table 9.1). A frequentist model and the corresponding Bayesian model can be expressed as follows:

A frequentist's model:

$$\begin{aligned}
y_{ij} &\sim \text{Poisson}(\mu_{ij}) \\
\log \mu_{ij} &= \log t_{ij} + \beta_0 + b_{0i} + \beta_1 x_{1i} + (\beta_2 + b_{1i}) x_{2ij} + \beta_3 x_{1i} x_{2ij} + w_1 \text{age} \\
b_{0i} &\sim N(0, \sigma_{B0}^2) \\
b_{1i} &\sim N(0, \sigma_{B1}^2)
\end{aligned}$$

A Bayesian model:

$$\begin{aligned}
y_{ij} &\sim \text{Poisson}(\mu_{ij}) \\
\log \mu_{ij} &= \log t_{ij} + \beta_0 + b_{0i} + \beta_1 x_{1i} + (\beta_2 + b_{1i}) x_{2ij} + \beta_3 x_{1i} x_{2ij} + w_1 \text{age} \\
\beta_k &\sim N(0, 10^4), \ k = 0, ..., 3 \\
w_1 &\sim N(0, 10^4) \\
b_{0i} &\sim N(0, \sigma_{b0}^2), \ i = 1, ..., N \\
b_{1i} &\sim N(0, \sigma_{b1}^2), \ i = 1, ..., N \\
\tau_{b0} &= 1/\sigma_{b0}^2 \sim \text{Gamma}(0.001, 0.001) \\
\tau_{b1} &= 1/\sigma_{b1}^2 \sim \text{Gamma}(0.001, 0.001)
\end{aligned}$$

TABLE 10.4
Respiratory Data: Comparison of the mixed-effects logistic regression Model IV and the corresponding Bayesian model.

Model	Mixed-effects model			Bayesian model		
		95% CI			95% CI	
Parameter	Estimate	Lower	Upper	Estimate	Lower	Upper
Intercept ($\hat{\beta}_0$)	-0.276	-1.955	1.404	-2.441	-4.896	-0.120
age	-0.030	-0.072	0.013	-0.031	-0.031	0.015
centre	1.996	0.855	3.137	2.124	0.910	3.454
gender	-0.408	-1.838	1.021	-0.434	-2.08	1.171
treatment ($\hat{\beta}_1$)	-0.176	-1.604	1.253	-0.164	-1.713	1.389
post ($\hat{\beta}_2$)	-0.103	-0.917	0.711	-0.109	-0.942	0.723
treatment*post ($\hat{\beta}_3$)	2.072	0.841	3.303	2.182	0.934	3.470
$\hat{\sigma}^2_{B0}$	5.745	(s.e. = 1.5994)		6.996	4.001	12.43

Program 10.5. **OpenBUGS code (1) for the Poisson Model Va**

```
model {
for(i in 1 : N) {
for(j in 1 : 5) {
log(mu[subject[5*(i-1) + j], j]) <- log(t[j]) + a0
+ b0[subject[5*(i-1) + j]]
+ b1[subject[5*(i-1) + j]] * post[j]
+ beta1*treatment[5*(i-1) + j]
+ beta2*post[j]
+ beta3*treatment[5*(i-1) + j]*post[j]
+ beta.age* (age[5*(i-1) + j] - age.bar)
#
seizure[5*(i-1) + j] ~ dpois(mu[subject[5*(i-1) + j], j])
          }
      }
#
for (i in 1:N){
b0[i] ~ dnorm(0.0, tau.b0)          # subject random effects
b1[i] ~ dnorm(0.0, tau.b1)          # subject random effects
   }
        age.bar <- mean(age[])
# priors:
a0 ~ dnorm(0.0,1.0E-4)
beta1 ~ dnorm(0.0,1.0E-4)
beta2 ~ dnorm(0.0,1.0E-4)
beta3 ~ dnorm(0.0,1.0E-4)
beta.age ~ dnorm(0.0,1.0E-4)
tau.b0 ~ dgamma(1.0E-3,1.0E-3)
tau.b1 ~ dgamma(1.0E-3,1.0E-3)
sigma2.b0  <- 1.0/  tau.b0
sigma2.b1  <- 1.0/  tau.b1
beta0<- a0 - age.bar*beta.age
}
```

Program 10.6. **OpenBUGS code (2) for the Poisson Model Va**

```
# Initial values
list(tau.b0 =1, tau.b1=1, a0=0, beta1=0, beta2=0, beta3=0, beta.age=0)
list(tau.b0 =3, tau.b1=2, a0=1, beta1=1, beta2=-2, beta3=-2, beta.age=0)

# Data
list(N=59, t=c(8,2,2,2,2), post=c(0,1,1,1,1))

no[] subject[] treatment[] visit[] seizure[] age[]
1          1  0          0      11        31
2          1  0          1       5        31
3          1  0          2       3        31
4          1  0          3       3        31
5          1  0          4       3        31
6          2  0          0      11        30
7          2  0          1       3        30
8          2  0          2       5        30
9          2  0          3       3        30
10         2  0          4       3        30
.....
```

The OpenBUGS code is shown in Program 10.5 and the corresponding `Initial values` and `Data` are shown in Program 10.6.

Here also, the variable `age` had *centering*, i.e., $(x - \bar{x})$. In this analysis also, we used two chains and so we gave two sets of initial values. Furthermore, we obtained the results after running the model on 2 chains for 50,000 iterations with a burn-in of 5,000 iterations. For checking the convergence, the `history` plots for several parameters are shown in Figure 10.9, where we can be reasonably confident that convergence has been achieved because the two chains appear to be overlapping one another. Figure 10.10 shows auto-correlations for all monitored parameters, where we can see that the three chains `beta.Age`, `beta.0`, and `beta.1`, have slightly higher autocorrelations but the auto-correlation reduces with the lag between iterations. For a more formal approach to convergence diagnosis, the BGR diagram for all monitored parameters are shown in Figure 10.11. Since this is a black and white book, you cannot see three lines in color. If the figure were in color, you can see that the red line has converged to 1 and the blue (= green) lines are both stable. In Figure 10.12, the `density` plots are shown for all parameters, from where we can estimate summary statistics of the monitored nodes, pooling over the chains selected. Summary statistics for the monitored parameters are shown in Table 10.5. Comparison of the estimates from the mixed-effects model Va and the corresponding Bayesian model are also shown in Table 10.6, which shows that both estimates are quite similar despite high auto-correlations observed for three parameters.

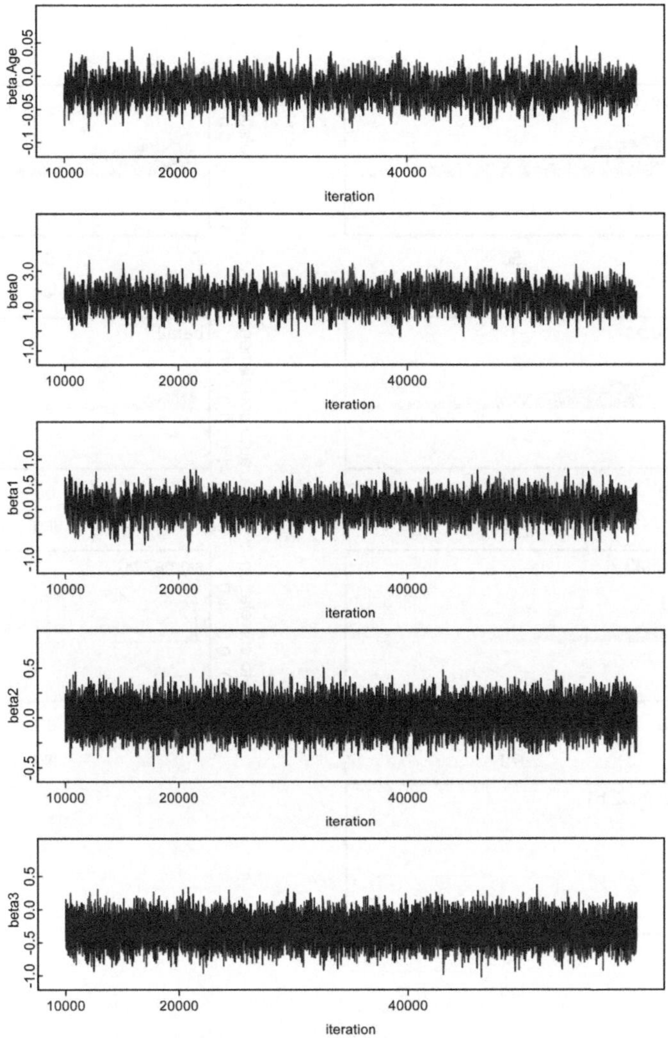

FIGURE 10.9
Epilepsy Data: History for some parameters of the Bayesian Poisson regression Model Va (2 chains are run for 50,000 iterations with a burn-in of 5,000 iterations).

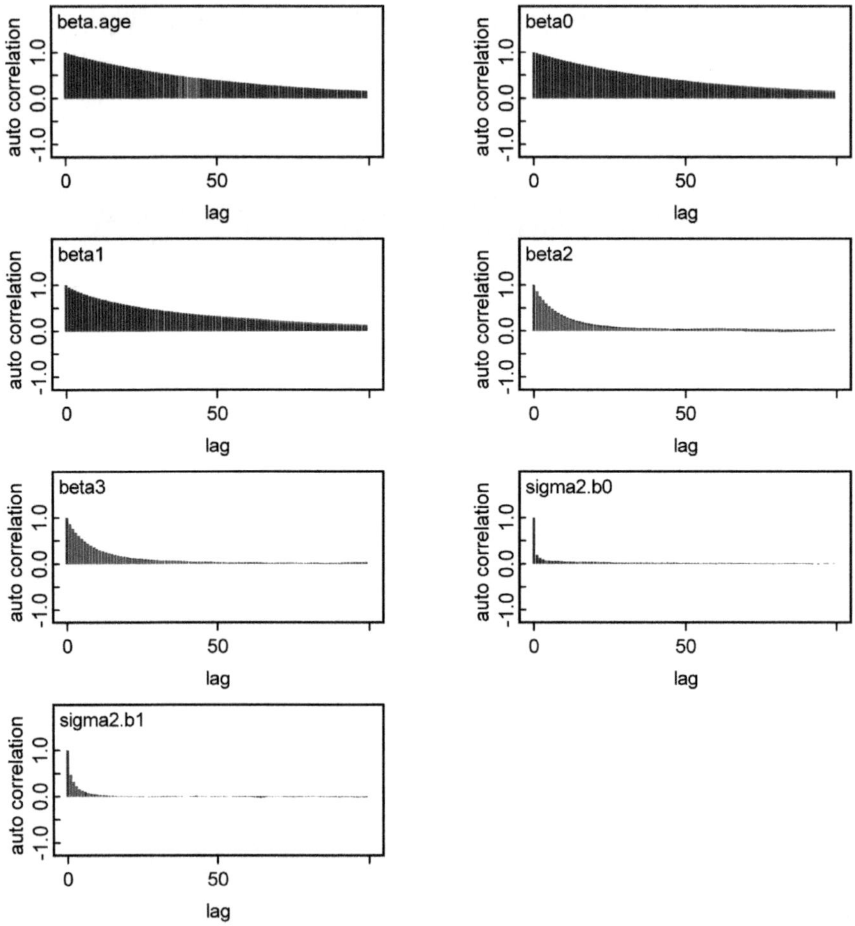

FIGURE 10.10
Epilepsy Data: Auto-correlation for all monitored parameters of the Bayesian Poisson regression Model Va.

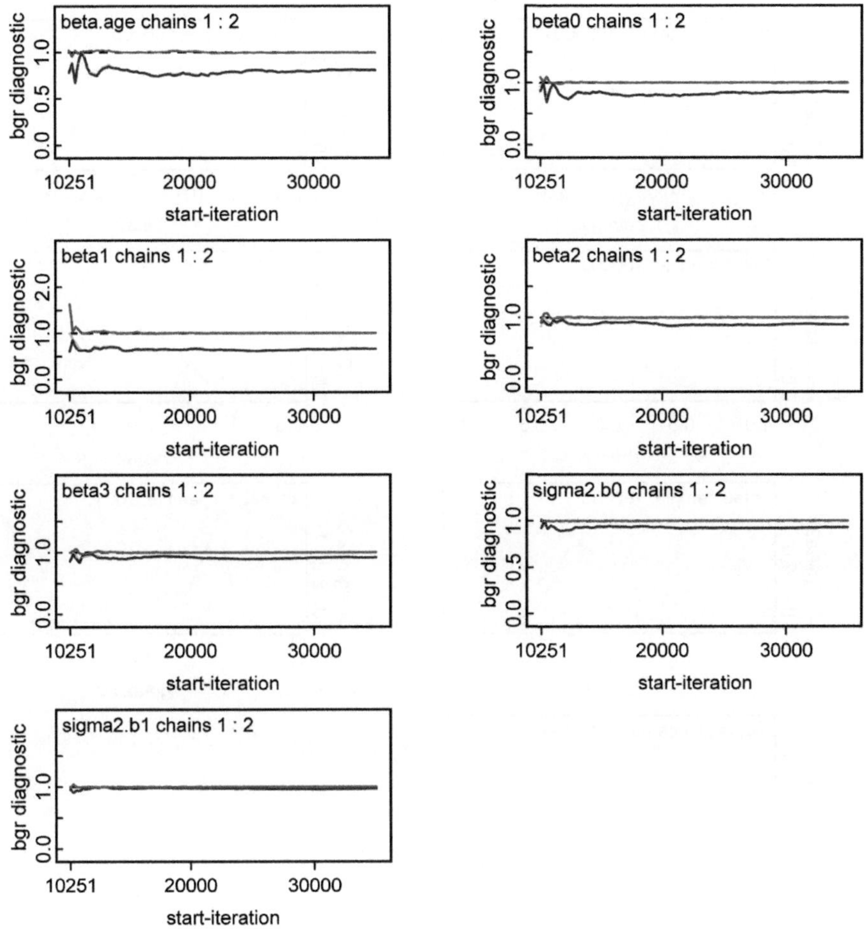

FIGURE 10.11
Epilepsy Data: BGR diagram for all monitored parameters of the Bayesian Poisson regression Model Va.

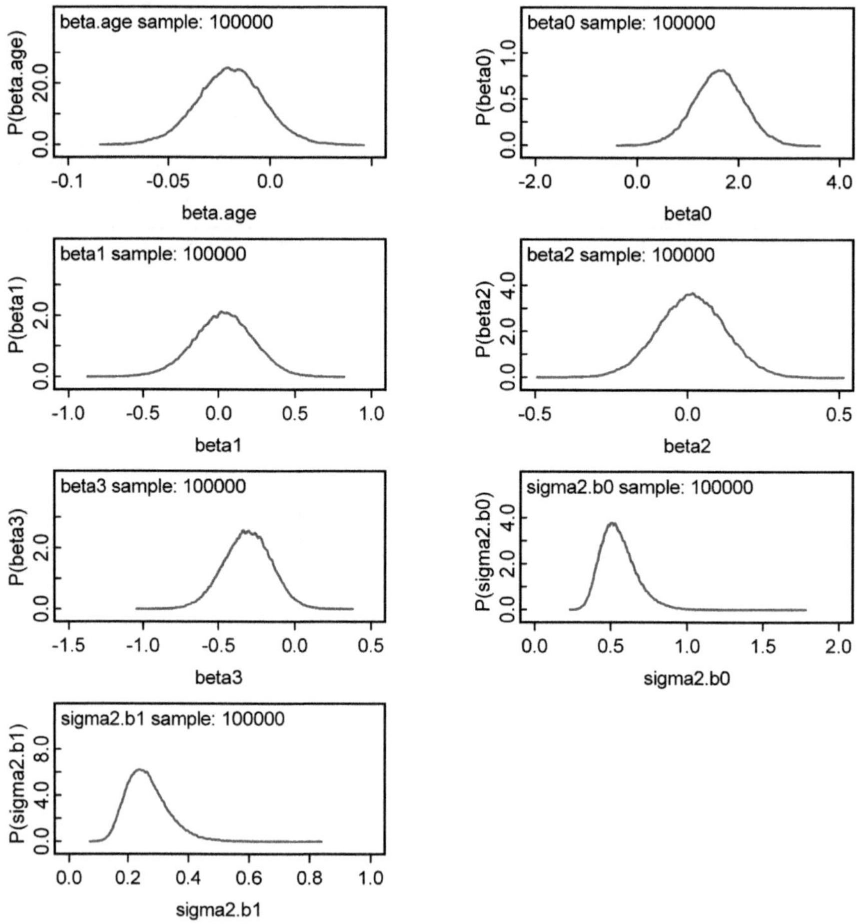

FIGURE 10.12
Epilepsy Data: Posterior densities for all parameters of the Bayesian Poisson regression Model Va.

TABLE 10.5
Epilepsy Data: Summary statistics of the Bayesian Model Va. 'Sample size" (= 100,000) is excluded for space.

Node	Mean	sd	MC error	2.5%	Median	97.5%	Start
beta.age	-0.020	0.016	4.77E-4	-0.050	-0.020	0.011	10001
beta0	1.628	0.480	0.0155	0.703	1.626	2.583	10001
beta1	0.029	0.205	0.00842	-0.378	0.0312	0.425	10001
beta2	0.014	0.115	0.00344	-0.205	0.0117	0.243	10001
beta3	-0.308	0.155	0.00472	-0.623	-0.306	-0.007	10001
sigma2.b0	0.551	0.117	8.15E-4	0.366	0.5362	0.821	10001
sigma2.b1	0.264	0.070	4.63E-4	0.154	0.2552	0.427	10001

TABLE 10.6
Epilepsy Data: Comparison of the mixed-effects Poisson regression Model Va and the corresponding Bayesian model.

Model	Mixed-effects model			Bayesian model		
		95% CI			95% CI	
Parameter	Estimate	Lower	Upper	Estimate	Lower	Upper
Intercept ($\hat{\beta}_0$)	1.630	0.690	2.569	1.628	0.703	2.583
age	-0.020	-0.050	0.011	-0.020	-0.050	0.011
treatment ($\hat{\beta}_1$)	0.027	-0.357	0.411	0.026	-0.378	0.425
post ($\hat{\beta}_2$)	0.012	-0.205	0.229	0.014	-0.205	0.243
treatment*post ($\hat{\beta}_3$)	-0.309	-0.611	-0.006	-0.308	-0.623	-0.007
$\hat{\sigma}^2_{B0}$	0.501	(s.e. = 0.100)		0.536	0.366	0.821
$\hat{\sigma}^2_{B1}$	0.242	(s.e. = 0.062)		0.255	0.154	0.427

11

Latent profile models: Classification of individual response profiles

The main focus of this book is to introduce the generalized linear mixed-effects models, which provide a flexible and powerful tool to deal with longitudinal data with heterogeneity or variability among subject-specific responses and missing data. In these mixed-effects models, the subject-specific response has been considered as a *random-effects* variable assumed to be normally distributed. Verbeke and Lesaffre (1996, 2001) proposed a linear mixed-effects model with heterogeneity for random effects by allowing the random effects to be taken from a mixture of several normal distributions with equal covariance matrix. Although these models have been developed for dealing with heterogeneity or variability among subject-specific responses, it seems to me that they are still based upon the "homogeneous" assumption in the sense that the *fixed-effects mean response profile within each treatment group is meaningful*, and thus the treatment effect is usually evaluated by the difference in mean response profiles or difference in means during the pre-specified evaluation periods near the end of follow-up. However, if the *subject by time interaction* within each treatment group is not negligible, the mean response profiles could be inappropriate measures for treatment effect.

For example, Figure 11.1 shows the subject-specific changes from baseline of log-transformed serum level of glutamate pyruvate transaminase (GPT) for each of treatment groups in a double-blinded placebo-controlled randomized trial of Gritiron for patients with chronic hepatitis (Yano et al., 1989). This data set is called here *Gritiron Data.* The result of this trial was summarized as the difference in median changes from baseline of log (GPT) as shown in Figure 11.2 and the difference at each evaluation time (4 weeks, 8 weeks, 12 weeks, and 16 weeks after randomization) was all statistically significant at $\alpha = 0.05$ by the two-tailed Bonferroni p-value adjusted Wilcoxon rank-sum test.

However, we can observe from this figure that, even if the subjects belong to the same treatment group, some are increasing, some are not changing, and some are decreasing. In this situation, one concern is that the mean response profile for each treatment group is really an appropriate summary statistic? To deal with the variability of the subject-specific response profiles, many authors, for example, Tango (1989, 1998), Skene and White (1992), Muthen and Shedden (1999), Lin, McCulloch, and Turnbull et al. (2000), and Lin,

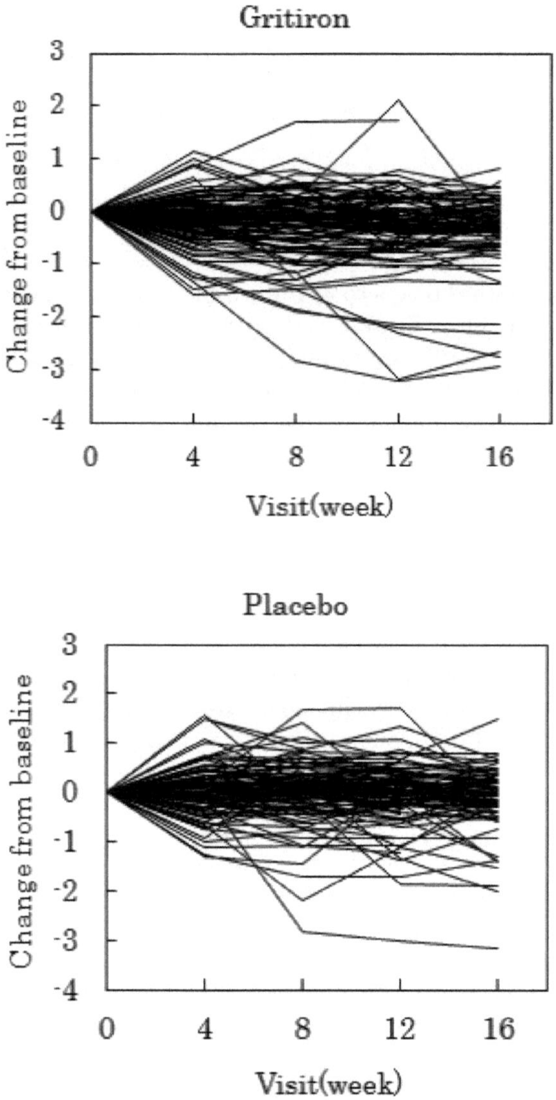

FIGURE 11.1
Gritiron Data: Subject-specific changes from baseline of log-transformed serum levels of GPT by treatment group in a double-blinded placebo-controlled randomized trial of Gritiron for patients with chronic hepatitis (Yano et al., 1989).

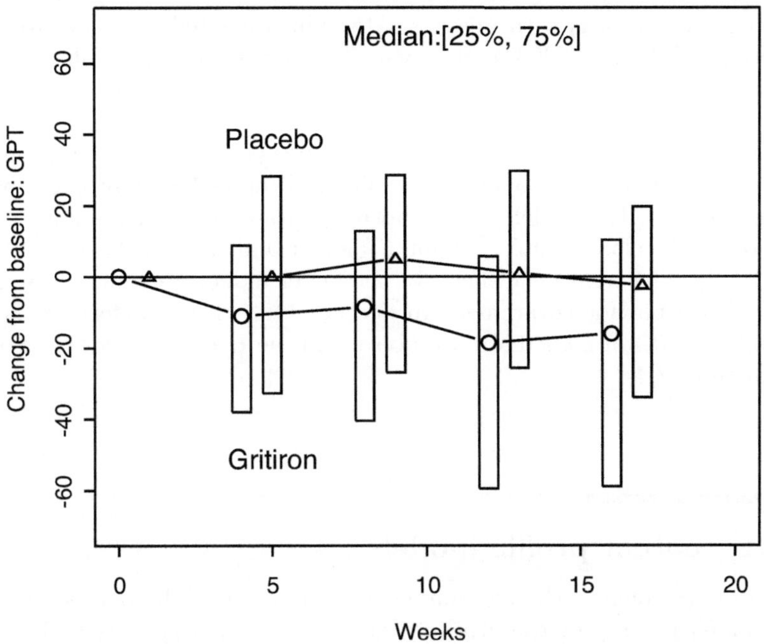

FIGURE 11.2
Gritiron Data: Median changes from baseline of log (GPT) by treatment group in a double-blinded placebo-controlled randomized trial of Gritiron for patients with chronic hepatitis patients. The difference at each evaluation time (4 weeks, 8 weeks, 12 weeks, and 16 weeks after randomization) was all statistically significant at $\alpha = 0.05$ by the two-tailed Bonferroni p-value adjusted Wilcoxon rank-sum test.

Turnbull, and McCulloch et al. (2002), have proposed several types of mixture models in which each treatment group consists of a mixture of several latent profiles (classes) of response variable.

Especially, Tango (1989) proposed a mixture model for the analysis of change from baseline in a randomized controlled trial assuming that (1) each treatment group consists of a mixture of several "ordered" latent profiles such as "improved," "unchanged," "worsened," (2) a low-degree polynomial can represent the mean response profile for each of latent profiles, and (3) the treatment effect can be characterized by the shape of the latent profiles and the difference in the mixing proportions of these latent profiles. Skene and White (1992) also proposed a similar mixture model but it is undesirable since it estimates unrealistic ragged profiles and it cannot cope with incomplete data that contains missing data or is measured at irregularly spaced intervals. Tango (1998) modified his model so that it can cope with improper longitudinal records with missing data, which is cited as a new approach by Everitt and Pickles (2004). However, Tango did not take both covariate adjustments and the nature of "ordered" classes into account in evaluating the treatment effect.

The purpose of this chapter is to introduce (1) Tango's latent profile model and (2) an extended model by combining Tango's latent profile model with proportional odds model to take both covariate adjustments and the nature of "ordered" classes into account (Taguchi and Tango, 2008; Nakamura et al., 2012). The treatment effect for the latter model is estimated by the odds ratio (adjusted for covariates). In Section 11.4, these models are illustrated with the *Gritiron Data* discussed above and the *Beat the Blues Data* discussed in Chapter 7.

11.1 Latent profile models

Let $y_{ij}(t_{ijk})$ denote the measurement made at the kth time point t_{ijk} ($k = 0, 1, ..., K_{ij}(\leq T)$) of the jth subject ($j = 1, 2, ..., n_j$) in the ith treatment group ($i = 1, 2$), where $y_{ij}(t_{ij0}) = y_{ij}(0)$ indicates the baseline level and the change from baseline is defined as $d_{ij}(t_{ijk}) = y_{ij}(t_{ijk}) - y_{ij}(0)$. Further assume the existence of M latent profiles of change from baseline that are common to all the treatment groups. Then, under the condition that the jth subject of the ith treatment group follows the mth latent profile ($m = 1, 2, ..., M$), it can be assumed that

$$d_{ij}(t) \mid m = \mu_m(t) + \varepsilon_{ij}(t), \quad \varepsilon_{ij}(t) \sim N(0, \sigma^2), \tag{11.1}$$

where $\mu_m(t)$ is the mean profile of the mth latent profile and it is assumed that the mth latent profile and $\varepsilon_{ij}(t)$ are, conditional on m, mutually independent. Regarding the latent profile, Tango (1989) proposed a smooth low-degree polynomial function of time, i.e.,

$$\mu_m(t) = \sum_{r=1}^{R} \beta_{mr} t^r, \tag{11.2}$$

where R is the degree of polynomial common to all the profiles except for the unchanged profile. Without loss of generality, let us assume here that the treatment effect is evaluated by the "decrease" from the baseline level. For example, when $M = 3$, we have

$$\mu(t) = \begin{cases} \mu_1(t) = \sum_{r=1}^{R} \beta_{1r} t^r (< 0) & \text{“}\textit{improved}\text{”} \\ \mu_2(t) = 0 & \text{“}\textit{unchanged}\text{”} \\ \mu_3(t) = \sum_{r=1}^{R} \beta_{3r} t^r (> 0) & \text{“}\textit{worsened.}\text{”} \end{cases} \tag{11.3}$$

When $M = 5$, we have

$$\mu(t) = \begin{cases} \mu_1(t) = \sum_{r=1}^{R} \beta_{1r} t^r (< \mu_2(t)) & \text{“}\textit{greatly improved}\text{”} \\ \mu_2(t) = \sum_{r=1}^{R} \beta_{2r} t^r (< 0) & \text{“}\textit{improved}\text{”} \\ \mu_3(t) = 0 & \text{“}\textit{unchanged}\text{”} \\ \mu_4(t) = \sum_{r=1}^{R} \beta_{4r} t^r (> 0) & \text{“}\textit{worsened}\text{”} \\ \mu_5(t) = \sum_{r=1}^{R} \beta_{5r} t^r (> \mu_3(t)) & \text{“}\textit{greatly worsened.}\text{”} \end{cases} \tag{11.4}$$

As M should be initially set as an odd number for symmetry, the middle, the $\frac{M+1}{2}$th latent profile, is “unchanged” class and $\beta_{(M+1)/2,r} = 0$, $\mu_{(M+1)/2}(t) = 0$. In this mixture model, the response profile for the jth subject of ith group $\boldsymbol{d}_{ij} = \left(d_{ij}(t_{ij1}), \cdots, d_{ij}(t_{ijK_{ij}})\right)^t$ has the following mixture density,

$$g_i\left(\boldsymbol{d}_{ij} \,|\, \boldsymbol{\phi}_1\right) = \sum_{m=1}^{M} p_{im} f_m(\boldsymbol{d}_{ij}), \tag{11.5}$$

where p_{im} denotes the mixing probability of the mth latent profile in the ith treatment group and $f_m(\cdot)$ denotes the density function of the mth latent profile, which is given by

$$f_m(\boldsymbol{d}_{ij}) = \left(\frac{1}{2\pi\sigma^2}\right)^{\frac{K_{ij}}{2}} \exp\left\{-\frac{1}{2\sigma^2} \sum_{k=1}^{K_{ij}} \left(d_{ij}(t_{ijk}) - \mu_m(t_{ijk})\right)^2\right\} \tag{11.6}$$

and $\boldsymbol{\phi}_1$ denotes the vector of parameters included in the model, i.e.,

$$\boldsymbol{\phi}_1 = (p_{11}, ..., p_{1M}, p_{21}, ..., p_{2M}, \beta_{11}, ..., \beta_{1R}, ..., \beta_{M1}, ..., \beta_{MR}, \sigma^2)^t.$$

In this mixture model, the comparison of treatment effect can be reduced to the test of the following null hypothesis

$$\begin{aligned} H_0 &: p_{11} = p_{21},\ ...,\ p_{1M} = p_{2M} \\ H_1 &: \text{not } H_0. \end{aligned} \tag{11.7}$$

Given the number of latent profiles M, the usual likelihood ratio test can be applied to test the above null hypothesis. Furthermore, this model provides us with a criterion of classification of subjects into one of the latent classes based on the maximum of the posterior probability that the jth subject of the dth treatment group comes from the mth latent profile

$$\hat{Q}_{ij}(m) = \frac{\hat{p}_{im} f_m(\boldsymbol{d}_{ij})}{g_i(\boldsymbol{d}_{ij}|\hat{\boldsymbol{\phi}}_1)}, \tag{11.8}$$

where $\hat{\boldsymbol{\phi}}_1$ denotes the maximum likelihood estimate. Goodness-of-fit of the model is investigated by observing each patient's response pattern classified according to the max $Q_{ij}(m)$ in relation to the estimated 95% region for each latent profile as shown below.

$$\hat{\mu}_m(t) \pm 2\hat{\sigma} \tag{11.9}$$

E-M algorithm

To obtain the maximum likelihood estimate of parameter $\boldsymbol{\phi}_1$, a Newton–Raphson algorithm and the EM algorithm have been used. Especially the use of the EM algorithm can be recommended for its easy implementation. Its solution, however, heavily depends on the initial values and then careful examination is necessary to assure that the global, rather than a local, maximum was attained. The EM algorithm is briefly outlined below:

1. Step 0: Give starting initial values of the posterior probability $Q_{ij}(m)$. One simple way to do this is to calculate the subject-specific total sum of d_{ij} adjusted for the number of missing data, i.e.,

$$S_{ij} = \frac{T}{K_{ij}} \sum_{k=1}^{K_{ij}} d_{ij}(t_{ijk}).$$

   Then, for example, in the case of $M = 3$, we can use the following classification rule

$$\begin{cases} Q_{ij}(1) = 1, & \text{if } S_{ij} < \text{ 25 percentile of } S_{ij} \\ Q_{ij}(2) = 1, & \text{if } S_{ij} \geq \text{ 75 percentile of } S_{ij} \\ Q_{ij}(0) = 1, & \text{otherwise.} \end{cases}$$

2. Step 1: M-step

   Given the $\hat{Q}_{ij}(m)$, the parameters p_{im} are easily calculated as

$$\hat{p}_{im} = \sum_{j=1}^{n_i} \hat{Q}_{ij}(m)/n_i \tag{11.10}$$

   and $\hat{\beta}_{mk}$ are obtained by using a weighted least squares procedure minimizing

$$\sum_{i=1}^{2}\sum_{j=1}^{n_i}\sum_{m=1}^{M} \hat{Q}_{ij}(m) \sum_{k=1}^{K_{ij}} (d_{ij}(t_{ijk}) - \mu_m(t_{ijk}))^2 \tag{11.11}$$

   and $\hat{\sigma}^2$ is obtained as

$$\hat{\sigma}^2 = \sum_{i=1}^{2}\sum_{j=1}^{n_i}\sum_{m=1}^{M} \hat{Q}_{ij}(m) \sum_{k=1}^{K_{ij}} (d_{ij}(t_{ijk}) - \hat{\mu}_m(t_{ijk}))^2 / \sum_{i=1}^{2}\sum_{j=1}^{n_i} K_{ij}. \tag{11.12}$$

3. Step 2: E-step Calculate the posteriori probability $\hat{Q}_{ij}(m)$ based on the estimates $\hat{\boldsymbol{\phi}}_1 = (\hat{p}_{im}, \hat{\beta}_{mk}, \hat{\sigma}^2)^t$ obtained in Step 1.

4. Step 3: Check to see if $\hat{\boldsymbol{\phi}}_1$ has converged; if not, repeat the M-step and E-step.

11.2 Latent profile plus proportional odds model

In Tango's mixture model, the treatment effect is evaluated by the difference in the mixing probabilities and thus even when the null hypothesis (11.7) is rejected, its interpretation is not always easy due to at most $(M - 1)$ degrees of freedom. Furthermore, Tango's model does not take both covariate adjustments and the nature of "ordered" latent classes into account. Therefore, we introduce here a new mixture model by combining Tango's model with a proportional odds model to take both covariate adjustments and the nature of "ordered" latent classes into account, where the treatment effect can be estimated by a covariate-adjusted odds ratio.

Here, let us get back to the notation of *repeated measures design* defined in Chapter 1, i.e., using the following notational change:

$$ij \to i, \; k \to j, \; K_{ij} \to K_i, \; d_{ij}(t) \to d_{ij}, t_{ijk} \to t_{ij}.$$

Furthermore, let $(w_{1i}, ..., w_{qi})$ denote the vector of covariates with fixed effects of the ith subject and the first covariate w_{1i} denotes the treatment group,

$$w_{1i} = 1 \text{ (New treatment)}, \; = 0 \text{ (Control treatment)}.$$

Then, the *latent profile plus proportional odds model* is defined as follows:

$$h\left(\boldsymbol{d}_i \,|\boldsymbol{\phi}_2\right) = \sum_{m=1}^{M} r_{im} f_m(\boldsymbol{d}_i) \tag{11.13}$$

$$\log\left(\frac{q_{im}}{1 - q_{im}}\right) = \theta_m + \sum_{s=1}^{q} \gamma_s w_{si} \quad (m = 1, \cdots, M-1), \tag{11.14}$$

where r_{im} denotes the probability that the ith subject comes from the mth latent profile and q_{im} denotes the cumulative probability up to and including the category m of the probability r_{im}, i.e.,

$$q_{im} = r_{i1} + \cdots + r_{im}, \tag{11.15}$$

and $\boldsymbol{\phi}_2$ denotes the vector of parameters included in the combined model, i.e.,

$$\boldsymbol{\phi}_2 = (\beta_{11}, ..., \beta_{1R}, ..., \beta_{M1}, ..., \beta_{MR}, \sigma^2, \gamma_1, ..., \gamma_I, \theta_1, ..., \theta_{M-1})^t.$$

The log-likelihood function is given by

$$l = \sum_{i=1}^{N} \log\left\{h\left(\boldsymbol{d}_i \,|\boldsymbol{\phi}_2\right)\right\}. \tag{11.16}$$

In the latent profile plus proportional odds model, the treatment effect is evaluated by testing the following null hypothesis:

$$H_0 : \gamma_1 = 0, \; H_1 : \gamma_1 > 0. \tag{11.17}$$

The estimated odds ratio $e^{\hat{\gamma}_1}$ will be interpreted as the **improvement odds ratio** of the new treatment to the control treatment.

For comparison with Tango's original latent profile model, consider a simple situation where we have only one covariate w_1 indicating the treatment group in the case of $M = 3$. Then, letting $\gamma = \gamma_1$, we have

$$\begin{aligned}
\log\left(\frac{r_{i1}}{1-r_{i1}}\right) &= \begin{cases} \theta_1, & \text{(control)} \\ \theta_1+\gamma, & \text{(new treatment)} \end{cases} \\
\log\left(\frac{r_{i1}+r_{i2}}{1-(r_{i1}+r_{i2})}\right) &= \begin{cases} \theta_2, & \text{(control)} \\ \theta_2+\gamma, & \text{(new treatment).} \end{cases}
\end{aligned}$$

In other words, the relationships between r_{im} (i means a subject) and p_{im} (i means a treatment group) are given by

$$\begin{aligned}
m=1: r_{i1}=r_1 &= \begin{cases} \frac{1}{1+e^{-\theta_1}}, & \text{(control)} \;\rightarrow p_{11} \\ \frac{1}{1+e^{-(\theta_1+\gamma)}}, & \text{(new treatment)} \;\rightarrow p_{21} \end{cases} \\
m=2: r_{i2}=r_2 &= \begin{cases} \frac{1}{1+e^{-\theta_2}} - \frac{1}{1+e^{-\theta_1}}, & \text{(control)} \;\rightarrow p_{12} \\ \frac{1}{1+e^{-(\theta_2+\gamma)}} - \frac{1}{1+e^{-(\theta_1+\gamma)}}, & \text{(new treatment)} \;\rightarrow p_{22} \end{cases} \\
m=3: r_{i3}=r_3 &= 1-r_1-r_2.
\end{aligned}$$

To examine the proportional odds assumption, let us consider the following non-proportional odds model

$$\log\left(\frac{q_{im}}{1-q_{im}}\right) = \theta_m + \sum_{s=1}^{q}(\gamma_s+\eta_{s(m)})w_{si}, \quad (\eta_{s(1)}=0). \tag{11.18}$$

Then, the null hypothesis for testing the proportional odds assumption will be

$$H_0: \eta_{s(m)} = 0, \quad s=1,...,q;\; m=2,...,M-1. \tag{11.19}$$

The log-likelihood for the parameters of the model (11.18) is

$$l = \sum_{i=1}^{N} \log\{h(\boldsymbol{d}_i \,|\phi_2, \boldsymbol{\eta})\}, \tag{11.20}$$

where $\boldsymbol{\eta} = (\eta_{1(2)}, ..., \eta_{q(M-1)})^t$. The efficient score for the log-likelihood (11.20) is

$$\begin{aligned} U(\boldsymbol{\phi}_2, \boldsymbol{\eta}) &= \left(\frac{\partial l}{\partial \beta_{11}}, \cdots, \frac{\partial l}{\partial \beta_{MR}}, \frac{\partial l}{\partial \sigma^2}, \frac{\partial l}{\partial \gamma_1}, \cdots, \frac{\partial l}{\partial \gamma_q}, \frac{\partial l}{\partial \theta_1}, \right. \\ & \left. \cdots \frac{\partial l}{\partial \theta_{M-1}}, \frac{\partial l}{\partial \eta_{1(2)}}, \cdots, \frac{\partial l}{\partial \eta_{q(M-1)}} \right)^t. \end{aligned}$$

Then, the proportional odds assumption can be tested by the following efficient score test,

$$X^2 = U(\hat{\boldsymbol{\phi}}_2, \boldsymbol{\eta} = 0)^t H^{-1}(\hat{\boldsymbol{\phi}}_2, \boldsymbol{\eta} = 0) U(\hat{\boldsymbol{\phi}}_2, \boldsymbol{\eta} = 0) \sim \chi^2_{(M-2)q}, \qquad (11.21)$$

where $\hat{\boldsymbol{\phi}}_2$ denotes the vector of the maximum likelihood estimates and $\hat{H}$ denotes the negative of the Hessian matrix (second derivative of the log-likelihood) evaluated under the null hypothesis (11.19). The maximum likelihood estimates of parameters can be obtained by the Newton–Raphson algorithm and/or the EM algorithm.

11.3 Number of latent profiles

It is well known that the classical asymptotic theory of distribution of likelihood ratio tests cannot be applied to testing the number of components in mixture models because it does not satisfy the regularity condition. Self and Liang (1987) discussed its theoretical issues and gave several examples in which the distribution can be expressed as mixtures of chi-squared distribution. However, its application to mixture models is difficult. Everitt (1981), Thord, Finch and Mendell (1988) conducted a simulation study to find the percentage points of the likelihood ratio test. McLachlan (1987) applied boostrapping methods. So far, the challenge to the distribution of the likelihood ratio test has never been successful. Therefore, especially in confirmatory trials such as phase III randomized controlled trials, the number of latent profiles should not be selected statistically but be carefully discussed before starting clinical trials and be specified in the protocol. Given the number, or the maximum number, of latent profiles, the problem becomes simple. Within the specified range of M, the optimal M can be chosen by applying the AIC or BIC (McLachlan and Peel, 2000) together with graphical investigation of the estimated 95% region for each latent profile and individual response profiles classified into the corresponding latent profile.

TABLE 11.1
Gritiron Data: A part of the data from the double-blinded placebo-controlled randomized trial of Gritiron for chronic patients. NA denotes missing data.

No.	subject	center	treatment	age	visit	gpt
1	1	1	1	76	0	52
2	1	1	1	76	4	76
3	1	1	1	76	8	81
4	1	1	1	76	12	77
5	1	1	1	76	16	70
6	2	1	1	54	0	51
7	2	1	1	54	4	74
8	2	1	1	54	8	86
9	2	1	1	54	12	66
10	2	1	1	54	16	83
11	3	1	1	66	0	91
12	3	1	1	66	4	138
13	3	1	1	66	8	147
14	3	1	1	66	12	74
15	3	1	1	66	16	90
16	4	1	1	24	0	164
17	4	1	1	24	4	116
18	4	1	1	24	8	80
19	4	1	1	24	12	94
20	4	1	1	24	16	NA

11.4 Application to the Gritiron Data

We shall illustrate the above-stated two kinds of latent profile models with a subset of the *Gritiron Data* shown in Figures 11.1 and 11.2 where $N = 212$ patients with chronic hepatitis who were randomly assigned to the Gritiron group ($n_2 = 106$ patients) and the placebo group ($n_1 = 106$ patients) in a multi-centered double-blinded randomized controlled trial (Yano et al., 1989). Laboratory data including GPT were scheduled to be measured at baseline and at 4-week intervals thereafter up to 16 weeks (*1:4* design). One of the primary endpoints is the change from the baseline of log-transformed GPT. In this trial, the effect of treatment can be observed as a "decrease" in levels of GPT as compared with baseline level, where the change from baseline should be negative. Coincidentally, the number of patients who have missing data is the same 23 for both groups. In this application, we shall consider the maximum number of latent profiles as set to 5 because several other ordinal categorical endpoints were evaluated by 5 ordered categories. Table 11.1 shows a part of the *Gritiron Data* [1] with long format where missing data is coded as "NA" and consists of the following six variables:

1. `subject`: a numeric factor indicating the patient ID.
2. `center`: a numeric factor indicating the center ID.
3. `treatment`: a binary variable indicating the treatment group (Gritiron=1, placebo=0).
4. `age`: a continuous variable for age.
5. `visit`: a numeric factor indicating the week of visit: takes 0 (baseline), 4, 8, 12, 16.
6. `gpt`: the primary endpoint of log-transformed GPT, $\log(GPT + 1.0)$.

Let us consider here the three models $M = 3, 4, 5$ for the number of latent profiles and a quadratic polynomial function of time, i.e., $R = 2$ for all the models, i.e.,

$$\mu_m(t) = \beta_{m1}t + \beta_{m2}t^2.$$

Cubic polynomial models with $R = 3$ did not bring significant improvement of the goodness-of-fit for most models. As a covariate, we consider the baseline level of log-transformed GPT.

11.4.1 Latent profile models

Regarding the estimates of the latent profile models, we first obtain the maximum likelihood estimates using an `R` or `S-Plus` code. Then, we also obtain the estimates of the Bayesian version of latent profile models using `OpenBUGS` code because *we are still facing the convergence problem of our program (*`R` *code) regarding the maximum likelihood estimates of the latent profile plus proportional odds model.*

First of all, the estimated latent profiles $\hat{\mu}_m(t)$, the 95% region of profiles $\hat{\mu}_m(t) \pm 2\hat{\sigma}$, and the patient-specific profiles classified into the corresponding latent profile of each of three models $M = 3, 4, 5$ are shown in Figures 11.3, 11.4 and 11.5, respectively. The classification of patients by each of three kinds ($M = 3, 4, 5$) of latent profile models are shown in Table 11.2. Furthermore, estimates of the mixing probabilities $\hat{p}_{im}$ and fixed-effects parameters of latent profiles $\hat{\beta}_{mr}$ are shown in Tables 11.3, 11.4, and 11.5, respectively.

For example, Figure 11.3 clearly shows that there are several patients classified into the latent profile "improved" who do not fit the model, i.e., their response profiles are out of the estimated 95% region of the profile, downward

[1] The *Gritiron Data* set cannot be open at present.

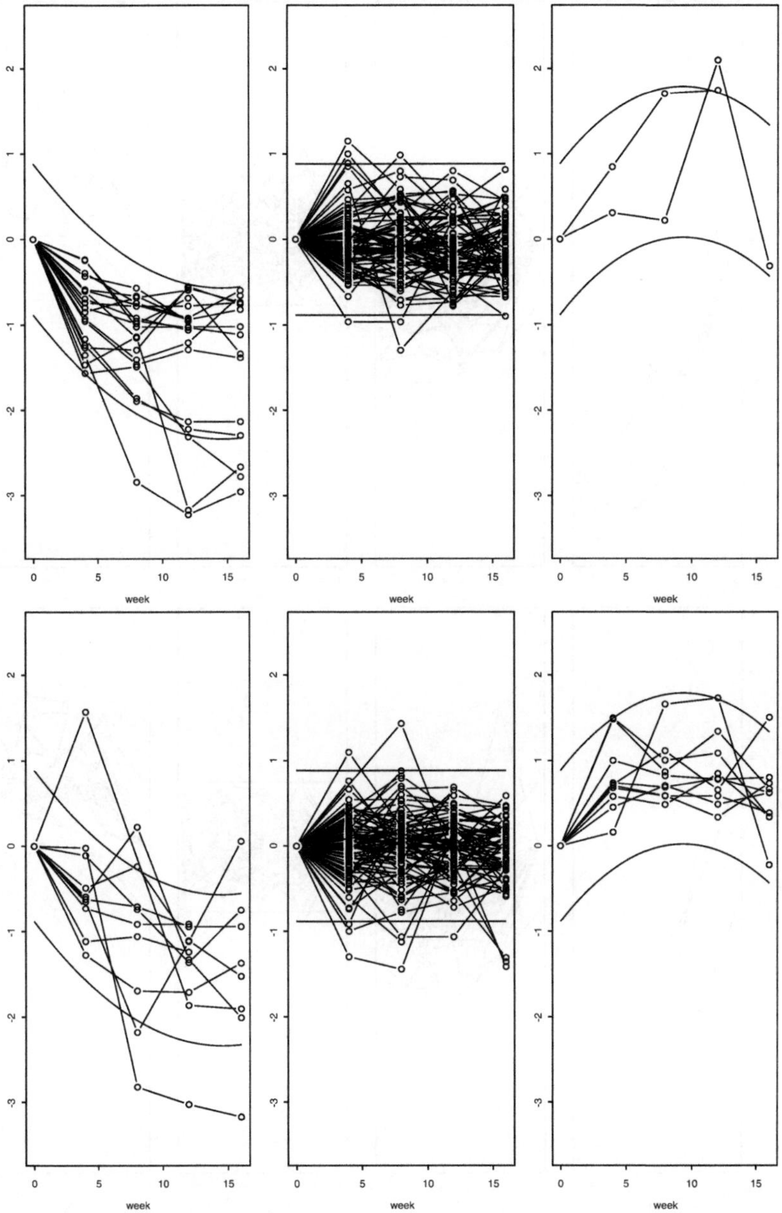

FIGURE 11.3
Gritiron Data with $M = 3$: Estimated latent profiles $\hat{\mu}_m(t)$, the 95% region of profiles $\hat{\mu}_m(t) \pm 2\hat{\sigma}$, and the subject-specific profiles classified into the corresponding latent profile. The upper profiles indicate the Gritiron group and the lower profiles, the placebo group.

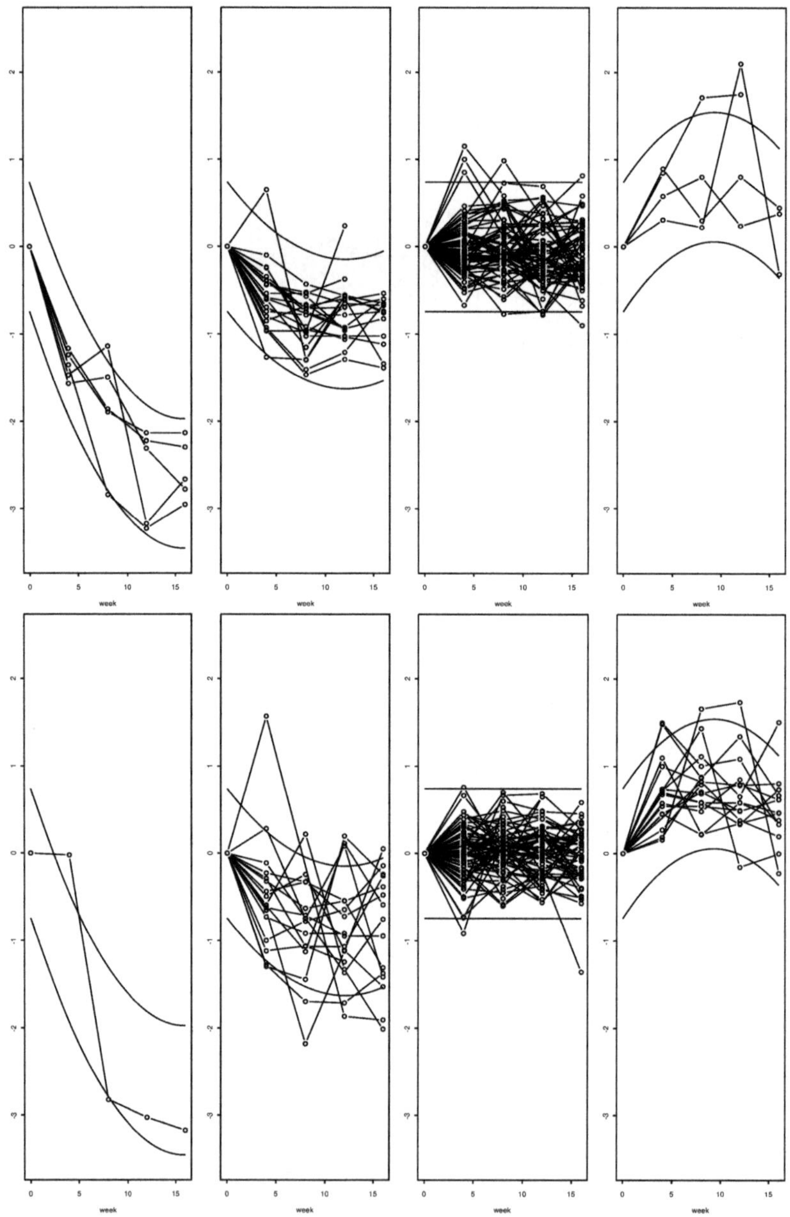

FIGURE 11.4
Gritiron Data with $M = 4$: Estimated latent profiles $\hat{\mu}_m(t)$, the 95% region of profiles $\hat{\mu}_m(t) \pm 2\hat{\sigma}$, and the subject-specific profiles classified into the corresponding latent profile. The upper profiles indicate the Gritiron group and the lower profiles, the placebo group.

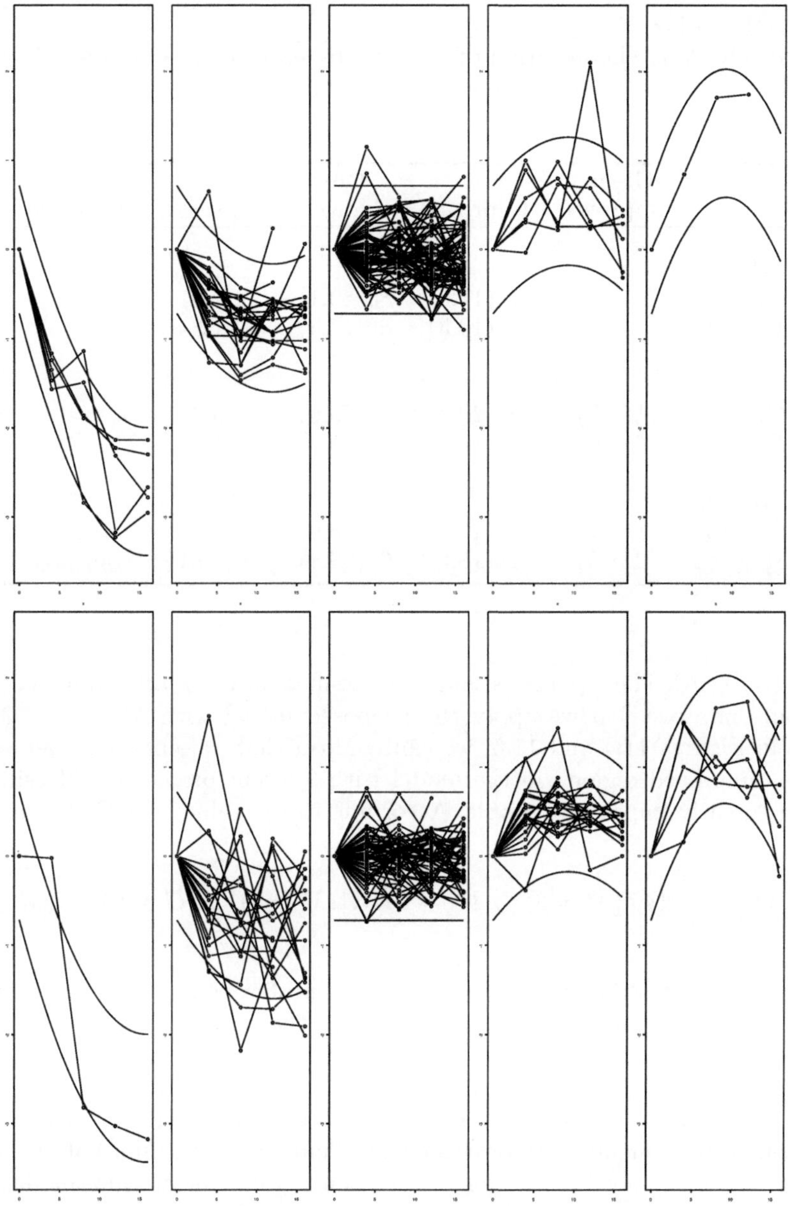

FIGURE 11.5
Gritiron Data with $M = 5$: Estimated latent profiles $\hat{\mu}_m(t)$, the 95% region of profiles $\hat{\mu}_m(t) \pm 2\hat{\sigma}$, and the subject-specific profiles classified into the corresponding latent profile. The upper profiles indicate the Gritiron group and the lower profiles, the placebo group.

TABLE 11.2
Gritiron Data: classification of patients by each of three kinds ($M = 3, 4, 5$) of latent profile models. The estimated mixing probabilities $\hat{p}_{im}$ are shown in parentheses.

	Grealty improved	Improved	Un-changed	Worsened	Greatly worsened	Total
$M = 3$						
Gritiron		19(17.0)	85(80.1)	2(2.9)		106
Placebo		10(10.3)	86(77.3)	10(12.4)		106
$M = 4$						
Gritiron	5(4.7)	21(20.4)	76(69.6)	4(5.3)		106
Placebo	1(1.0)	17(16.1)	71(65.5)	17(17.4)		106
$M = 5$						
Gritiron	5(4.7)	22(20.8)	72(66.0)	6(7.4)	1(1.0)	106
Placebo	1(1.0)	18(16.5)	62(59.1)	20(19.1)	5(4.3)	106

and outward. These patients could be classified into "Greatly improved" rather than "improved" if we apply the proposed model with $M = 4$ or $M = 5$. From Figures 11.4 and 11.5, we can confirm that patients who were outside the "improved region" in the model with 3 latent profiles are classified into the "greatly improved" profile. According to the value of AIC, we have

$$AIC = 1214.4(M = 3),\ AIC = 1037.1(M = 4),\ AIC = 1028.4(M = 5),$$

which indicates the model with five latent profiles is the best.

As a second step of analysis, we applied the Bayesian version of the latent profile model with non-informative priors, and the resultant estimates are also shown in the same Tables 11.3, 11.4, and 11.5. We can observe that these two kinds of estimates are shown to be quite similar for each of three latent profile models. As described in Chapter 11, an information criterion DIC (10.4) cannot be used for comparison of different mixture models. So in these tables, the value of deviance ($= -2 \log L$) is shown.

11.4.2 R, S-Plus, and OpenBUGS programs

The `R` or `S-Plus` programs used to obtain the maximum likelihood estimates of the latent profile models are available upon request. However, they cannot be of general use because the interface with a data file such as the *Gritiron Data*

TABLE 11.3
Gritiron Data with $M = 3$: Parameter estimates and standard errors from 4 kinds of latent profile models. The *unchanged profile* is defined as the profile $m = 2$ with $\beta_{21} = \beta_{22} = 0$.

	Latent profile model		Latent profile + proportional odds model	
Parameter	MLE	Bayesian	MLE	Bayesian
$-2\log L$	1196.4	1176.0	1136.1	1128.0
AIC	1214.4		1154.1	
p_{11}	0.103	0.109 (0.030)		
p_{12}	0.773	0.779 (0.047)		
p_{13}	0.124	0.113 (0.039)		
p_{21}	0.170	0.170 (0.038)		
p_{22}	0.801	0.799 (0.042)		
p_{23}	0.029	0.031 (0.018)		
β_{11}	- 0.199	-0.200 (0.018)	-0.195 (0.017)	-0.200 (0.017)
β_{12}	0.007	0.007 (0.001)	0.007 (0.001)	0.007 (0.001)
β_{31}	0.194	0.210 (0.030)	0.185 (0.028)	0.205 (0.027)
β_{32}	-0.010	-0.011 (0.002)	-0.010 (0.002)	-0.011 (0.002)
σ	0.451	0.453 (0.012)	0.452 (0.011)	0.451 (0.011)
γ_1: treatment effect			0.896 (0.435)	0.890 (0.431)
γ_1: 95%CI			[0.043, 1.749]	[0.060, 1.755]
γ_2: baseline data			2.474 (0.409)	2.394 (0.379)
γ_2: 95%CI			[1.672, 3.276]	[1.687, 3.165]
θ_1			-12.858 (2.160)	-14.38 (2.030)
θ_2			-6.860 (1.744)	-7.982 (1.599)

TABLE 11.4
Gritiron Data with $M = 4$: Parameter estimates and standard errors from 4 kinds of latent profile models. The *unchanged profile* is defined as the profile $m = 3$ with $\beta_{31} = \beta_{32} = 0$.

	Latent profile model		Latent profile + proportional odds model	
Parameter	MLE	Bayesian	MLE	Bayesian
$-2 \log L$	1011.1	989.8	936.7	928.5
AIC	1037.1		960.7	
p_{11}	0.009	0.018 (0.013)		
p_{12}	0.161	0.160 (0.037)		
p_{13}	0.655	0.652 (0.053)		
p_{14}	0.174	0.169 (0.042)		
p_{21}	0.047	0.055 (0.022)		
p_{22}	0.203	0.199 (0.041)		
p_{23}	0.696	0.690 (0.048)		
p_{24}	0.053	0.056 (0.025)		
β_{11}	- 0.343	-0.343 (0.028)	-0.343 (0.029)	-0.343 (0.029)
β_{12}	0.011	0.011 (0.002)	0.011 (0.002)	0.011 (0.002)
β_{21}	-0.147	-0.151 (0.013)	-0.146 (0.013)	-0.151 (0.013)
β_{22}	0.006	0.006 (0.001)	0.006 (0.001)	0.006 (0.001)
β_{41}	0.172	0.178 (0.019)	0.171 (0.020)	0.178 (0.018)
β_{42}	-0.009	-0.010 (0.001)	-0.009 (0.001)	-0.010 (0.001)
σ	0.378	0.378 (0.010)	0.379 (0.008)	0.378 (0.010)
γ_1: treatment effect			0.811 (0.359)	0.811 (0.359)
γ_1: 95%CI			[0.107, 1.515]	[0.126, 1.529]
γ_2: baseline data			2.454 (0.346)	2.423 (0.327)
γ_2: 95%CI			[1.776, 3.132]	[1.806, 3.097]
θ_1			-15.319 (2.042)	-16.86 (1.929)
θ_2			-12.164 (1.801)	-13.71 (1.690)
θ_3			-7.302 (1.492)	-8.662 (1.369)

TABLE 11.5
Gritiron Data with $M = 5$: Parameter estimates and standard errors from 4 kinds of latent profile models. The *unchanged profile* is defined as the profile $m = 3$ with $\beta_{31} = \beta_{32} = 0$.

	Latent profile model		Latent profile + proportional odds model	
Parameter	MLE	Bayesian	MLE	Bayesian
$-2 \log L$	994.4	941.7		883.0
AIC	1028.4			
p_{11}	0.010	0.018 (0.013)		
p_{12}	0.165	0.163 (0.037)		
p_{13}	0.591	0.600 (0.055)		
p_{14}	0.191	0.174 (0.045)		
p_{15}	0.043	0.045 (0.022)		
p_{21}	0.047	0.054 (0.022)		
p_{22}	0.208	0.202 (0.041)		
p_{23}	0.660	0.656 (0.052)		
p_{24}	0.074	0.069 (0.030)		
p_{25}	0.010	0.018 (0.013)		
β_{11}	- 0.343	-0.347 (0.028)		-0.344 (0.028)
β_{12}	0.011	0.011 (0.002)		0.011 (0.002)
β_{21}	-0.146	-0.148 (0.013)		-0.148 (0.013)
β_{22}	0.006	0.006 (0.001)		0.006 (0.001)
β_{41}	0.117	0.128 (0.017)		0.126 (0.016)
β_{42}	-0.006	-0.006 (0.001)		-0.006 (0.001)
β_{51}	0.285	0.311 (0.042)		0.317 (0.042)
β_{52}	-0.016	-0.017 (0.003)		-0.018 (0.003)
σ	0.366	0.367 (0.010)		0.367 (0.010)
γ_1: treatment effect				0.833 (0.339)
γ_1: 95%CI				[0.183, 1.524]
γ_2: baseline data				2.340 (0.307)
γ_2: 95%CI				[1.768, 2.972]
θ_1				-16.42 (1.824)
θ_2				-13.24 (1.577)
θ_3				-8.753 (1.318)
θ_4				-6.315 (1.352)

including missing data is not yet generalized. Furthermore, we often face the problem of non-convergence of the `R` or `S-Plus` program for the latent profile plus proportional odds model. So, we consider the following steps to obtain the parameter estimates:

1. First, obtain the MLE for *a latent profile model* using our `R` or `S-Plus` program.

2. Second, obtain the Bayesian estimates for the corresponding *latent profile model* using `OpenBUGS`, in which some of the MLEs are used as the initial values.

3. Similarly. obtain the Bayesian estimates for the corresponding *latent profile plus proportional odds model* using `OpenBUGS`, in which some of the MLEs are used as the initial values.

Programs 11.1 and 11.2 show OpenBUGS code for the latent profile plus proportional odds model with three latent profiles ($M = 3$). It should be noted that in all our programs, the data record including missing data must be deleted in advance.

Program 11.1 OpenBUGS code (1) for the *latent profile plus proportional odds model* with $M = 3$

```
model {
  for(i in 1:N){
     T[i] ~ dcat( P[i, 1:3] )
     for(j in 1:nr[i]){
        lgbase[ ne[i]+j-1 ] <- log( base[ne[i]+j-1] + 1)
        cfb[i, j] <- log(gpt[ne[i]+j-1]+1) - log(base[ne[i]+j-1]+1)
        cfb[i, j] ~ dnorm(mu[ T[i], visit[ne[i]+j-1] ], tau)
    }
   P[i,1] <- 1/(1+exp( - (theta11 + gam1*treatment[ne[i]]
                    + gam2*(lgbase[ne[i]] - base.bar) )))
   P[i,2] <- 1/(1+exp( - (theta22 + gam1*treatment[ne[i]]
                    +  gam2*(lgbase[ne[i]] - base.bar) )))   -  P[i,1]
   P[i,3]<-  1 - P[i,1] - P[i,2]
   }
   for (k in 1:4){
      mu[1, time[k]]< -beta11* time[k] + beta12 * time[k]*time[k]
      mu[3, time[k]]<- (beta11+alp31)* time[k]
                           + (beta12+alp32) * time[k]*time[k]
      mu[2, time[k]]<- 0
   }
   base.bar <- mean( lgbase[] )
# priors
beta11 ~ dnorm(0.0,1.0E-4)
beta12 ~ dnorm(0.0,1.0E-4)
theta11 ~ dnorm(0.0,1.0E-4)
theta22 ~ dnorm(0.0,1.0E-4)
alp31 ~ dnorm(0.0,1.0E-4)
alp32 ~ dnorm(0.0,1.0E-4)
gam1 ~ dnorm(0.0,1.0E-4)
gam2 ~ dnorm(0.0,1.0E-4)
tau ~ dgamma(1.0E-3,1.0E-3)
sigma  <- 1.0/  sqrt(tau)
#
        beta31<-beta11+alp31
        beta32<-beta12+alp32
        theta1<-theta11 - gam2*base.bar
        theta2<-theta22 - gam2*base.bar
}
```

A brief account of OpenBUGS code (1) and (2)

- `N` denotes the number of patients.
- `T[i]` denotes the profile number m to which the patient i belongs. In this program, we set `T=c( 2, NA, 2, 2, 2, 1, ...)` as input data using a `list` statement. This means that, when the estimated posterior probability $\hat{Q}_{ij}(m)$ (11.8) of the latent profile model is quite large such as "larger than 0.9," then the patient i is forcibly assigned to the latent profile m. Otherwise, assigned to "NA."
- `P[i,1]`, `P[i,2]`, `P[i,3]` denote the probability $r_{im}, (m = 1, 2, 3)$.
- `nr[i]` denotes the number of observed data (≤ 4) of the patient i.

• `ne[i]` denotes the index number of the data record in which the patient i's data first appears.
• `beta11, beta12` denotes β_{11}, β_{12}.
• `theta1, theta2` denotes θ_1, θ_2.
• `gam1, gam2` denotes γ_1, γ_2.

Program 11.2. OpenBUGS code (2) for the *latent profile plus proportional odds model* with $M = 3$

```
# Initial values
list(tau =4,  beta11=-0.2, beta12=0.1, alp31= 0.5,
alp32= -0.01, theta11=0,theta22=1, gam1=0, gam2=0)
list(tau =5,  beta11=-0.3, beta12=0.04, alp31=0.35,
alp32=-0.02, theta11=1, theta22=2, gam1=1, gam2=1)

#Data
list(N=212,  time=c(4,8,12,16),
nr=c(4,   4,   4,   3,   4,     4,   4,   4,   4,   4,
      4,   4,   4,   4,   4,     4,   3,   4,   4,   4,
      4,   4,   4,   4,   4,     3,   4,   4,   4,   4,
      4,   3,   4,   1,   4,     3,   3,   2,   4,   3,
      2,   4,   2,   3,   4,     4,   3,   4,   4,   4,
      ...... ),
ne=c(1,   5,   9,  13,  16,  20,  24,  28,  32,  36,  40,
  44,  48,  52,  56,  60,  64,  67,  71,  75,  79,  83,  87,
  91,  95,  99, 102, 106, 110, 114, 118, 122, 125, 129, 130,
 134, 137, 140, 142, 146, 149, 151, 155, 157, 160, 164, 168,
 171, 175, 179, 183, 187, 191, 194, 198, 202, 206, 210, 214,
  ....) ,
T=c( 2, NA, 2, 2, 2, 1, 1, NA, 2, 2, 2, 2, 2, 2, 2, NA, 2, 2, 2, 2,
   2, 2, NA, NA, NA, 2, 2, 2, 2, 2, 2, 2, 2, 2, 2, 2, 2, 2, NA, 3,
   NA, 1, 2, 2, 2, NA, 2, 2, 2, 2, ....)
)

# data records including missing data must be deleted in advance

id[] center[] treatment[] age[] visit[] gpt[] base[]
1     1         1          76       4     76      52
1     1         1          76       8     81      52
1     1         1          76      12    77     52
1     1         1          76      16    70     52
2     1         1          54       4     74      51
2     1         1          54       8     86      51
2     1         1          54      12     66     51
2     1         1          54      16     83     51
3     1         1          66       4    138     91
....
END
```

11.4.3 Latent profile plus proportional odds models

First, we shall add the results from fitting the latent profile plus proportional odds model with $M = 3$ and $M = 4$ to the *Gritiron Data* by Nakamura et al. (2012) in Tables 11.3 and 11.4. They devised the SAS program based on a Newton–Raphson algorithm. In the same tables, the estimates from the corresponding Bayesian model are also added for comparison. From these two tables, you can see the following:

1. Four kinds of estimates of the latent profiles β_{m1}, β_{m2}, and the standard deviation σ are quite similar.

2. Two kinds of estimates of the parameters $(\gamma_1, \gamma_2, \theta_1, \theta_2, \theta_3)$ of the latent profile plus proportional odds models are also similar.

The next observation not shown in these tables is the test results for the proportional odds assumption (11.21). In the model with $M = 3$ and the model with $M = 4$, the test results are not statistically significant, i.e.,:

1. For the case of $M = 3$, we have $X^2 = 1.16, df = 2, p = 0.44$.

2. For the case of $M = 4$ we have $X^2 = 4.40, df = 4, p = 0.65$.

Furthermore, comparison with the latent profile models, the model fit of the latent profile plus proportional odds models are far improved based on the value of the AICs. For example, the values of the AICs of the latent profile models are

$$AIC = 1214.4\ (M = 3),\ \ AIC = 1037.1\ (M = 4)$$

and the values of AICs of the latent profile plus proportional odds models are

$$AIC = 1154.1\ (M = 3),\ \ AIC = 960.7\ (M = 4).$$

Regarding the treatment effect e^{γ_1}, we have the following estimates

1. MLE:

$$M = 3:\ \ 2.45\ (95\%CI : 1.04, 5.74),\ \ p = 0.039$$

$$M = 4:\ \ 2.25\ (95\%CI : 1.11, 4.55),\ \ p = 0.024$$

2. Bayesian estimate:

$$M = 3:\ \ 2.44\ (95\%CI : 1.06, 5.78)$$

$$M = 4:\ \ 2.25\ (95\%CI : 1.13, 4.61)$$

TABLE 11.6
Average treatment effect during 16-week treatment period estimated by the six kinds of mixed-effects linear normal regression models.

Model	Estimate (s.e.)	p-value	AIC (ML)
Repeated measures model			
IIa	-0.2247 (0.0719)	0.0031	1541.1
III	-0.2255 (0.0766)	0.0036	1459.0
Va	-0.2230 (0.0721)	0.0022	1549.5
ANCOVA-type model			
VIIIa	-0.1834 (0.0642)	0.0047	1086.0
VIIIb	-0.1903 (0.0649)	0.0038	1025.9
IX	-0.1817 (0.0641)	0.0051	1095.3

For the case of $M = 5$, Nakamura et al. (2012) did not report the result. So, here, we shall show the estimates from the corresponding Bayesian model. The results are added to Table 11.5. Here also, we can observe that in the three kinds of estimates of the latent profiles β_{m1}, β_{m2}, the standard deviation σ are quite similar. The treatment effect is estimated as 2.30 ($95\%CI : 1.20, 4.59$), similar to the results of the case of $M = 4$.

11.4.4 Comparison with the mixed-effects normal regression models

For comparison with the mixed-effects normal regression model discussed in Chapter 7, let us apply several kinds of mixed-effects models to the *Gritiron Data* to estimate the *average treatment effect*. Especially, we select three repeated measures models, Model IIa, III, and Va, and the corresponding ANCOVA-type models, Model VIIIa, VIIIb, and IX. The resultant estimated treatment effect and the value of AIC (ML) based on the maximum likelihood estimates (3.27) are shown in Table 11.6. Needless to say, we cannot use the value of AIC to compare the model fits between repeated measures models and ANCOVA-type model because the data structure is different.

As in the case of the *Beat the Blues Data* illustrated in Chapter 7, compared with the ANCOVA-type models, the repeated measures model tends to give larger treatment effect and smaller p-values, all of which are statistically significant at $\alpha = 0.05$.

Now, the goodness-of-fit of the latent profile plus proportional odds models can be compared with ANCOVA-type models with the response variable $y_{ij} - y_{i0}$. The minimum value of AIC was 1025.9 for the Model IIIb and the AIC of the latent profile plus proportional odds model with $M = 4$ is 960.7, indicating

TABLE 11.7
The *Beat the Blues Data*: Classification of patients by each of three kinds ($M = 3, 4, 5$) of latent profile models. The estimated mixing probabilities $\hat{p}_{im}$ are shown in parentheses.

	Improved (+++)	Improved (++)	Improved (+)	Unchanged	Worsened	Total
$M = 3$						
BtheB		7(15.3)	37(65.5)	3(19.2)		52
TAU		3(7.3)	23(50.9)	19(41.8)		45
$M = 4$						
BtheB		7(15.5)	36(63.3)	9(21.1)	0(0.0)	52
TAU		3(7.3)	25(54.0)	13(28.8)	4(9.8)	45
$M = 5$						
BtheB	2 (4.0)	6(13.1)	31(57.2)	13(25.8)	0(0.0)	52
TAU	2(4.2)	1(3.4)	24(51.4)	14(31.1)	4(9.8)	45

that the latter model is far better than the former. Bayesian estimates for the model with $M = 5$ show some improvement over the model with $M = 4$, indicating that the latent profile plus proportional odds models are better than the mixed-effects models in estimating the mean response profile by treatment groups in the case of the *Gritiron Data*.

11.5 Application to the Beat the Blues Data

In this section, we shall apply the latent profile models and the latent profile plus proportional odds models to the *Beat the Blues Data* illustrated in Chapter 7. First, using the latent profile models without covariates, the estimated latent profiles $\hat{\mu}_m(t)$, the 95% region of profiles $\hat{\mu}_m(t) \pm 2\hat{\sigma}$, and the subject-specific profiles classified into the corresponding latent profile of each of three models $M = 3, 4, 5$ are shown in Figures 11.6, 11.7, and 11.8, respectively. And, the classification of patients by each of three kinds ($M = 3, 4, 5$) of latent profile models and the estimated mixing probabilities $\hat{p}_{im}$ are shown in Table 11.7. The values of AIC for each of three models are

$$AIC = 1950.7\ (M = 3), 1946.4\ (M = 4), 1936.2\ (M = 5),$$

TABLE 11.8
Maximum likelihood estimates (MLE) for three kinds of latent profile models and Bayesian estimates for the corresponding three kinds of latent profile plus proportional odds models. Standard errors are shown in parentheses.

	$M=3$		$M=4$		$M=5$	
	MLE	Bayesian	MLE	Bayesian	MLE	Bayesian
AIC	1950.7		1946.4		1936.2	
$-2\log L$	1932.7		1920.4		1902.2	
deviance		1900.0		1887.0		1864.0
β_{11}	- 11.92	-11.6 (0.73)	-11.91	-11.7 (0.71)	-15.17	-15.25 (1.10)
β_{12}	1.08	1.04 (0.11)	1.07	1.05 (0.10)	1.39	1.40 (0.16)
β_{21}	-3.45	-3.37 (0.41)	-3.43	-3.26 (0.40)	-9.74	-9.92 (0.84)
β_{22}	0.24	0.23 (0.06)	0.24	0.22 (0.05)	0.86	0.88 (0.12)
β_{31}	0.00	0.00	0.00	0.00	-3.53	-3.52 (0.39)
β_{32}	0.00	0.00	0.00	0.00	0.25	0.24 (0.05)
β_{41}			4.29	4.40 (1.16)	0.00	0.00
β_{42}			-0.45	-0.47 (0.17)	0.00	0.00
β_{51}					4.38	4.43 (1.02)
β_{52}					-0.47	-0.47 (0.15)
γ_1(treatment)		1.78 (0.71)		1.67 (0.66)		1.45 (0.61)
γ_2(baseline)		0.18 (0.04)		0.16 (0.04)		0.14 (0.03)
γ_3(drug)		0.90 (0.73)		0.89 (0.74)		0.60 (0.59)
γ_4(length)		-0.89 (0.67)		-0.81 (0.60)		-0.62 (0.53)
θ_1		-8.35 (1.67)		-7.67 (1.48)		-8.78 (1.51)
θ_2		-3.14 (0.00)		-2.53 (0.92)		-6.84 (1.29)
θ_3				0.10 (0.92)		-2.52 (0.80)
θ_4						0.25 (0.83)
σ	6.31	6.38 (0.29)	5.99	6.12 (0.29)	5.57	5.68 (0.27)

indicating that the model fit tends to get better as the number of latent profiles gets larger.

Next, we applied each of the three corresponding Bayesian latent profile plus proportional odds models with four covariates, `treatment`, `bdi0`, `drug` and `length`, to the *Beat the Blues Data* and the resultant parameter estimates are shown in Table 11.8 together with the maximum likelihood estimates of the latent profile models. The covariate-adjusted treatment effect is estimated as

1. $M=3: 5.99(95\% CI: 1.56, 27.36)$,

2. $M=4: 5.31(95\% CI: 1.53, 21.26)$, and

3. $M=5: 4.28(95\% CI: 1.38, 15.36)$,

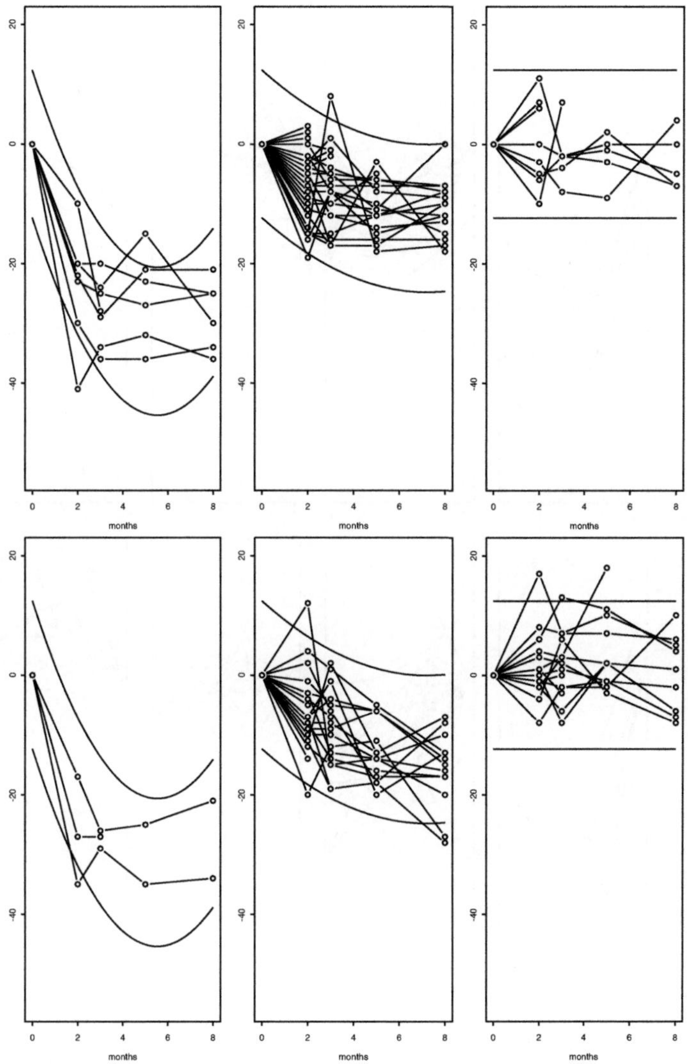

FIGURE 11.6
The *Beat the Blues Data* with $M = 3$: Estimated latent profiles $\hat{\mu}_m(t)$, the 95% region of profiles $\hat{\mu}_m(t) \pm 2\hat{\sigma}$, and the subject-specific profiles classified into the corresponding latent profile. The upper profiles indicate the BtheB group and the lower profiles, the TAU group.

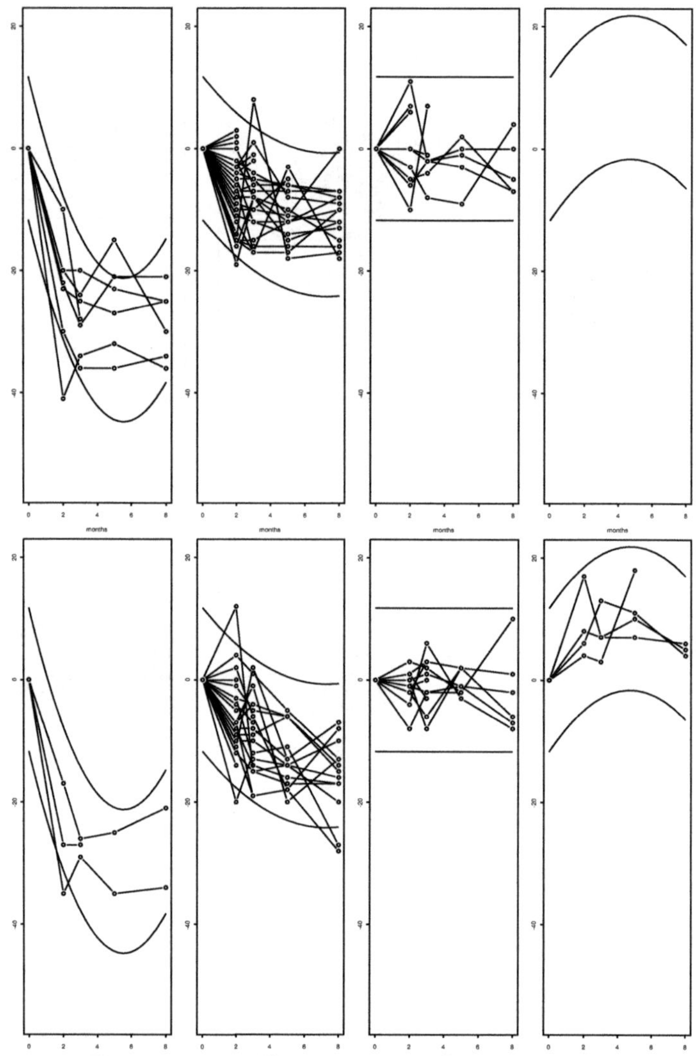

FIGURE 11.7
The *Beat the Blues Data* with $M = 4$: Estimated latent profiles $\hat{\mu}_m(t)$, the 95% region of profiles $\hat{\mu}_m(t) \pm 2\hat{\sigma}$, and the subject-specific profiles classified into the corresponding latent profile. The upper profiles indicate the BtheB group and the lower profiles, the TAU group.

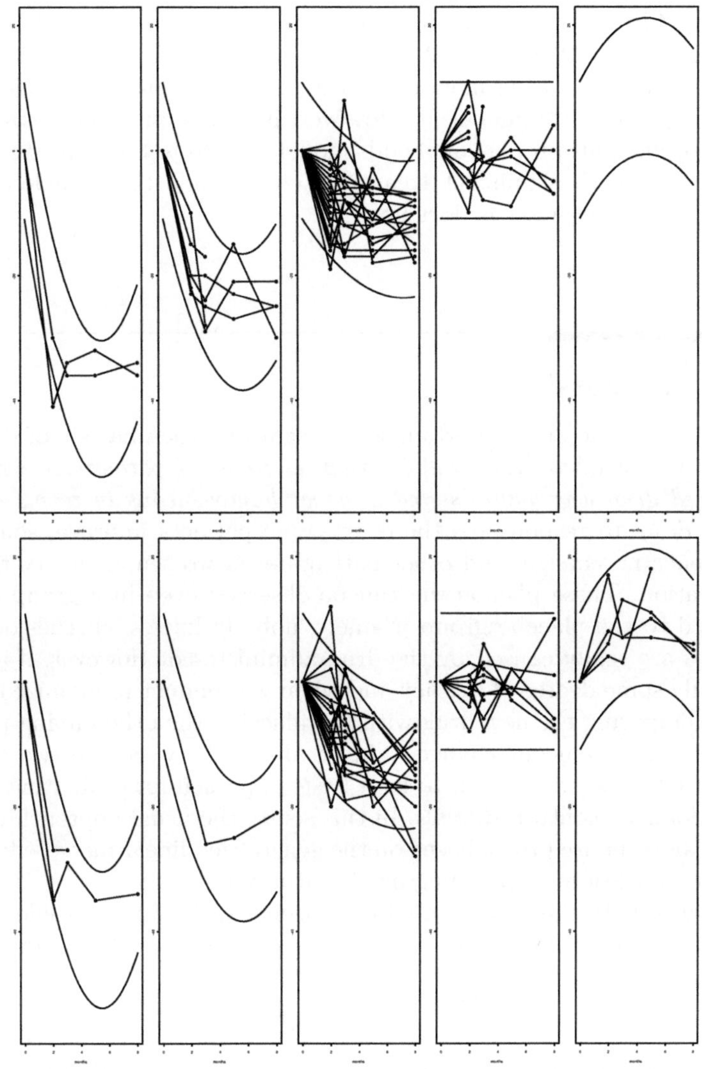

FIGURE 11.8
The *Beat the Blues Data* with $M = 5$: Estimated latent profiles $\hat{\mu}_m(t)$, the 95% region of profiles $\hat{\mu}_m(t) \pm 2\hat{\sigma}$, and the subject-specific profiles classified into the corresponding latent profile. The upper profiles indicate the BtheB group and the lower profiles, the TAU group.

respectively. In terms of the goodness-of-fit of the model, the AIC values based on the maximum likelihood estimates (3.27) of the ANCOVA-type mixed-effects model are within the range 1893.6 (Model VIIIa) $\sim$ 1907.7 (Model IX) and the AIC of the latent profile plus proportional odds model is expected to be less than 1936.2, which is the value of the AIC of the latent profile model with $M = 5$ without covariates. So, we cannot say which model is better regarding the model fit. However, it seems quite interesting that the latent profile plus proportional odds model applied to the *Beat the Blues Data* provides us with significant treatment effect while the mixed-effects linear normal regression models does not.

11.6 Discussion

One of the basic and important ideas regarding the analysis of data in randomized controlled trials will be that *a group of patients to which a new approved drug was administered is never homogeneous in terms of response to the drug.* In response to the drug, some patients improve, some patients experience no change, and other patients even worsen, contrary to patients' expectation. These phenomena can be observed even in a group of patients assigned to the placebo group. Namely, nobody knows whether or not these changes are really caused by the drug administered. However, if a new drug has truly some degree of efficacy and when we conduct randomized controlled trials comparing the new drug with the placebo, then the mixing proportions of these heterogeneous changes will be altered between the two groups. We think that these ideas seem to be a basic approach for evaluating the results of randomized controlled trials. In this sense, the usual approach to estimate the mean response profile based on the generalized linear mixed-effects models could be misleading depending on the situation.

To deal with the above-stated heterogeneity, the latent profile models and the latent profile plus proportional odds models could be useful alternative approaches.

12

Applications to other trial designs

So far, we have considered generalized linear mixed-effects models and their related models for parallel group randomized controlled trials for comparing two treatment groups. In this chapter, we shall present some generalized linear mixed-effects models for other trial designs such as

- trials for comparing multiple treatments,
- three-arm non-inferiority trials including a placebo, and
- cluster randomized trials

within the framework of the $S{:}T$ repeated measures design by taking for example Model V, a random intercept plus slope model for the average treatment effects. Unfortunately, however, I do not know of any real data on the above trials adopting the $S{:}T$ design with $S > 1$ that is available. So, in this chapter, I shall mainly introduce generalized linear mixed-effects models with the $S{:}T$ repeated measures design for each of the trial designs.

12.1 Trials for comparing multiple treatments

The random intercept plus slope model with the random intercept b_{0i} and the random slope b_{1i} for the average treatment effect comparing K treatment groups in a parallel group randomized controlled trial is expressed as

$$
g\{E(y_{ij} \mid b_{0i}, b_{1i})\} = \begin{cases} \beta_0 + b_{0i} + \boldsymbol{w}_i^t \boldsymbol{\xi},\ i = 1, ..., n_1 \text{ (treatment group 1)} \\ \beta_0 + b_{0i} + \beta_{12} + \boldsymbol{w}_i^t \boldsymbol{\xi}, \\ \quad i = n_1 + 1, ..., n_1 + n_2 \text{ (treatment group 2)} \\ \cdots\cdots\cdots\cdots \\ \beta_0 + b_{0i} + \beta_{1K} + \boldsymbol{w}_i^t \boldsymbol{\xi}, \\ \quad i = n_1 + \cdots + n_{K-1} + 1, ..., n_1 + \cdots + n_K \\ \qquad \text{(treatment group } K) \end{cases}
$$

$$
j = -S + 1, .., 0
$$

$$
g\{E(y_{ij} \mid b_{0i}, b_{1i})\} = \begin{cases} \beta_0 + b_{0i} + b_{1i} + \beta_2 + \boldsymbol{w}_i^t \boldsymbol{\xi},\ i = 1, ..., n_1 \\ \qquad \text{(treatment group 1)} \\ \beta_0 + b_{0i} + b_{1i} + \beta_{12} + \beta_2 + \beta_{32} + \boldsymbol{w}_i^t \boldsymbol{\xi}, \\ \quad i = n_1 + 1, ..., n_1 + n_2 \text{ (treatment group 2)} \\ \cdots\cdots\cdots\cdots \\ \beta_0 + b_{0i} + b_{1i} + \beta_{1K} + \beta_2 + \beta_{3K} + \boldsymbol{w}_i^t \boldsymbol{\xi}, \\ \quad i = n_1 + \cdots + n_{K-1} + 1, ..., n_1 + \cdots + n_K \\ \qquad \text{(treatment group } K) \end{cases}
$$

$$
j = 1, .., T,
$$

Interpretations of the fixed-effects parameters $\boldsymbol{\beta}$ newly introduced here are as follows:

- β_{1k} denotes the mean difference in unit of $g(\mu)$ between the treatment group k and the treatment group 1 at the baseline period.
- β_2 denotes the mean change from the baseline in units of $g(\mu)$ in treatment group 1.
- $\beta_2 + \beta_{3k}$ denotes the mean change from the baseline in units of $g(\mu)$ in treatment group k.
- Therefore, β_{3k} denotes the difference in these two means, i.e., the effect size of treatment k compared with treatment 1.

The above model is re-expressed as

$$
\begin{aligned} g\{y_{ij} \mid (b_{0i}, b_{1i})\} &= \beta_0 + b_{0i} + \sum_{k=2}^{K} \beta_{1k} x_{1ki} + (\beta_2 + b_{1i}) x_{2ij} \\ &\quad + \sum_{k=2}^{K} \beta_{3k} x_{1ki} x_{2ij} + \boldsymbol{w}_i^t \boldsymbol{\xi} \qquad (12.1) \\ &\quad j = -S + 1, .., 0, 1, .., T \\ \boldsymbol{b}_i &= (b_{0i}, b_{1i}) \sim N(0, \Phi), \\ \boldsymbol{\Phi} &= \begin{pmatrix} \sigma_{B0}^2 & \rho_B \sigma_{B0} \sigma_{B1} \\ \rho_B \sigma_{B0} \sigma_{B1} & \sigma_{B1}^2 \end{pmatrix}, \end{aligned}
$$

where $(x_{12i}, x_{13i}, ..., x_{1Ki})$ are the sets of $(K-1)$ dummy variables such that

$$x_{1ki} = \begin{cases} 1, & \text{if the } i\text{th subject is assigned to the treatment group } k \\ 0, & \text{otherwise} \end{cases} \tag{12.2}$$

and

$$x_{2ij} = \begin{cases} 1, & \text{for } j \geq 1 \\ 0, & \text{for } j \leq 0. \end{cases} \tag{12.3}$$

Needless to say, some sort of statistical procedures for handling multiplicity due to multiple treatment comparisons consisting of at least $(K-1)$ comparisons, $(\beta_{32}, ..., \beta_{3K})$, are needed to control the overall type I error rate in confirmatory trials.

12.2 Three-arm non-inferiority trials including a placebo

In this section, we shall consider the three-arm non-inferiority trials including a placebo, which is a recent hot topic in clinical trials and a special case of multiple treatment comparisons.

12.2.1 Background

In non-inferiority trials, a new experimental treatment is compared to an active reference treatment to demonstrate that the experimental treatment is not inferior to the reference treatment by more than a small amount. This trial design is usually known as the two-arm non-inferiority trial (D'Agostino et al., 2003). The amount $\Delta(>0)$, called *the non-inferiority margin*, has been defined as *the maximum clinically irrelevant difference between treatments* and must be prespecified in the trial protocol. Recently, the FDA (Food and Drug Administration) published draft guidance on non-inferiority trials (FDA, 2011). The key elements in the design of a non-inferiority trial are "*the choice of the non-inferiority margin*" and "*the establishment of assay sensitivity*" (ICH, 1998; ICH, 2000; European Medicines Agency, 2009). The selection of margin has been discussed in many articles or guidelines without achieving consensus. On the other hand, assay sensitivity is a property of a clinical trial and is defined as the ability to distinguish an effective treatment from a less effective or ineffective treatment (ICH, 2000). The choice of margin and the decision on whether a trial will have assay sensitivity are based on three considerations: (1) HESDE, or *historical evidence of sensitivity to drug effects*, (2) CS, or *constancy assumption*, and (3) *quality of the new trial* (ICH, 2000; FDA , 2011). That is, the value of interest in determining the non-inferiority margin is the effect size of the reference treatment to the placebo in past placebo controlled trials, and it is necessary for the reference treatment to be shown consistently superior to the placebo (HESDE). CS requires that the new non-inferiority trial should be sufficiently similar to the past studies with respect to all important aspects of the trial. However, these requirements cannot be adequately assessed in the usual two-arm non-inferiority trials because they do not include a placebo. Thus, it is strongly recommended to conduct a three-arm non-inferiority trial including a placebo, the so-called *gold standard* non-inferiority design, as a useful approach for assessing assay sensitivity and internal validation (ICH, 2000; European Medicines Agency, 2009). However, there seems to be some confusion, misunderstanding, and debate in the literature on the appropriate design of three-arm non-inferiority trials. For example, see Koch and Tangen (1999), Pigeot *et al.* (2003), Koch and Röhmel (2004), Röhmel and Pigeot (2010, 2011), Hida and Tango (2011a, 2011b, 2013), Stuck and Kieser (2012), and Kwong et al. (2012).

12.2.2 Hida–Tango procedure

In this section, we introduce the procedures proposed by Tango (2003) and Hida and Tango (2011a, 2013), which seem to me statistically the most sound method under the current definition of *superiority* (1.16). Let us assume here that the primary endpoints under an experimental treatment (E), an active reference treatment (R), and a placebo (P) are mutually independent and normally distributed with the expected value, μ_E, μ_R, and μ_P, respectively. Needless to say, any type of endpoints, such as a binary, count, and survival endpoints, may be used. Assume also that larger mean values indicate greater benefits.

In this framework, Tango (2003) and Hida and Tango (2011a) proposed that the gold standard non-inferiority trial can be termed successful if and only if the relationship among μ_E, μ_R and μ_P satisfied the following inequality

$$\mu_P < \mu_R - \Delta < \mu_E, \tag{12.4}$$

where Δ denotes the non-inferiority margin. The inequality (12.4) is expressed by the following two sets of hypothesis tests:

$$\begin{aligned} H_0 &: \mu_E \le \mu_R - \Delta, \text{ v.s. } H_1 : \mu_E > \mu_R - \Delta, & (12.5)\\ K_0 &: \mu_R \le \mu_P + \Delta, \text{ v.s. } K_1 : \mu_R > \mu_P + \Delta, & (12.6) \end{aligned}$$

where both null hypotheses H_0 and K_0 must be simultaneously rejected by one-tailed test at the $\alpha/2$ significance level, respectively. Equivalently, this condition can be expressed by the two confidence intervals: *the lower limit of the* $100(1-\alpha)\%$ *confidence interval for* $\mu_E - \mu_R$ *is larger than* $-\Delta$ *and that of the* $100(1-\alpha)\%$ *confidence interval for* $\mu_R - \mu_P$ *is larger than* Δ.

12.2.3 Generalized linear mixed-effects models

The Model V with the random intercept b_{0i} and the random slope b_{1i} for the average treatment effects within the framework of the Hida–Tango procedure is expressed as

$$
\begin{aligned}
g\{E(y_{ij} \mid b_{0i}, b_{1i})\} &= \begin{cases} \beta_0 + b_{0i} + \boldsymbol{w}_i^t \boldsymbol{\xi}, \ i = 1, ..., n_1 \text{ (placebo)} \\ \beta_0 + b_{0i} + \beta_{12} + \boldsymbol{w}_i^t \boldsymbol{\xi}, \\ \quad i = n_1 + 1, ..., n_1 + n_2 \text{ (reference treatment)} \\ \beta_0 + b_{0i} + \beta_{13} + \boldsymbol{w}_i^t \boldsymbol{\xi}, \\ \quad i = n_1 + n_2 + 1, ..., n_1 + n_2 + n_3 \text{ (new treatment)} \end{cases} \\
& j = -S + 1, .., 0 \\
g\{E(y_{ij} \mid b_{0i}, b_{1i})\} &= \begin{cases} \beta_0 + b_{0i} + b_{1i} + \beta_2 + \boldsymbol{w}_i^t \boldsymbol{\xi}, \ i = 1, ..., n_1 \text{ (placebo)} \\ \beta_0 + b_{0i} + b_{1i} + \beta_{12} + \beta_2 + \beta_{32} + \boldsymbol{w}_i^t \boldsymbol{\xi}, \\ \quad i = n_1 + 1, ..., n_1 + n_2 \text{ (reference treatment)} \\ \beta_0 + b_{0i} + b_{1i} + \beta_{13} + \beta_2 + \beta_{33} + \boldsymbol{w}_i^t \boldsymbol{\xi}, \\ \quad i = n_1 + n_2 + 1, ..., n_1 + n_2 + n_3 \text{ (new treatment)} \end{cases} \\
& j = 1, .., T,
\end{aligned}
$$

which is re-expressed as

$$
\begin{aligned}
g\{y_{ij} \mid (b_{0i}, b_{1i})\} &= \beta_0 + b_{0i} + \sum_{k=2}^{3} \beta_{1k} x_{1ki} + (\beta_2 + b_{1i}) x_{2ij} \\
& \quad + \sum_{k=2}^{3} \beta_{3k} x_{1ki} x_{2ij} + \boldsymbol{w}_i^t \boldsymbol{\xi} \qquad (12.7) \\
& \quad j = -S + 1, .., 0, 1, .., T \\
\boldsymbol{b}_i &= (b_{0i}, b_{1i}) \sim N(0, \Phi), \\
\boldsymbol{\Phi} &= \begin{pmatrix} \sigma_{B0}^2 & \rho_B \sigma_{B0} \sigma_{B1} \\ \rho_B \sigma_{B0} \sigma_{B1} & \sigma_{B1}^2 \end{pmatrix}.
\end{aligned}
$$

In terms of the generalized linear mixed-effects models, the two sets of hypothesis tests (12.5) and (12.6) can be replaced as follows:

Three-arm non-inferiority hypotheses

If a positive β_{3k} indicates benefits, the hypotheses are

$$H_0 \;:\; \beta_{33} \le \beta_{32} - \Delta, \text{ v.s. } H_1 : \beta_{33} > \beta_{32} - \Delta, \tag{12.8}$$
$$K_0 \;:\; \beta_{32} \le \Delta, \text{ v.s. } K_1 : \beta_{32} > \Delta. \tag{12.9}$$

If a negative β_{3k} indicates benefits, the hypotheses should be

$$H_0 \;:\; \beta_{33} \ge \beta_{32} + \Delta, \text{ v.s. } H_1 : \beta_{33} < \beta_{32} + \Delta, \tag{12.10}$$
$$K_0 \;:\; \beta_{32} \ge -\Delta, \text{ v.s. } K_1 : \beta_{32} < -\Delta. \tag{12.11}$$

Both null hypotheses H_0 and K_0 must be simultaneously rejected by one-tailed test at the $\alpha/2$ significance level, respectively. Equivalently, this condition can be expressed by the two confidence intervals. For example, if a positive β_{3k} indicates benefits, *the lower limit of the* $100(1-\alpha)\%$ *confidence interval for* $\beta_{33} - \beta_{32}$ *is larger than* $-\Delta$ *and that of the* $100(1-\alpha)\%$ *confidence interval for* β_{32} *is larger than* Δ.

For the logistic model and the Poisson model, we have to replace Δ with

$$\Delta \Longrightarrow -\log\{1 - \Delta^* \text{sign}(\beta_{3k})\}, \tag{12.12}$$

where Δ^* is the non-inferiority margin defined in the unit of the *ORR, odds ratio ratio*, and the *RRR, rate ratio ratio*, respectively.

12.3 Cluster randomized trials

In this section, we consider a three-level (hierarchically structured) cluster randomized trial (e.g., Donner and Klar, 2000; Hayes and Moulton, 2009; Eldridge and Kerry, 2012; Campbell and Walters, 2014) where two kinds of interventions or treatments are randomly assigned to study centers or clinics, called "clusters" in general and the response profile repeated measures within the framework of the *S:T* design are denoted by y_{kij} for the $j(=-S,-S+1,...,0,1,...,T)$th measurement (the level 1 unit) of the $i(=1,...,n_{1k}+n_{2k})$th subject (the level 2 unit) nested within the $k(=1,...,2I)$th center (the level 3 unit). To analyze these data, we shall introduce some three-level generalized linear mixed-effects models.

12.3.1 Three-level models for the average treatment effect

We shall consider here the following three-level mixed-effects model that has (1) random intercept $b_{0i(k)}$ and the random slope $b_{1i(k)}$ for the ith subject and (2) random intercept c_{0k} for the kth center (cluster) reflecting the intra-center variability at the baseline period as follows:

$$
g\{E(y_{kij} \mid c_{0k}, b_{0i(k)}\} \sim \begin{cases} \beta_0 + c_{0k} + b_{0i(k)} + \boldsymbol{w}_i^t\boldsymbol{\xi}, \ i = 1, ..., n_{1k} \\ \qquad\qquad\qquad\qquad (\text{Control}) \\ \beta_0 + c_{0k} + b_{0i(k)} + \beta_1 + \boldsymbol{w}_i^t\boldsymbol{\xi}, \\ i = n_{1k} + 1, ..., n_{1k} + n_{2k} \ (\text{New treatment}) \end{cases}
$$
$$
j = -S + 1, .., 0
$$
$$
g\{E(y_{kij} \mid c_{0k}, \boldsymbol{b}_{i(k)}\} \sim \begin{cases} \beta_0 + c_{0k} + b_{0i(k)} + b_{1i(k)} + \beta_2 + \boldsymbol{w}_i^t\boldsymbol{\xi}, \\ \qquad i = 1, ..., n_{1k} \ (\text{Control}) \\ \beta_0 + c_{0k} + b_{0i(k)} + b_{1i(k)} + \beta_1 + \beta_2 + \beta_3 + \boldsymbol{w}_i^t\boldsymbol{\xi}, \\ i = n_{1k} + 1, ..., n_{1k} + n_{2k} \ (\text{New treatment}) \end{cases}
$$
$$
j = 1, ..., T,
$$

which is re-expressed as

$$
\begin{aligned}
g\{y_{kij} \mid c_{0k}, b_{0i(k)}, b_{1i(k)}\} &= \beta_0 + c_{0k} + b_{0i(k)} + \beta_1 x_{1i} + (\beta_2 + b_{1i(k)}) x_{2ij} \\
&\quad + \beta_3 x_{1i} x_{2ij} + \boldsymbol{w}_i^t\boldsymbol{\xi} \qquad (12.13) \\
c_{0k} &\sim N(0, \sigma_{C0}^2), \\
\boldsymbol{b}_{i(k)} &= (b_{0i(k)}, b_{1i(k)}) \sim N(0, \Phi), \\
\boldsymbol{\Phi} &= \begin{pmatrix} \sigma_{B0}^2 & \rho_B \sigma_{B0} \sigma_{B1} \\ \rho_B \sigma_{B0} \sigma_{B1} & \sigma_{B1}^2 \end{pmatrix} \\
& \quad k = 1, ..., 2I, i = 1, ..., n_{1k} + n_{2k}; \\
& \quad j = -S, -S + 1, ..., 0, 1, ..., T,
\end{aligned}
$$

where these random components c_{0k} and $\boldsymbol{b}_{i(k)}$ are assumed to be mutually independent. Furthermore it is assumed that $\boldsymbol{b}_{i(k)}$ are independent conditional on c_{0k} while c_{0k} are unconditionally independent of each other.

Especially, let us consider the following normal mixed-effects model

$$
\begin{aligned}
y_{kij} \mid (c_{0k}, \boldsymbol{b}_{i(k)}) &= \beta_0 + c_{0k} + b_{0i(k)} + \beta_1 x_{1i} + (\beta_2 + b_{1i(k)}) x_{2ij} \\
&\quad + \beta_3 x_{1i} x_{2ij} + \boldsymbol{w}_i^t \boldsymbol{\xi} + \epsilon_{kij} \qquad (12.14) \\
c_{0k} &\sim N(0, \sigma_{C0}^2), \ \ \epsilon_{kij} \sim N(0, \sigma_E^2) \\
\boldsymbol{b}_{i(k)} &= (b_{0i(k)}, b_{1i(k)}) \sim N(0, \Phi), \\
\boldsymbol{\Phi} &= \begin{pmatrix} \sigma_{B0}^2 & \rho_B \sigma_{B0} \sigma_{B1} \\ \rho_B \sigma_{B0} \sigma_{B1} & \sigma_{B1}^2 \end{pmatrix} \\
& k = 1, ..., 2I, i = 1, ..., n_{1k} + n_{2k}; \\
& j = -S, -S+1, ..., 0, 1, ..., T
\end{aligned}
$$

where the three random components c_{0k}, $\boldsymbol{b}_{i(k)}$, and ϵ_{kij} are assumed to be mutually independent. Furthermore, it is assumed that ϵ_{kij} are independent of each other conditional on both c_{0k} and $\boldsymbol{b}_{i(k)}$. In this model, the parameter of interest is also β_3 and the corresponding null and alternative hypotheses for superiority will be

$$
H_0 \ : \ \beta_3 \geq 0, \text{ versus } \ H_1 : \beta_3 < 0 \qquad (12.15)
$$

in the case that a negative β_3 indicates benefits. If a positive β_3 indicates benefits, then they are

$$
H_0 \ : \ \beta_3 \leq 0, \text{ versus } \ H_1 : \beta_3 > 0. \qquad (12.16)
$$

Then, we have

$$
\begin{aligned}
E(y_{kij}) &= \beta_0 + \beta_1 x_{1i} \ (j \leq 0) \\
E(y_{kij}) &= \beta_0 + \beta_1 x_{1i} + \beta_2 + \beta_3 x_{1i} \ (j > 0) \\
E(d_{kij}) &= \beta_2 + \beta_3 x_{1i} \\
Var(d_{kij}) &= \sigma_{B1}^2 + 2\sigma_E^2 \\
Var(y_{kij}) &= \sigma_{C0}^2 + \sigma_{B0}^2 + \sigma_E^2 \ (j \leq 0) \\
Var(y_{kij}) &= \sigma_{C0}^2 + \sigma_{B0}^2 + \sigma_{B1}^2 + 2\rho_B \sigma_{B0} \sigma_{B1} + \sigma_E^2 \ (j > 0) \\
Cov(y_{kij_1}, y_{kij_2}) &= \sigma_{C0}^2 + \sigma_{B0}^2 \ \ (\text{for } j_1, j_2 \leq 0) \\
Cov(y_{kij_1}, y_{kij_2}) &= \sigma_{C0}^2 + \sigma_{B0}^2 + \rho_B \sigma_{B0} \sigma_{B1} \ \ (\text{for } j_1 \leq 0, \ j_2 > 0) \\
Cov(y_{kij_1}, y_{kij_2}) &= \sigma_{C0}^2 + \sigma_{B0}^2 + \sigma_{B1}^2 + 2\rho_B \sigma_{B0} \sigma_{B1} \ \ (\text{for } j_1, j_2 > 0) \\
Cov(y_{ki_1j_1}, y_{ki_2j_2}) &= \sigma_{C0}^2.
\end{aligned}
$$

Hence, the center-level ICC (intra-cluster correlation) among data on subjects (level 2) can be written for $i_1 \neq i_2$ as

$$
Corr(y_{ki_1j_1}, y_{ki_2j_2}) = \frac{\sigma_{C0}^2}{\sqrt{Var(y_{ki_1j_1}) Var(y_{ki_2j_2})}} \qquad (12.17)
$$

and the subject-level ICC among data on repeated measures (level 1) can be written for $j_1 \neq j_2$ as

$$Corr(y_{kij_1}, y_{kij_2}) = \frac{Cov(y_{kij_1}, y_{kij_2})}{\sqrt{Var(y_{kij_1})Var(y_{kij_2})}}. \quad (12.18)$$

Extension to the four-level models where centers are the level 4 unit and nurses nested within each center are the level 3 unit is straightforward.

Now, let us fit the model (12.14) to the *Beat the Blues Data* using SAS procedure `PROC MIXED` assuming that this trial is a multi-center cluster randomized trial. Let the variable `centerid` denote the center id. Then the SAS program is similar to Model Va or Vb shown in Program 7.2 and is shown in Program 12.1. The key difference between this code and the code used in Program 7.2 is the use of two `RANDOM` statements. The first `RANDOM` is specifying center as the subject at level 3 and the second `RANDOM` statement specifies the subject as subject nested within centers at level 2, i.e., `subject=subject(centerid)`.

Program 12.1: SAS procedure `PROC MIXED` for the model (12.14)

```
  proc mixed data=dbb method=reml covtest;
  class centerid subject visit/ ref=first ;
  model bdi =  drug length treatment post treatment*post /s cl ddfm=sat ;

/* Model Va  */
  random intercept        / type=simple subject= centerid g gcorr;
  random intercept post / type=simple subject= subject(centerid) g gcorr ;

/* Model Vb */
  random intercept        / type=simple subject= centerid g gcorr;
  random intercept post / type=un subject= subject(centerid) g gcorr ;

  repeated visit / type = simple subject = subject r  rcorr ;
 run ;
```

Regarding the SAS program for the three-level mixed-effects logistic regression and Poisson regression model, similar steps can be easily made using the SAS procedure `PROC GLIMMIX`.

12.3.2 Three-level models for the treatment by linear time interaction

Here also, we shall consider the following three-level mixed-effects model that has (1) random intercept $b_{0i(k)}$ and the random slope $b_{1i(k)}$ for the ith subject and (2) random intercept c_{0k} for the kth center (cluster) reflecting the intra-center variability at the baseline period as follows:

$$g\{E(y_{kij} \mid c_{0k}, b_{0i(k)}\} \sim \begin{cases} \beta_0 + c_{0k} + b_{0i(k)} + \boldsymbol{w}_i^t \boldsymbol{\xi}, \\ \qquad i = 1, ..., n_{1k} \quad \text{(Control)} \\ \beta_0 + c_{0k} + b_{0i(k)} + \beta_1 + \boldsymbol{w}_i^t \boldsymbol{\xi}, \\ i = n_{1k} + 1, ..., n_{1k} + n_{2k} \quad \text{(New treatment)} \end{cases}$$
$$j = -S + 1, .., 0$$
$$g\{E(y_{kij} \mid c_{0k}, \boldsymbol{b}_{i(k)}\} \sim \begin{cases} \beta_0 + c_{0k} + b_{0i(k)} + (b_{1i(k)} + \beta_2) t_j + \boldsymbol{w}_i^t \boldsymbol{\xi}, \\ \qquad i = 1, ..., n_{1k} \quad \text{(Control)} \\ \beta_0 + c_{0k} + b_{0i(k)} + \beta_1 \\ \qquad + (b_{1i(k)} + \beta_2 + \beta_3) t_j + \boldsymbol{w}_i^t \boldsymbol{\xi}, \\ i = n_{1k} + 1, ..., n_{1k} + n_{2k} \quad \text{(New treatment)} \end{cases}$$
$$j = 1, ..., T,$$

which is re-expressed as

$$\begin{aligned} g\{y_{kij} \mid c_{0k}, \boldsymbol{b}_{i(k)}\} &= \beta_0 + c_{0k} + b_{0i(k)} + \beta_1 x_{1i} \\ &\quad + (\beta_2 + \beta_3 x_{1i} + b_{1i(k)}) t_j + \boldsymbol{w}_i^t \boldsymbol{\xi} \qquad (12.19) \\ c_{0k} &\sim N(0, \sigma_{C0}^2), \\ \boldsymbol{b}_i &= (b_{0i(k)}, b_{1i(k)}) \sim N(0, \Phi), \\ \boldsymbol{\Phi} &= \begin{pmatrix} \sigma_{B0}^2 & \rho_B \sigma_{B0} \sigma_{B1} \\ \rho_B \sigma_{B0} \sigma_{B1} & \sigma_{B1}^2 \end{pmatrix} \\ & \quad k = 1, ..., 2I, i = 1, ..., n_{1k} + n_{2k}; \\ & \quad j = -S, -S + 1, ..., 0, 1, ..., T, \end{aligned}$$

where these random components c_{0k} and $\boldsymbol{b}_{i(k)}$ are assumed to be mutually independent. Furthermore, it is assumed that $\boldsymbol{b}_{i(k)}$ are independent conditional on c_{0k}, while c_{0k} are unconditionally independent of each other.

Especially, let us consider the following normal mixed-effects model

$$\begin{aligned} y_{kij} \mid c_{0k}, \boldsymbol{b}_{i(k)} &= \beta_0 + c_{0k} + b_{0i(k)} + \beta_1 x_{1i} + (\beta_2 + \beta_3 x_{1i} + b_{1i(k)}) t_j \\ &\quad + \boldsymbol{w}_i^t \boldsymbol{\xi} + \epsilon_{kij} \qquad (12.20) \\ c_{0k} &\sim N(0, \sigma_{C0}^2), \quad \epsilon_{kij} \sim N(0, \sigma_E^2) \\ \boldsymbol{b}_i &= (b_{0i(k)}, b_{1i(k)}) \sim N(0, \Phi), \\ \boldsymbol{\Phi} &= \begin{pmatrix} \sigma_{B0}^2 & \rho_B \sigma_{B0} \sigma_{B1} \\ \rho_B \sigma_{B0} \sigma_{B1} & \sigma_{B1}^2 \end{pmatrix} \\ & \quad k = 1, ..., 2I, i = 1, ..., n_{1k} + n_{2k}; \\ & \quad j = -S, -S + 1, ..., 0, 1, ..., T, \end{aligned}$$

where these three random components c_{0k}, $\boldsymbol{b}_{i(k)}$, and ϵ_{kij} are assumed to be mutually independent. Furthermore, it is assumed that ϵ_{kij} are independent of each other conditional on both c_{0k} and $\boldsymbol{b}_i$. In this model, the parameter of interest is also β_3 and the corresponding null and alternative hypotheses for superiority, for example, are the same as (12.15) and (12.15).

It should be noted that the SAS program for the model (12.20) fitted to the *Beat the Blues Data* assuming that this trial is a multi-center cluster randomized trial is quite similar to that of Program 12.1 where Model Va and Model Vb should be replaced by Model VIIa and Model VIIb. Therefore, we omit the program here. Furthermore, similar steps on the SAS program for the three-level mixed-effects logistic regression and Poisson regression model can be easily made using the SAS procedure `PROC GLIMMIX`.

Appendix A

Sample size

The sample size calculations for longitudinal data analysis in the literature are based on the *basic 1:T design* where the baseline data, if any, is used as a covariate (for example, Hedeker, Gibbons, Waternaux, 1999; Diggle et al., 2002; Fitzmaurice, Laird and Ware, 2011; Amatya et al., 2013; Kapur et al., 2014.)

In this section, we shall present the sample size (the number of subjects) calculations for the *random intercept model* (1.11) and the *random intercept plus slope model* (1.12) **for the average treatment effect** within the framework of the $S : T$ *repeated measures design* separately for continuous, binary, and count responses (Tango, 2016a). As the parameter β_3 is of primary interest in these models, the pair of hypotheses of interest here takes the form

$$H_0 \quad : \quad \beta_3 = 0, \text{ versus } H_1 : \beta_3 \neq 0, \tag{A.1}$$

which is **a test for superiority trials** (1.16).

First, consider the *random intercept model* (1.11) where there exists a sufficient statistic for the random effects b_{0i} (Diggle et al., 2002; Liang and Zeger, 2000). Namely, the conditional likelihood approach can provide sample size formulas that are invariant to the distributional assumption on b_{0i} except for the case of the logistic regression model. For the normally distributed response, we can also derive the sample size formula for the *random intercept plus slope* model (1.12). For the logistic regression models and the *random intercept plus slope* Poisson regression model, we can obtain Monte Carlo simulated sample sizes.

A.1 Normal linear regression model

Let us define θ_{1i} and θ_{2ij} as

$$\theta_{1i} \quad = \quad \beta_0 + b_{0i} + \beta_1 x_{1i} + \boldsymbol{w}_i^t \boldsymbol{\xi} \tag{A.2}$$

$$\theta_{2ij} \quad = \quad \begin{cases} 0, & \text{for } j = -S+1, ..., 0 \\ \beta_2 + \beta_3 x_{1i}, & \text{for } j = 1, ..., T. \end{cases} \tag{A.3}$$

Then, the subject i's contribution to the likelihood of the *random-intercept model* (1.11) is given by

$$\begin{aligned} p(\boldsymbol{y}_i \mid b_{0i}) &= (2\pi\sigma_E^2)^{-(S+T)/2} \exp\left\{ -\frac{1}{2\sigma_E^2} \{-2\theta_{1i} y_{i+} \right. \\ &\quad \left. + \sum_{j=-S}^{T} [y_{ij}^2 - 2\theta_{2ij} y_{ij} + (\theta_{1i} + \theta_{2ij})^2] \} \right\}, \end{aligned}$$

where $\phi(.)$ denotes the probability density function of the standard normal distribution $N(0,\ 1)$ and $y_{i+} = \sum_{j=-S+1}^{T} y_{ij}$. Namely, y_{i+} is the minimal sufficient statistic for θ_{1i}. Then the conditional likelihood for (β_2, β_3) given y_{i+} is

$$L_C(\beta_2, \beta_3 \mid y_{i+}) \propto \exp\left\{ -\frac{ST}{2(S+T)\sigma_E^2} (d_i(S,T) - \beta_2 - \beta_3 x_{1i})^2 \right\} \quad \text{(A.4)}$$

where

$$d_i(S,T) = \bar{y}_{i+(post)} - \bar{y}_{i+(pre)} \quad \text{(A.5)}$$

$$\bar{y}_{i+(post)} = \frac{1}{T} \sum_{j=1}^{T} y_{ij}, \quad \text{(A.6)}$$

$$\bar{y}_{i+(pre)} = \frac{1}{S} \sum_{j=-S+1}^{0} y_{ij}. \quad \text{(A.7)}$$

Then, the conditional maximum likelihood estimator $\hat{\beta}_{3C}$ of treatment effect β_3 is given by the difference in means of change from baseline, i.e.,

$$\hat{\beta}_{3C} = \frac{1}{n_2} \sum_{i=1}^{N} d_i(S,T) x_{1i} - \frac{1}{n_1} \sum_{i=1}^{N} d_i(S,T)(1 - x_{1i}), \quad \text{(A.8)}$$

and is equal to $\hat{\beta}_3$, the maximum likelihood estimator of the *random intercept* normal linear regression model (1.11). The variance of $\hat{\beta}_{3C}$ or $\hat{\beta}_3$ is

$$\text{Var}(\hat{\beta}_3) = \frac{n_1 + n_2}{n_1 n_2} \left(\frac{S+T}{ST} \right) \sigma_E^2. \quad \text{(A.9)}$$

In general, the *random intercept* model fits worse than the *random intercept plus slope* model (1.12) in the case of normal linear regression models. Although the conditional likelihood approach cannot be applied, the maximum likelihood estimator $\hat{\beta}_3$ of the *random intercept and slope* model is also given by the same form as (A.8) and its variance is given by

$$\text{Var}(\hat{\beta}_3) = \frac{n_1 + n_2}{n_1 n_2} \left\{ \sigma_{B1}^2 + \left(\frac{S+T}{ST} \right) \sigma_E^2 \right\}, \quad \text{(A.10)}$$

which includes the variance (A.9) as a special case. The covariance structure of the *random intercept plus slope* model is given by

$$\begin{aligned}
Var(y_{ij} \mid j \leq 0) &= \sigma_{B0}^2 + \sigma_E^2 \\
Var(y_{ij} \mid j > 0) &= \sigma_{B0}^2 + \sigma_{B1}^2 + 2\rho_B\sigma_{B0}\sigma_{B1} + \sigma_E^2 \\
Cov(y_{ij}, y_{ij'} \mid j \leq 0, j' \leq 0) &= \sigma_{B0}^2 \\
Cov(y_{ij}, y_{ij'} \mid j \leq 0, j' > 0) &= \sigma_{B0}^2 + \rho_B\sigma_{B0}\sigma_{B1} \\
Cov(y_{ij}, y_{ij'} \mid j > 0, j' > 0) &= \sigma_{B0}^2 + \sigma_{B1}^2 + 2\rho_B\sigma_{B0}\sigma_{B1}.
\end{aligned}$$

Then, the sample size (the number of subjects) formula with two equally sized groups ($n_1 = n_2 = n$) to detect an effect size β_3 under the *random intercept plus slope* model with two-sided significance level α and power $100(1-\phi)\%$ for the *1:1 design* is given by

$$n_{S=1,T=1} = 2(Z_{\alpha/2} + Z_\phi)^2 \times \frac{\sigma_{B1}^2 + 2\sigma_E^2}{\beta_3^2}, \quad \text{(A.11)}$$

where Z_α denotes the upper $100\alpha\%$ percentile of the standard normal distribution. Then, we have the following sample size $n_{S,T}$ for the *S:T design*:

$$n_{S,T} = n_{S=1,T=1}\frac{\sigma_{B1}^2 + \left(\frac{S+T}{ST}\right)\sigma_E^2}{\sigma_{B1}^2 + 2\sigma_E^2}. \quad \text{(A.12)}$$

Namely, compared with the *1:1 design*, the percent reduction $r_{S,T}$ in sample size is given by

$$r_{S,T} = 1 - \frac{n_{S,T}}{n_{S=1,T=1}} = \frac{\left(2 - \frac{S+T}{ST}\right)\sigma_E^2}{\sigma_{B1}^2 + 2\sigma_E^2}. \quad \text{(A.13)}$$

The validity of the proposed sample size formula has been shown via a Monte Carlo simulation study using estimates based on real data (Tango, 2016a).

It should be noted that the sample size formulas for longitudinal data analysis described in some textbooks (for example, Diggle et al., 2002; Fitzmaurice, Laird and Ware, 2011) are different from those above and are based on the following repeated measures model for the *1:T design* where the baseline data is usually used as a covariate:

$$\begin{aligned}
y_{ij} \mid b_{2i} &= \beta_0 + b_{2i} + \beta_3^* x_{1i} + \boldsymbol{w}_i^t \boldsymbol{\xi} + \epsilon_{ij},\ j = 1, ..., T \\
b_{2i} = b_{0i} + b_{1i} &\sim N(0, \sigma_{B2}^2),\ \sigma_{B2}^2 = \sigma_{B0}^2 + \sigma_{B1}^2 + 2\rho_B\sigma_{B0}\sigma_{B1} \\
\epsilon_{ij} &\sim N(0, \sigma_E^2),
\end{aligned}$$

where β_3^* denotes the difference in means of average treatment effects during the evaluation period, which is expected to be equal to β_3 in RCT, i.e.,

$$\hat{\beta_3^*} = \frac{1}{n_2}\sum_{i=1}^{N} \bar{y}_{i+(post)} x_{1i} - \frac{1}{n_1}\sum_{i=1}^{N} \bar{y}_{i+(post)}(1 - x_{1i})$$

and

$$\text{Var}(\hat{\beta}_3^*) = \frac{n_1+n_2}{n_1 n_2}\left(\sigma_{B0}^2 + \sigma_{B1}^2 + 2\rho_B\sigma_{B0}\sigma_{B1} + \frac{1}{T}\sigma_E^2\right).$$

Namely, the sample size formula is

$$\begin{aligned} n_T &= 2(Z_{\alpha/2}+Z_\beta)^2 \times \frac{\sigma_{B2}^2 + \sigma_E^2/T}{\beta_3^2} \\ &= \frac{2(Z_{\alpha/2}+Z_\beta)^2\sigma^2}{\beta_3^2}\cdot\frac{1+(T-1)\rho}{T}, \end{aligned} \quad \text{(A.14)}$$

where $\sigma^2 = \text{Var}(y_{ij}) = \sigma_{B2}^2 + \sigma_E^2$ and covariance $\text{Cov}(y_{ij}, y_{ij'})$ has a compound symmetry with a correlation coefficient ρ given by

$$\rho = \frac{\sigma_{B0}^2 + \sigma_{B1}^2 + 2\rho_B\sigma_{B0}\sigma_{B1}}{\sigma_{B0}^2 + \sigma_{B1}^2 + 2\rho_B\sigma_{B0}\sigma_{B1} + \sigma_E^2}. \quad \text{(A.15)}$$

A.2 Poisson regression model

Here also, we can express subject i's contribution to the likelihood in the *random intercept* model (1.11) as

$$p(\boldsymbol{y}_i \mid \boldsymbol{b}_i) = \exp(\theta_{1i}y_{i+} + \sum_{j=-S+1}^{T} y_{ij}\theta_{2ij}) \prod_{j=-S+1}^{T} \frac{\exp(-\exp(\theta_{1i}+\theta_{2ij}))}{y_{ij}!}$$

and y_{i+} is shown to be the minimal sufficient statistic for θ_{1i}. Then, the conditional distribution for (β_2, β_3) given $y_{i+} = t$ $(= 1, 2, ..., S+T)$ is a multinomial distribution

$$\Pr\{y_{i(-S+1)}, ..., y_{i0}, y_{i1}, ..., y_{iT}) \mid y_{i+}\} = \text{Multinomial}(y_{i+}, \boldsymbol{p}), \quad \text{(A.16)}$$

where

$$\begin{aligned} \boldsymbol{p} &= (p_{i(-S+1)}, ..., p_{i0}, p_{i1}, ..., p_{iT})^t, \\ p_{ij}(j \le 0) &= \begin{cases} \frac{1}{S+Te^{\beta_2}}, & i = 1, ..., n_1, \text{ (control group)} \\ \frac{1}{S+Te^{\beta_2+\beta_3}}, & i = n_1+1, ..., n_1+n_2, \text{ (new treatment group)} \end{cases} \\ p_{ij}(j > 0) &= \begin{cases} \frac{e^{\beta_2}}{S+Te^{\beta_2}}, & i = 1, ..., n_1, \text{ (control group)} \\ \frac{e^{\beta_2+\beta_3}}{S+Te^{\beta_2+\beta_3}}, & i = n_1+1, ..., n_1+n_2, \text{ (new treatment group).} \end{cases} \end{aligned}$$

Then, the conditional likelihood is

$$L_C(\beta_2, \beta_3) \propto \prod_{i=n_1+1}^{n_1+n_2} \left(\frac{1}{S+Te^{\beta_2+\beta_3}}\right)^{\sum_{j=0}^{S-1} y_{i(-j)}} \left(\frac{e^{\beta_2+\beta_3}}{S+Te^{\beta_2+\beta_3}}\right)^{\sum_{j=1}^{T} y_{ij}}$$
$$\times \prod_{i=n_1}^{n_1} \left(\frac{1}{S+Te^{\beta_2}}\right)^{\sum_{j=0}^{S-1} y_{i(-j)}} \left(\frac{e^{\beta_2}}{S+Te^{\beta_2}}\right)^{\sum_{j=1}^{T} y_{ij}}. \quad \text{(A.17)}$$

Then, the conditional maximum likelihood estimator of e^{β_3} is given by

$$e^{\hat{\beta}_{3C}} = \frac{y_{+1}^{(2)} y_{+0}^{(1)}}{y_{+0}^{(2)} y_{+1}^{(1)}}, \quad \text{(A.18)}$$

where

$$y_{+0}^{(1)} = \sum_{i=1}^{n_1} \sum_{j(\le 0)} y_{ij}, \quad y_{+1}^{(1)} = \sum_{i=1}^{n_1} \sum_{j(>0)} y_{ij},$$

$$y_{+0}^{(2)} = \sum_{i=n_1+1}^{n_1+n_2} \sum_{j(\le 0)} y_{ij}, \quad y_{+1}^{(2)} = \sum_{i=n_1+1}^{n_1+n_2} \sum_{j(>0)} y_{ij}.$$

It should be noted that $e^{\hat{\beta}_{3C}}$ is equal to $e^{\hat{\beta}_3}$, the maximum likelihood estimator of the *random intercept* Poisson regression model (1.11). Its standard error is approximated by

$$S.E.(e^{\hat{\beta}_{3C}}) = \sqrt{\frac{1}{y_{+0}^{(2)}} + \frac{1}{y_{+1}^{(2)}} + \frac{1}{y_{+0}^{(1)}} + \frac{1}{y_{+1}^{(1)}}}. \quad \text{(A.19)}$$

Then, we can consider the sample size calculation based on the conditional efficient score test for testing the null hypothesis $H_0 : \beta_{3C} = 0$ derived as

$$Z = \frac{\sqrt{s_+}(y_{+1}^{(2)} y_{+0}^{(1)} - y_{+0}^{(2)} y_{+1}^{(1)})}{\sqrt{m_0 m_1 s_2 s_1}} \sim N(0,1). \quad \text{(A.20)}$$

Before going to the sample size calculation, let us assume here that $(b_{01}, \ldots, b_{0(2n)})$ is a sequence of $2n$ independent, identically distributed random variables having mean μ_b (expected counts) in each unit baseline period $(j = -S+1, ..., 0)$. Then, the sample size formula with two equally sized groups $(n_1 = n_2 = n)$ to detect an effect size e^{β_3} with power $100(1-\phi)\%$ at two-sided significance level α assuming *no period effect*, $\beta_2 = 0$, is given by

$$n_{S,T} = \frac{1}{\mu_b(e^{\beta_3}-1)^2} \left(z_{\alpha/2} \sqrt{\frac{2(S+T)(e^{\beta_3}+1)(S+Te^{\beta_3})}{ST\{2S+T(e^{\beta_3}+1)\}}} + \right.$$
$$\left. z_\phi \sqrt{\frac{(S+T)^3 e^{\beta_3} + (S+Te^{\beta_3})^3}{ST(S+T)(S+Te^{\beta_3})}} \right)^2, \quad \text{(A.21)}$$

which is an extension of Tango's sample size formula for the case $S = T = 1$ (Tango, 2009). From this formula, we can find the following relationship, i.e., sample size reduction to a considerable extent,

$$n_{T,T} = \frac{1}{T} n_{S=1,T=1}, \tag{A.22}$$

where

$$n_{S=1,T=1} = \frac{1}{\mu_b (e^{\beta_3} - 1)^2} \left(z_{\alpha/2} \sqrt{\frac{4(e^{\beta_3} + 1)^2}{(e^{\beta_3} + 3)}} + z_\phi \sqrt{\frac{8e^{\beta_3} + (1 + e^{\beta_3})^3}{2(1 + e^{\beta_3})}} \right)^2 . \tag{A.23}$$

The validity of the sample size formula $n_{S=1,T=1}$ has been examined via a Monte Carlo simulation study by Tango (2009). However, as in the case of normal linear regression models, the *random intercept* model sometimes fits worse than the *random intercept plus slope* model. For the latter model, we can obtain Monte Carlo simulated sample sizes.

A.3 Logistic regression model

In a similar manner to the Poisson regression model, the conditional efficient score test for testing the null hypothesis $H_0 : \beta_{3C} = 0$ can be derived. For illustrative purposes, let us consider a randomized controlled trial to compare the two treatments, a new treatment and a control treatment to improve the respiratory status. So, y_{ij} denotes the binary responses such that $y_{ij} = 1$ if subject i's respiratory status is "good" and $y_{ij} = 0$ the status is "poor." In a similar manner to the case of the normal linear regression model, we can express subject i's contribution to the likelihood in the *random intercept* model (1.11) as

$$\begin{aligned} p(\boldsymbol{y}_i \mid \boldsymbol{b}_i) &= \prod_{j=-S+1}^{T} \frac{(\exp(b_{0i} + \beta_0 + \boldsymbol{x}_{ij}^t \boldsymbol{\beta}))^{y_{ij}}}{1 + \exp(b_{0i} + \beta_0 + \boldsymbol{x}_{ij}^t \boldsymbol{\beta})} \\ &= \exp(y_{i+}\theta_{1i} + \sum_{j=-S+1}^{T} y_{ij}\theta_{2ij}) \\ &\quad \times \prod_{j=-S+1}^{T} \frac{1}{1 + \exp(\exp(b_{0i} + \beta_0 + \boldsymbol{x}_{ij}^t \boldsymbol{\beta})}. \end{aligned} \tag{A.24}$$

Namely, here also, y_{i+} is the minimal sufficient statistic for θ_{1i}. Then, the conditional likelihood for (β_2, β_3) given $y_{i+} = t$ $(= 1, 2, ..., S + T)$ is of the

TABLE A.1
Matched-pair 2 × 2 contingency table for change of respiratory status from baseline period to post randomization by treatment group.

Before randomization ($j = 0$)	Post randomization ($j = 1$)		Total
	good	poor	
New treatment (2)			
good		$y_{gp}^{(2)}$	
poor	$y_{pg}^{(2)}$		
total			n_2
Control treatment (1)			
good		$y_{gp}^{(1)}$	
poor	$y_{pg}^{(1)}$		
total			n_1

form

$$L_{iC}(\beta_2, \beta_3 \mid y_{i+} = t) \quad \propto \quad \frac{\exp(\sum_{j=-S+1}^{T} y_{ij}\theta_{2ij})}{\sum_{(j_{-S+1},\ldots,j_T)\in R(t)} \exp(\sum_{j\in(j_{-S+1},\ldots,j_T)} y_{ij}\theta_{2ij})}, \tag{A.25}$$

where $R(t)$ denotes the set of all possible combinations $(j_{-S+1}, \ldots, j_T)$ such that $y_{i+} = t$. Different from the normal linear regression models, it will be quite cumbersome to derive the sample size formula for a general *S:T design.* So, here, we shall consider the sample size for the simple *1:1 design.*

In this simplest case, we have only to consider the case of $y_{i+} = y_{i0} + y_{i1} = 1$ because the case $y_{i+} = 0$ or $y_{i+} = 2$ does not contribute the conditional likelihood. Then, the conditional likelihood given $y_{i+} = 1$ is

$$L_C(\beta_2, \beta_3 \mid t = 1) \quad = \quad \prod_{i:y_{i+}=1} \frac{\exp\{y_{i1}(\beta_2 + \beta_3 x_{1i})\}}{1 + \exp\{\beta_2 + \beta_3 x_{1i}\}} \tag{A.26}$$

and the conditional log-likelihood function is

$$l_C(\beta_2, \beta_3 \mid t = 1) \quad = \quad \sum_{i:y_{i+}=1} \{y_{i1}(\beta_2 + \beta_3 x_{1i}) - \log(1 + \exp(\beta_2 + \beta_3 x_{1i}))\}. \tag{A.27}$$

Then, the conditional maximum likelihood estimators of (β_2, β_3) are given by

TABLE A.2
2 × 2 contingency table between treatment groups and the type of transition from baseline to post treatment.

Group	Type of transition		Total
	poor → good	good → poor	
New treatment (2)	$y_{pg}^{(2)}$	$y_{gp}^{(2)}$	s_2
Control treatment (1)	$y_{pg}^{(1)}$	$y_{gp}^{(1)}$	s_1
Total	m_1	m_0	s_+

$$\hat{\beta}_{2C} = \log\left(\frac{y_{pg}^{(1)}}{y_{gp}^{(1)}}\right) \tag{A.28}$$

$$\hat{\beta}_{3C} = \log\left\{\left(\frac{y_{pg}^{(2)}}{y_{gp}^{(2)}}\right) / \left(\frac{y_{pg}^{(1)}}{y_{gp}^{(1)}}\right)\right\} = \log\left(\frac{y_{pg}^{(2)} y_{gp}^{(1)}}{y_{gp}^{(2)} y_{pg}^{(1)}}\right), \tag{A.29}$$

where $y_{pg}^{(k)}$ and $y_{gp}^{(k)}$ denote the number of subjects whose respiratory status improved ("poor" → "good") and got worse ("good" → "poor") from the baseline to the observation time point 1 in the treatment group k, respectively. When we tabulate these counts in Table A.1, we can see that the conditional maximum likelihood estimator $e^{\hat{\beta}_{2C}}$ implies the matched-pair odds ratio of improvement ("poor" → "good") in the control group and the conditional maximum likelihood estimator $e^{\hat{\beta}_{3C}}$ of treatment effect implies the ratio of the improvement odds ratio in the new treatment group to the improvement odds ratio in the control treatment group.

Furthermore, when we tabulate these four counts in the form of Table A.2, where $s_1 = y_{pg}^{(1)} + y_{gp}^{(1)}$ and $s_2 = y_{pg}^{(2)} + y_{gp}^{(2)}$, then we can see that the treatment effects are equal to the odds ratio of this 2 × 2 contingency table and so, its standard error is approximated by

$$S.E.(e^{\hat{\beta}_{3C}}) = \sqrt{\frac{1}{y_{gp}^{(2)}} + \frac{1}{y_{pg}^{(2)}} + \frac{1}{y_{gp}^{(1)}} + \frac{1}{y_{pg}^{(1)}}}. \tag{A.30}$$

Then, the conditional efficient score test for testing the null hypothesis $H_0 : \beta_{3C} = 0$ is derived as

$$Z = \frac{\sqrt{s_+}(y_{pg}^{(2)} y_{gp}^{(1)} - y_{gp}^{(2)} y_{pg}^{(1)})}{\sqrt{m_0 m_1 s_2 s_1}} \sim N(0, 1). \tag{A.31}$$

However, the conditional approach uses only the non-diagonal frequencies, and consequently, the standard error of treatment effects tends to be larger than in a mixed-effects model and the derived sample size formula (omitted here) tends to overestimate the sample size actually required. So, for logistic regression models, we have to rely on Monte Carlo simulated sample sizes.

Appendix B

Generalized linear mixed models

In this chapter, we present the theory for the three kinds of generalized linear mixed (or mixed-effects) models (GLMMs), normal linear, logistic and Poisson regression models, within the framework of the $S{:}T$ repeated measures design briefly introduced in Chapter 1. A general formulation of GLMM is presented and estimation methods for GLMM, based on the likelihood or the restricted likelihood of the parameters, are described together with the computational methods for the numerical integration to evaluate the integral included in the likelihood.

B.1 Likelihood

B.1.1 Normal linear regression model

For the $S{:}T$ repeated measures design introduced in (1.4), i.e.,

$$\boldsymbol{y}_i^t = (y_{i(-S+1)}, ..., y_{i0}, \ y_{i1}, ..., y_{iT}), \ i = 1, ..., N \tag{B.1}$$

and, given the random effects $\boldsymbol{b}_i$ $(q \times 1)$, the normal linear regression model in general can be expressed as

$$\begin{aligned} y_{ij} \mid \boldsymbol{b}_i &= \beta_0 + \boldsymbol{x}_{ij}^t \boldsymbol{\beta} + \boldsymbol{z}_{ij}^t \boldsymbol{b}_i + \epsilon_{ij}, \ i = 1, ..., N & \text{(B.2)} \\ \epsilon_{ij} &\sim N(0, \sigma_E^2) & \text{(B.3)} \\ \boldsymbol{b}_i &\sim N(0, \boldsymbol{\Phi}), & \text{(B.4)} \end{aligned}$$

where

$$\begin{aligned} \boldsymbol{x}_{ij} &= (x_{1ij}, ..., x_{kij})^t & \text{(B.5)} \\ \boldsymbol{\beta} &= (\beta_1, ..., \beta_k)^t & \text{(B.6)} \\ \boldsymbol{z}_{ij} &= (z_{1ij}, ..., z_{qij})^t & \text{(B.7)} \end{aligned}$$

and the errors ϵ_{ij} are assumed to be independent of each other. In other words, given the random effects $\boldsymbol{b}_i$, the subject-specific repeated measures $(y_{i(-S+1)}, ..., y_{i0}, y_{i1} ..., y_{iT})$ are *mutually independent.* Therefore, subject i's contribution to the likelihood is

$$p(\boldsymbol{y}_i \mid \boldsymbol{b}_i) = \prod_{j=0}^{T} \phi(y_{ij} \mid \beta_0 + \boldsymbol{x}_{ij}^t \boldsymbol{\beta} + \boldsymbol{z}_{ij}^t \boldsymbol{b}_i, \sigma_E^2), \tag{B.8}$$

where

$$\phi(x \mid \mu, \sigma_E^2) = \frac{1}{\sqrt{2\pi}} \exp\left\{ -\frac{(x-\mu)^2}{2\sigma_E^2} \right\} \tag{B.9}$$

and the probability density function of the random effects $\boldsymbol{b}_i$ is

$$f(\boldsymbol{b}_i \mid \boldsymbol{\Phi}) = \frac{1}{(2\pi)^{q/2}\sqrt{\mid \boldsymbol{\Phi} \mid}} \exp\left\{ -\frac{\boldsymbol{b}_i^t \boldsymbol{\Phi}^{-1} \boldsymbol{b}_i}{2} \right\}. \tag{B.10}$$

Therefore, the likelihood is given by

$$\begin{aligned} L(\boldsymbol{\beta}, \Phi, \sigma_E^2) &= \prod_{i=1}^{N} \int_{-\infty}^{\infty} p(\boldsymbol{y}_i \mid \boldsymbol{b}_i) f(\boldsymbol{b}_i \mid \boldsymbol{\Phi}) d\boldsymbol{b}_i \\ &= \prod_{i=1}^{N} \int_{-\infty}^{\infty} \left\{ \prod_{j=-S+1}^{T} \phi(y_{ij} \mid \beta_0 + \boldsymbol{x}_{ij}^t \boldsymbol{\beta} + \boldsymbol{z}_{ij}^t \boldsymbol{b}_i, \sigma_E^2) \right\} \\ &\qquad \times f(\boldsymbol{b}_i \mid \boldsymbol{\Phi}) d\boldsymbol{b}_i \end{aligned} \tag{B.11}$$

Especially, for the *random intercept model* (1.11), i.e., $\boldsymbol{b}_i = b_{0i}, \boldsymbol{z} = z_{1ij} = 1$ and

$$b_{0i} \sim N(0, \sigma_{B0}^2), \tag{B.12}$$

the likelihood is given by

$$(2\pi\sigma_{B0}^2)^{-N/2} \prod_{i=1}^{N} \int_{-\infty}^{\infty} \left\{ \prod_{j=-S+1}^{T} \phi(y_{ij} \mid \beta_0 + \boldsymbol{x}_{ij}^t \boldsymbol{\beta} + u, \sigma_E^2) \right\} \exp\{-\frac{u^2}{2\sigma_{B0}^2}\} du.$$

B.1.2 Logistic regression model

In the logistic regression model for binary endpoint y_{ij}, we have

$$y_{ij} \mid \boldsymbol{b}_i \sim \text{Bernoulli}(p_{ij}) \tag{B.13}$$

$$\text{logit } p(y_{ij} \mid \boldsymbol{b}_i) = \text{logit} \Pr\{y_{ij} = 1 \mid \boldsymbol{b}_i\} = \beta_0 + \boldsymbol{x}_{ij}^t \boldsymbol{\beta} + \boldsymbol{z}_{ij}^t \boldsymbol{b}_i \tag{B.14}$$

$$\boldsymbol{b}_i \sim N(0, \boldsymbol{\Phi}) \tag{B.15}$$

and

$$
\begin{aligned}
p(\boldsymbol{y}_i \mid \boldsymbol{b}_i) &= \prod_{j=-S+1}^{T} \left(\frac{\exp(\beta_0 + \boldsymbol{x}_{ij}^t \boldsymbol{\beta} + \boldsymbol{z}_{ij}^t \boldsymbol{b}_i)}{1 + \exp(\beta_0 + \boldsymbol{x}_{ij}^t \boldsymbol{\beta} + \boldsymbol{z}_{ij}^t \boldsymbol{b}_i)} \right)^{y_{ij}} \\
&\quad \times \left(\frac{1}{1 + \exp(\beta_0 + \boldsymbol{x}_{ij}^t \boldsymbol{\beta} + \boldsymbol{z}_{ij}^t \boldsymbol{b}_i)} \right)^{1-y_{ij}} \\
&= \prod_{j=-S+1}^{T} \frac{(\exp(\beta_0 + \boldsymbol{x}_{ij}^t \boldsymbol{\beta} + \boldsymbol{z}_{ij}^t \boldsymbol{b}_i))^{y_{ij}}}{1 + \exp(\beta_0 + \boldsymbol{x}_{ij}^t \boldsymbol{\beta} + \boldsymbol{z}_{ij}^t \boldsymbol{b}_i)}. \qquad \text{(B.16)}
\end{aligned}
$$

Therefore, the likelihood is

$$
\begin{aligned}
L(\boldsymbol{\beta}, \Phi) &= \prod_{i=1}^{N} \int_{-\infty}^{\infty} p(\boldsymbol{y}_i \mid \boldsymbol{b}_i) f(\boldsymbol{b}_i \mid \boldsymbol{\Phi}) d\boldsymbol{b}_i \\
&= \prod_{i=1}^{N} \int_{-\infty}^{\infty} \prod_{j=0}^{T} \frac{(\exp(\beta_0 + \boldsymbol{x}_{ij}^t \boldsymbol{\beta} + \boldsymbol{z}_{ij}^t \boldsymbol{b}_i))^{y_{ij}}}{1 + \exp(\beta_0 + \boldsymbol{x}_{ij}^t \boldsymbol{\beta} + \boldsymbol{z}_{ij}^t \boldsymbol{b}_i)} f(\boldsymbol{b}_i \mid \boldsymbol{\Phi}) d\boldsymbol{b}_i. \qquad \text{(B.17)}
\end{aligned}
$$

Especially, for the *random intercept model* (1.11), the likelihood is

$$
\begin{aligned}
L(\boldsymbol{\beta}, \Phi) &= (2\pi\sigma_{B0}^2)^{-N/2} \prod_{i=1}^{N} \int_{-\infty}^{\infty} \left\{ \prod_{j=-S+1}^{T} \frac{(\exp(\beta_0 + \boldsymbol{x}_{ij}^t \boldsymbol{\beta} + u))^{y_{ij}}}{1 + \exp(\beta_0 + \boldsymbol{x}_{ij}^t \boldsymbol{\beta} + u)} \right\} \\
&\quad \exp\{-\frac{u^2}{2\sigma_{B0}^2}\} du. \qquad \text{(B.18)}
\end{aligned}
$$

B.1.3 Poisson regression model

In the Poisson regression mode for the *count* endpoint y_{ij}, we have

$$
\begin{aligned}
y_{ij} \mid \boldsymbol{b}_i &\sim \text{Poisson}(\lambda_{ij}) \qquad \text{(B.19)} \\
\log \lambda_{ij} &= \log E(y_{ij} \mid \boldsymbol{b}_i) = \beta_0 + \boldsymbol{x}_{ij}^t \boldsymbol{\beta} + \boldsymbol{z}_{ij}^t \boldsymbol{b}_i \qquad \text{(B.20)} \\
p(y_{ij} \mid \boldsymbol{b}_i) &= \frac{(\lambda_{ij})^{y_{ij}}}{y_{ij}!} \exp(-\lambda_{ij}) \qquad \text{(B.21)} \\
\boldsymbol{b}_i &\sim N(0, \boldsymbol{\Phi}) \qquad \text{(B.22)}
\end{aligned}
$$

and

$$
\begin{aligned}
p(\boldsymbol{y}_i \mid \boldsymbol{b}_i) &= \prod_{j=-S+1}^{T} \frac{\exp(y_{ij}(\beta_0 + \boldsymbol{x}_{ij}^t \boldsymbol{\beta} + \boldsymbol{z}_{ij}^t \boldsymbol{b}_i))}{y_{ij}!} \\
&\quad \times \exp(-\exp(\beta_0 + \boldsymbol{x}_{ij}^t \boldsymbol{\beta} + \boldsymbol{z}_{ij}^t \boldsymbol{b}_i)). \qquad \text{(B.23)}
\end{aligned}
$$

Therefore, the likelihood is

$$\begin{aligned} L(\boldsymbol{\beta}, \Phi) &= \prod_{i=1}^{N} \int_{-\infty}^{\infty} p(\boldsymbol{y}_i \mid \boldsymbol{b}_i) f(\boldsymbol{b}_i \mid \boldsymbol{\Phi}) d\boldsymbol{b}_i \\ &= \prod_{i=1}^{N} \int_{-\infty}^{\infty} \prod_{j=-S+1}^{T} \frac{\exp(y_{ij}(\beta_0 + \boldsymbol{x}_{ij}^t \boldsymbol{\beta} + \boldsymbol{z}_{ij}^t \boldsymbol{b}_i))}{y_{ij}!} \\ &\quad \exp(-\exp(\beta_0 + \boldsymbol{x}_{ij}^t \boldsymbol{\beta} + \boldsymbol{z}_{ij}^t \boldsymbol{b}_i)) f(\boldsymbol{b}_i \mid \boldsymbol{\Phi}) d\boldsymbol{b}_i. \end{aligned} \tag{B.24}$$

Especially, for the *random intercept model* (1.11), the likelihood is

$$\begin{aligned} L(\boldsymbol{\beta}, \Phi) &= (2\pi\sigma_{B0}^2)^{-N/2} \prod_{i=1}^{N} \int_{-\infty}^{\infty} \\ &\left\{ \prod_{j=-S+1}^{T} \frac{\exp(y_{ij}(\beta_0 + \boldsymbol{x}_{ij}^t \boldsymbol{\beta} + u))}{y_{ij}!} \exp(-\exp(\beta_0 + \boldsymbol{x}_{ij}^t \boldsymbol{\beta} + u)) \right\} \\ &\exp\{-\frac{u^2}{2\sigma_{B0}^2}\} du. \end{aligned} \tag{B.25}$$

It should be noted that the likelihood function for the *random intercept model*, for example, in both the logistic regression and the Poisson regression models, has the integral of the form

$$\int_{-\infty}^{\infty} h_i(u \mid \boldsymbol{\xi}) \exp\{-\frac{u^2}{2\sigma_{B0}^2}\} du. \tag{B.26}$$

where $h_i(.)$ includes the parameters of interest $\boldsymbol{\xi}$. So, we need some numerical integration methods to assess the integral.

B.2 Maximum likelihood estimate

In this section, we shall change the notation as follows:

$$\begin{cases} \boldsymbol{x}_{ij} \leftarrow (1, x_{1ij}, ..., x_{kij})^t = (1, \boldsymbol{x}_{ij}^t)^t \\ \boldsymbol{\beta} \leftarrow (\beta_0, \beta_1, ..., \beta_k) = (\beta_0, \boldsymbol{\beta}^t)^t. \end{cases} \tag{B.27}$$

B.2.1 Normal linear regression model

The model (B.2) can be re-expressed as

$$\begin{aligned} \boldsymbol{y}_i \mid \boldsymbol{b}_i &= \boldsymbol{X}_i^t \boldsymbol{\beta} + \boldsymbol{Z}_i^t \boldsymbol{b}_i + \boldsymbol{\epsilon}_i & \text{(B.28)} \\ &= \boldsymbol{X}_i^t \boldsymbol{\beta} + \boldsymbol{\epsilon}_i^*, & \text{(B.29)} \end{aligned}$$

where

$$\begin{aligned} \boldsymbol{\epsilon}_i^* &\sim N(0, \boldsymbol{\Sigma}_i), && \text{(B.30)} \\ \boldsymbol{X}_i &= (\boldsymbol{x}_{i0}, \boldsymbol{x}_{i1}, ..., \boldsymbol{x}_{iT})^t, \ ((T+1) \times (k+1)) && \text{(B.31)} \\ \boldsymbol{Z}_i &= (\boldsymbol{z}_{i0}, \boldsymbol{z}_{i1}, ..., \boldsymbol{z}_{iT})^t, \ ((T+1) \times q) && \text{(B.32)} \\ \boldsymbol{\Sigma}_i &= \sigma_E^2 \boldsymbol{I} + \boldsymbol{Z}_i \boldsymbol{\Phi} \boldsymbol{Z}_i^t. && \text{(B.33)} \end{aligned}$$

Using these expressions, the likelihood (B.11) can be re-expressed as

$$\begin{aligned} L(\boldsymbol{\beta}, \boldsymbol{\Sigma}_i) &= \prod_{i=1}^N \int_{-\infty}^{\infty} p(\boldsymbol{y}_i \mid \boldsymbol{b}_i) f(\boldsymbol{b}_i \mid \boldsymbol{\Phi}) d\boldsymbol{b}_i \\ &= \prod_{i=1}^N (2\pi)^{-\frac{T+1}{2}} \exp\left\{ -\frac{(\boldsymbol{y}_i - \boldsymbol{X}_i\boldsymbol{\beta})^t \boldsymbol{\Sigma}_i^{-1} (\boldsymbol{y}_i - \boldsymbol{X}_i\boldsymbol{\beta})}{2} \right\} \mid \boldsymbol{\Sigma}_i \mid^{-\frac{1}{2}} \end{aligned} \quad \text{(B.34)}$$

and the log-likelihood is

$$\begin{aligned} l(\boldsymbol{\beta}, \boldsymbol{\Sigma}_i) &= -\frac{T+1}{2} \log(2\pi) - \frac{1}{2} \log(\mid \boldsymbol{\Sigma}_i \mid) \\ &\quad + \sum_{i=1}^N \left\{ -\frac{(\boldsymbol{y}_i - \boldsymbol{X}_i\boldsymbol{\beta})^t \boldsymbol{\Sigma}_i^{-1} (\boldsymbol{y}_i - \boldsymbol{X}_i\boldsymbol{\beta})}{2} \right\}. \end{aligned} \quad \text{(B.35)}$$

Then, given the covariance matrix $\boldsymbol{\Sigma}_i$, the maximum likelihood estimate $\hat{\boldsymbol{\beta}}$ is given by the general form

$$\hat{\boldsymbol{\beta}}(\boldsymbol{\Sigma}_i) = \left(\sum_{i=1}^N \boldsymbol{X}_i^t \boldsymbol{\Sigma}_i^{-1} \boldsymbol{X}_i \right)^{-1} \sum_{i=1}^N \boldsymbol{X}_i^t \boldsymbol{\Sigma}_i^{-1} \boldsymbol{y}_i \quad \text{(B.36)}$$

and its covariance matrix is given by

$$\text{Var}(\hat{\boldsymbol{\beta}}(\boldsymbol{\Sigma}_i)) = \left(\sum_{i=1}^n \boldsymbol{X}_i^t \boldsymbol{\Sigma}_i^{-1} \boldsymbol{X}_i \right)^{-1}. \quad \text{(B.37)}$$

Estimation of the covariance matrix $\boldsymbol{\Sigma}_i$, on the other hand, is usually based on the REML (restricted maximum likelihood) estimator to be described below because the maximum likelihood estimate of $\boldsymbol{\Sigma}_i$ is known to be *biased downward* in finite samples. The restricted maximum likelihood function of $\boldsymbol{\Sigma}_i$ is

$$L_{\text{REML}}(\boldsymbol{\Sigma}_i) = \int_{-\infty}^{\infty} L(\boldsymbol{\beta}, \boldsymbol{\Sigma}_i) d\boldsymbol{\beta}. \quad \text{(B.38)}$$

By taking the relationship

$$\boldsymbol{y}_i - \boldsymbol{X}_i\boldsymbol{\beta} = (\boldsymbol{y}_i - \boldsymbol{X}_i\hat{\boldsymbol{\beta}}) - \boldsymbol{X}_i(\boldsymbol{\beta} - \hat{\boldsymbol{\beta}}),$$

the likelihood function (B.38) can be re-expressed as

$$\begin{aligned}
L_{\text{REML}}(\boldsymbol{\Sigma}_i) &= \int_{-\infty}^{\infty} \prod_{i=1}^{N} (2\pi)^{-\frac{T+1}{2}} \exp\left\{-\frac{(\boldsymbol{y}_i - \boldsymbol{X}_i\hat{\boldsymbol{\beta}})^t \boldsymbol{\Sigma}_i^{-1}(\boldsymbol{y}_i - \boldsymbol{X}_i\hat{\boldsymbol{\beta}})}{2}\right\} \\
&\quad \times \exp\left\{-\frac{(\boldsymbol{\beta} - \hat{\boldsymbol{\beta}})^t \boldsymbol{X}_i^t \boldsymbol{\Sigma}_i^{-1} \boldsymbol{X}_i(\boldsymbol{\beta} - \hat{\boldsymbol{\beta}})}{2}\right\} \mid \boldsymbol{\Sigma}_i \mid^{-\frac{1}{2}} d\boldsymbol{\beta} \\
&= \prod_{i=1}^{N} (2\pi)^{-\frac{T+1-k}{2}} \exp\left\{-\frac{(\boldsymbol{y}_i - \boldsymbol{X}_i\hat{\boldsymbol{\beta}})^t \boldsymbol{\Sigma}_i^{-1}(\boldsymbol{y}_i - \boldsymbol{X}_i\hat{\boldsymbol{\beta}})}{2}\right\} \\
&\quad \times \mid \sum_{i=1}^{N} \boldsymbol{X}_i^t \boldsymbol{\Sigma}_i \boldsymbol{X}_i \mid^{-\frac{1}{2}} \mid \boldsymbol{\Sigma}_i \mid^{-\frac{1}{2}} \\
&= \text{constant} \cdot L(\hat{\beta}(\boldsymbol{\Sigma}_i), \boldsymbol{\Sigma}_i) \cdot \mid \sum_{i=1}^{N} \boldsymbol{X}_i^t \boldsymbol{\Sigma}_i \boldsymbol{X}_i \mid^{-\frac{1}{2}}. \qquad \text{(B.39)}
\end{aligned}$$

Namely, the REML estimator can be obtained by maximizing the following so-called REML log-likelihood function

$$l_{\text{REML}}(\boldsymbol{\Sigma}_i) = l(\hat{\beta}(\boldsymbol{\Sigma}_i), \boldsymbol{\Sigma}_i) + \log(\mid \sum_{i=1}^{N} \boldsymbol{X}_i^t \boldsymbol{\Sigma}_i \boldsymbol{X}_i \mid^{-\frac{1}{2}}). \qquad \text{(B.40)}$$

Now, the estimated covariance or the standard errors (B.37) do not take the variability introduced in estimating $\boldsymbol{\Sigma}_i$ into account and then they also tend to be *biased downward* in estimating $\boldsymbol{\beta}$. So, the Wald test statistics based on the estimated standard errors, (B.36) and (B.37), tend to be more significant than it is. In the literature, to resolve this downward bias, several approximate t-statistics or F-statistics have been proposed for testing hypotheses about $\boldsymbol{\beta}$. Among other things, Satterthwaite-type approximation (Satterthwaite, 1941) has often been used in practice. For example, for the null hypothesis $H_0 : \beta_k = 0$, by setting the linear contrast as $\beta_k = \boldsymbol{c}^t\boldsymbol{\beta}$, the ordinary Wald test statistic is given by

$$z = \frac{\boldsymbol{c}^t\hat{\boldsymbol{\beta}}}{\sqrt{\boldsymbol{c}^t(\sum_{i=1}^{N} \boldsymbol{X}_i^t \boldsymbol{\Sigma}_i^{-1} \boldsymbol{X}_i)^{-1}\boldsymbol{c}}} \sim N(0,1). \qquad \text{(B.41)}$$

Satterthwaite's approximate t-statistic, on the other hand, adopts the following degrees of freedom

$$\nu = \frac{2(\boldsymbol{c}^t(\sum_{i=1}^{N} \boldsymbol{X}_i^t \boldsymbol{\Sigma}_i^{-1} \boldsymbol{X}_i)^{-1}\boldsymbol{c})^2}{\boldsymbol{g}^t \text{Cov}(\hat{\boldsymbol{\theta}})\boldsymbol{g}}, \qquad \text{(B.42)}$$

where $\boldsymbol{\theta} = (\sigma_E^2, \sigma_{B0}^2, ...)^t$ is the vector of parameters included in $\boldsymbol{\Sigma}_i$ and

$$\boldsymbol{g} = \frac{\partial\ \boldsymbol{c}^t(\sum_{i=1}^{N} \boldsymbol{X}_i^t \boldsymbol{\Sigma}_i^{-1} \boldsymbol{X}_i)^{-1}\boldsymbol{c}}{\partial\boldsymbol{\theta}} \Big|_{\boldsymbol{\theta}=\hat{\boldsymbol{\theta}}} \cdot$$

Although Kenward and Roger (1997) proposed alternative approximate degrees of freedom that can be used in SAS, we shall use Satterthwaite's approximation in this book.

B.2.2 Logistic regression model

Here also, let us consider the *random intercept model* (1.11). By noting the change of notation (B.27), the log-likelihood function is

$$l(\boldsymbol{\beta}, \Phi) = -\frac{N}{2}\log(2\pi\sigma_{B0}^2) + \sum_{i=1}^{N}\sum_{j=0}^{T} y_{ij}\boldsymbol{x}_{ij}^t\boldsymbol{\beta} + \sum_{i=1}^{N}\log\int_{-\infty}^{\infty} e^{g_i(u|\boldsymbol{\beta},\sigma_{B0}^2)}du, \tag{B.43}$$

where

$$g_i(u \mid \boldsymbol{\beta}, \sigma_{B0}^2) = \sum_{j=0}^{T} y_{ij}u - \sum_{j=0}^{T}\log[1+\exp(\boldsymbol{x}_{ij}^t\boldsymbol{\beta}+u)] - \frac{u^2}{2\sigma_{B0}^2}. \tag{B.44}$$

Further, we have

$$\frac{\partial g_i}{\partial \beta_s} = -\sum_{j=0}^{T}\frac{x_{sij}\exp(\boldsymbol{x}_{ij}^t\boldsymbol{\beta}+u)}{1+\exp(\boldsymbol{x}_{ij}^t\boldsymbol{\beta}+u)} \tag{B.45}$$

$$\frac{\partial^2 g_i}{\partial \beta_s \beta_t} = \sum_{j=0}^{T}\frac{x_{sij}x_{tij}\exp(\boldsymbol{x}_{ij}^t\boldsymbol{\beta}+u)}{[1+\exp(\boldsymbol{x}_{ij}^t\boldsymbol{\beta}+u)]^2} \tag{B.46}$$

$$\frac{\partial g_i}{\partial \sigma_{B0}^2} = \frac{u^2}{2\sigma_{B0}^4}. \tag{B.47}$$

Then, the partial derivatives of l with respect to the parameters $\boldsymbol{\beta}, \sigma_{B0}^2$ are given by

$$\frac{\partial l}{\partial \beta_s} = \sum_{i=1}^{N}\sum_{j=0}^{T} y_{ij}\boldsymbol{x}_{ij}^t + \sum_{i=1}^{N}\frac{J_{i1s}}{J_{i0}} \tag{B.48}$$

$$\frac{\partial^2 l}{\partial \beta_s \beta_t} = \sum_{i=1}^{N}\frac{J_{i3st}}{J_{i0}} - \sum_{i=1}^{N}\frac{J_{i1s}J_{i1t}}{J_{i0}^2} \tag{B.49}$$

$$\frac{\partial l}{\partial \sigma_{B0}^2} = -\frac{N}{2\sigma_{B0}^2} + \frac{1}{2\sigma_{B0}^4}\sum_{i=1}^{N}\frac{J_{i2}}{J_{i0}}, \tag{B.50}$$

where

$$
\begin{aligned}
J_{i0} &= \int_{-\infty}^{\infty} e^{g_i(u|\boldsymbol{\beta},\sigma_{B0}^2)} du && \text{(B.51)} \\
J_{i1s} &= \int_{-\infty}^{\infty} \frac{\partial g_i}{\partial \beta_s} e^{g_i(u|\boldsymbol{\beta},\sigma_{B0}^2)} du && \text{(B.52)} \\
J_{i2} &= \int_{-\infty}^{\infty} u^2 e^{g_i(u|\boldsymbol{\beta},\sigma_{B0}^2)} du && \text{(B.53)} \\
J_{i3st} &= \int_{-\infty}^{\infty} \frac{\partial^2 g_i}{\partial \beta_s \beta_t} e^{g_i(u|\boldsymbol{\beta},\sigma_{B0}^2)} du. && \text{(B.54)}
\end{aligned}
$$

Therefore, the MLE of the parameters $\boldsymbol{\gamma} = (\boldsymbol{\beta}^t, \sigma_{B0}^2)^t$ is obtained by using the following Newton–Raphson algorithm.

$$
\hat{\boldsymbol{\gamma}}^{(k+1)} = \hat{\boldsymbol{\gamma}}^{(k)} - \left(\frac{\partial^2 l}{\partial \boldsymbol{\gamma}^2} \right)^{-1}_{\hat{\boldsymbol{\gamma}}^{(k)}} \left(\frac{\partial l}{\partial \boldsymbol{\gamma}} \right)_{\hat{\boldsymbol{\gamma}}^{(k)}} \qquad \text{(B.55)}
$$

However, regarding the variance parameter σ_{B0}^2, we can consider the following updating method according to the equation (B.50):

$$
\hat{\sigma}_{B0}^{2(k+1)} = \frac{1}{N} \sum_{i=1}^{N} \left(\frac{\hat{J}_{i2}}{\hat{J}_{i0}} \right)_{\hat{\boldsymbol{\beta}}^{(k)}}. \qquad \text{(B.56)}
$$

B.2.3 Poisson regression model

Here also, let us consider the *random intercept model* (1.11). By noting the change of notation (B.27), the log-likelihood function is

$$
\begin{aligned}
l(\boldsymbol{\beta}, \Phi) &= -\frac{N}{2} \log(2\pi\sigma_{B0}^2) + \sum_{i=1}^{N} \sum_{j=0}^{T} (-\log y_{ij}! + y_{ij} \boldsymbol{x}_{ij}^t \boldsymbol{\beta}) \\
&\quad + \sum_{i=1}^{N} \log \int_{-\infty}^{\infty} e^{g_i(u|\boldsymbol{\beta},\sigma_{B0}^2)} du, && \text{(B.57)}
\end{aligned}
$$

where

$$
g_i(u \mid \boldsymbol{\beta}, \sigma_{B0}^2) = u \sum_{j=0}^{T} y_{ij} - \sum_{j=0}^{T} \exp(\boldsymbol{x}_{ij}^t \boldsymbol{\beta} + u) - \frac{u^2}{2\sigma_{B0}^2}. \qquad \text{(B.58)}
$$

Then, the partial derivatives of g with respect to the parameters $\boldsymbol{\beta}, \sigma_{B0}^2$ are given by

$$\frac{\partial g_i}{\partial \beta_s} = -\sum_{j=0}^{T} y_{ij} x_{sij} \exp(\boldsymbol{x}_{ij}^t \boldsymbol{\beta} + u) \tag{B.59}$$

$$\frac{\partial^2 g_i}{\partial \beta_s \beta_t} = -\sum_{j=0}^{T} y_{ij} x_{sij} x_{tij} \exp(\boldsymbol{x}_{ij}^t \boldsymbol{\beta} + u) \tag{B.60}$$

$$\frac{\partial g_i}{\partial \sigma_{B0}^2} = \frac{u^2}{2\sigma_{B0}^4}. \tag{B.61}$$

Therefore, the MLE of the parameters $\boldsymbol{\gamma} = (\boldsymbol{\beta}^t, \sigma_{B0}^2)^t$ is obtained by using the Newton–Raphson algorithm within a similar process as (B.48)–(B.56) in the case of logistic regression models.

B.3 Evaluation of integral

In this section, we discuss several approximations for evaluating integrals included in the log-likelihood function. For example, the *random intercept model* (1.11) for the logistic and Poisson regression models, by employing the variable transformation $x = u/(\sqrt{2}\sigma_{B0})$, the integral included in the log-likelihood function is expressed as the special case of the following general form

$$\int_{-\infty}^{\infty} f(x) e^{-x^2} dx = \int_{-\infty}^{\infty} e^{\log f(x) - x^2} dx = \int_{-\infty}^{\infty} e^{g(x)} dx. \tag{B.62}$$

So, let us consider here some approximations for this integral for any function $f(x)$ or $g(x)$ (Demidenko, 2013; Press et al., 2007).

B.3.1 Laplace approximation

The Laplace approximation is based on a quadratic approximation at the point $x = x_{max}$ where the integrand takes its maximum. Using the Taylor series expansion of the second order at the point $x = a$, we approximate

$$g(x) \approx \tilde{g}(x \mid a) = g(a) + (x-a)g'(a) + \frac{1}{2}(x-a)^2 g''(a). \tag{B.63}$$

Then, substituting this expression into the equation (B.62), we obtain

$$\begin{aligned} \int_{-\infty}^{\infty} e^{g(x)} dx &\approx e^{g(a)} \int_{-\infty}^{\infty} \exp\left\{(x-a)g'(a) + \frac{1}{2}(x-a)^2 g''(a)\right\} dx \\ &= \sqrt{\frac{2\pi}{-g''(a)}} \exp\left\{g(a) - \frac{(g'(a))^2}{2g''(a)}\right\}. \end{aligned} \tag{B.64}$$

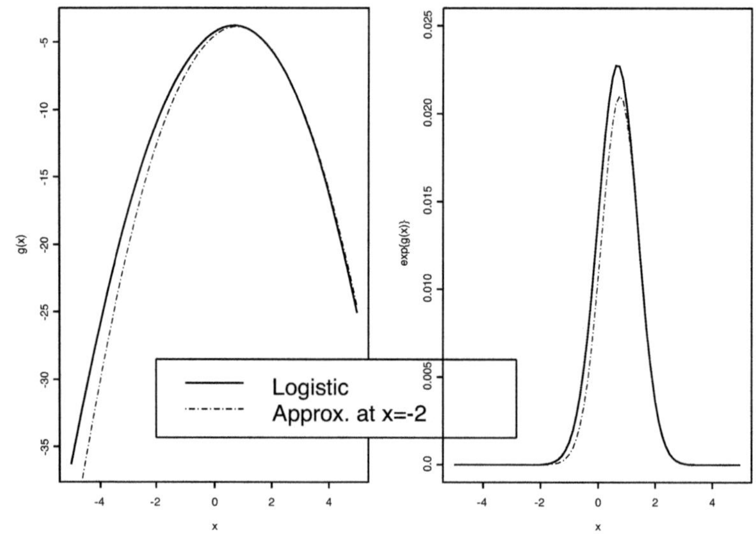

FIGURE B.1
Approximation $\tilde{g}(x \mid x = 2)$ (left) and $e^{\tilde{g}(x|x=2)}$ (right) of the function $g(x)$ (B.68).

When the function $g(x)$ is unimodal, we can easily see that this approximation takes its maximum at $x = x_{max}$, where $g^{'}(x_{max}) = 0$. Hence, by using the following approximation,

$$g(x) \quad \approx \quad \tilde{g}(x \mid x_{max}) = g(x_{max}) + \frac{1}{2}(x - x_{max})^2 g^{''}(x_{max}). \tag{B.65}$$

The Laplace approximation is defined as

$$\int_{-\infty}^{\infty} e^{g(x)} dx \quad \approx \quad \sqrt{-\frac{2\pi}{g^{''}(x_{max})}} e^{g(x_{max})}, \tag{B.66}$$

where $g^{''}(x_{max}) < 0$.

To illustrate the Laplace approximation, let us consider the following integral, which is a simple example of a mixed-effects logistic regression model

$$\int_{-\infty}^{\infty} \frac{\exp(\sqrt{2}(x-3))}{1+\exp(\sqrt{2}(x-3))} e^{-x^2} dx \quad = \quad \int_{-\infty}^{\infty} e^{g(x)} dx, \tag{B.67}$$

where

$$g(x) \quad = \quad \sqrt{2}(x-3) - \log\{1 + \exp(\sqrt{2}(x-3))\} - x^2 \tag{B.68}$$

and the derivatives needed for the approximation are given by

$$g^{'}(x) \quad = \quad \sqrt{2} - \sqrt{2}\frac{\exp(\sqrt{2}(x-3))}{1+\exp(\sqrt{2}(x-3))} - 2x \tag{B.69}$$

$$g^{''}(x) \quad = \quad -2\frac{\exp(\sqrt{2}(x-3))}{(1+\exp(\sqrt{2}(x-3)))^2} - 2. \tag{B.70}$$

Using the Newton–Raphson algorithm, we have $x_{max} = 0.6814$, the solution for $g^{'}(x) = 0$. Then, let us compare the results of different approximations: one is based on the approximation (B.63) at $x = 2$ and the other based on the Laplace approximation, i.e., at $x_{max} = 0.6814$. Figure B.1 shows the approximation $\tilde{g}(x \mid x = 2)$ and $e^{\tilde{g}(x|x=2)}$ of the function $g(x)$ (B.68). Similarly, Figure B.2 shows the Laplace approximation $\tilde{g}(x \mid x = x_{max})$ and $e^{\tilde{g}(x|x=x_{max})}$. From these two figures, we can see that the Laplace approximation is better.

Based on the Laplace approximation (B.66), we have

$$\int_{-\infty}^{\infty} e^{g(x)}dx = 0.03975172.$$

To check the accuracy of this integral, let us apply the following trapezoid formula

$$Q = \int_{-\infty}^{\infty} e^{g(x)}dx = \quad \approx \quad h\left\{\frac{1}{2}e^{g(L)} + \sum_{k=1}^{K-1} e^{g(x_k)} + \frac{1}{2}e^{g(U)}\right\}, \tag{B.71}$$

where we set

$$L = -5, U = 5, h = (U-L)/K,\ x_k = L + (k-1)h,\ (k = 1, ..., K).$$

When $K = 10, 100, 1000$, we have $Q = 0.03963643,\ 0.03963724,\ 0.03963724$ indicating that the Laplace approximation is proved to be quite accurate.

B.3.2 Gauss–Hermite quadrature

On the other hand, it is well known that the numerical integration or the numerical quadrature method is expressed as

$$\int_{-\infty}^{\infty} f(x)dx \quad \approx \quad \int_a^b f(x)dx \approx \sum_{m=1}^{M} w_m f(x_m), \tag{B.72}$$

where $a = x_1 < \cdots < x_M = b$ are the nodes or abscissas and w_m denote the positive weights. Its special case includes the above-stated trapezoid formula (B.71). As a numerical integration method used for the generalized linear mixed-effects models assuming the random effects to be distributed with a

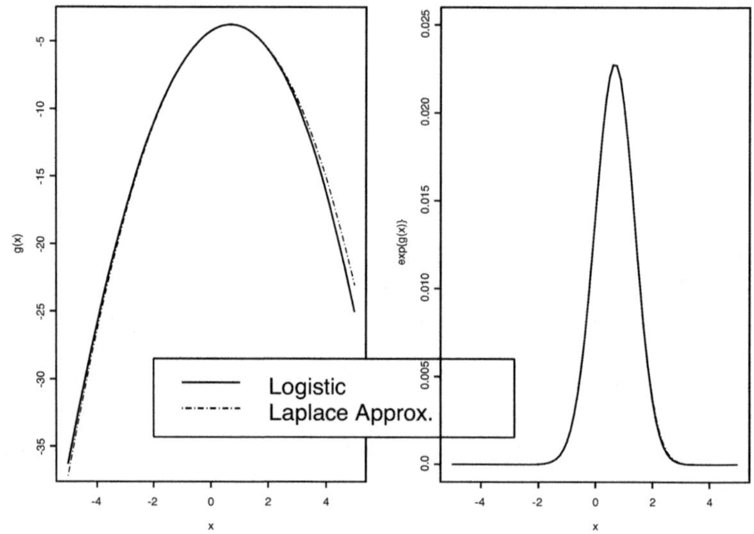

FIGURE B.2
The Laplace approximation $\tilde{g}(x \mid x = x_{max})$ (left) and $e^{\tilde{g}(x|x=x_{max})}$ (right) of a function $g(x)$ (B.68).

normal distribution, the following Gauss–Hermite quadrature formula is well known:

$$\int_{-\infty}^{\infty} f(x)e^{-x^2}dx \quad \approx \quad \sum_{m=1}^{M} w_m f(x_m). \tag{B.73}$$

This type of integral is called an integral with a Gaussian kernel $\exp(-x^2)$. An algorithm to compute the nodes and weights for any M is given by Press et al. (2007). In Table B.1, the nodes and weights (x_m, w_m), $m = 1, ..., 15$ are given. These imply that (1) the farther the value is from zero, the lower the weights, and (2) nodes are symmetrical around zero and have the same weight. As the weights approach zero rapidly with $M \to \infty$, the number of nodes greater than 15 is unlikely to improve the precision of the approximation.

Now, let us apply the Gauss–Hermite quadrature with $M = 15$ to the evaluation of the integral (B.67). We obtained as follows:

$$\begin{aligned}\int_{-\infty}^{\infty} \frac{\exp(\sqrt{2}(x-3))}{1+\exp(\sqrt{2}(x-3))}e^{-x^2}dx &= \int_{-\infty}^{\infty} (e^{g(x)+x^2})e^{-x^2}dx \\ &= \sum_{m=1}^{13} w_m e^{g(x_m)+x_m^2} \\ &= 0.03963724,\end{aligned}$$

which is equal to the value from the trapezoid formula (B.71).

TABLE B.1
The nodes and weights for $M = 15$ of the Gauss–Hermite quadrature formula.

No.	x_m	w_m
1, 9	$\pm$ 4.499990707	1.5224758E-9
2,10	$\pm$ 3.669950373	1.05911555E-6
3,11	$\pm$ 2.967166928	1.000044412E-4
4,12	$\pm$ 2.325732486	0.002778068843
5,13	$\pm$ 1.719992575	0.0307800339
6,14	$\pm$ 1.136115585	0.158488916
7,15	$\pm$ 0.565069583	0.412028687
8	0	0.564100309

B.3.3 Adaptive Gauss–Hermite quadrature

When we applied the Gauss–Hermite quadrature to the integral (B.67), which is a simple function, the Gauss–Hermite quadrature gave a result identical to the true value. However, it cannot in general. So, we shall introduce an extended method that might have an improved approximation. The Gauss–Hermite quadrature is an approximate method that is carried out around the origin, i.e., $x = 0$, for any function $f(x)$. However, as in the case of the Laplace approximation, the better method should be carried out around the maximum value of the integrand, i.e., $x = x_{max}$. Furthermore, the *minus* second derivative of a function g at the maximum point $x = x_{max}$ could be considered as the degrees of *kurtosis* of g around the maximum point. In other words, it can be considered as the *variance* of g around the maximum point. So, by letting

$$\hat{\sigma} = [-g''(x_{max})]^{-1/2}, \tag{B.74}$$

let us consider the following *normalization* around x_{max}

$$y = \frac{x - x_{max}}{\sqrt{2}\hat{\sigma}}, \tag{B.75}$$

where the constant $\sqrt{2}$ implies that, as in the case of (B.18) and (B.25), the random effects are assumed to be normally distributed. Namely, in the *adaptive* Gauss–Hermite quadrature, we approximate

$$
\begin{aligned}
\int_{-\infty}^{\infty} f(x)e^{-x^2}dx &= \int_{-\infty}^{\infty} e^{g(x)}dx \\
&= \sqrt{2}\hat{\sigma}\int_{-\infty}^{\infty} e^{g(x_{max}+\sqrt{2}\hat{\sigma}x)}dx \\
&= \sqrt{2}\hat{\sigma}\int_{-\infty}^{\infty} e^{g(x_{max}+\sqrt{2}\hat{\sigma}x)+x^2}e^{-x^2}dx \\
&\approx \sqrt{2}\hat{\sigma}\sum_{m=1}^{M} w_m \exp\{g(x_{max}+\sqrt{2}\hat{\sigma}x_m)+x_m^2\}.
\end{aligned}
\tag{B.76}
$$

It should be noted that the adaptive Gauss–Hermite quadrature with $M = 1$ is identical to the Laplace approximation (B.65) because $(x_1 = 0, w_1 = \sqrt{\pi})$.

Now let us apply the adaptive Gauss–Hermite quadrature to the integral (B.67). Then we have

$$
\begin{aligned}
\int_{-\infty}^{\infty} \frac{\exp(\sqrt{2}(x-3))}{1+\exp(\sqrt{2}(x-3))}e^{-x^2}dx &= \int_{-\infty}^{\infty} e^{g(x)}dx \\
&= \sqrt{2}\hat{\sigma}\int_{-\infty}^{\infty} e^{g(x_{max}+\sqrt{2}\hat{\sigma}x)+x^2}e^{-x^2}dx \\
&= \sqrt{2}\hat{\sigma}\sum_{m=1}^{15} w_m e^{g(x_{max}+\sqrt{2}\hat{\sigma}x_m)+x_m^2} \\
&= 0.03963724,
\end{aligned}
$$

which is also shown to be identical to the true value.

B.3.3.1 An application

As a more practical example, let us consider here the mixed-effects logistic regression Model IV applied to the *Respiratory Data* shown in Table 8.1.

$$
\begin{aligned}
\text{logit}\,\Pr(y_{ij} = 1 \mid b_{0i}) &= \beta_0 + b_{0i} + \beta_1 x_{1i} + \beta_2 x_{2ij} \\
&\qquad + \beta_3 x_{1i} x_{2ij} + \boldsymbol{w}_i^t \boldsymbol{\xi} \\
&= \beta_0 + \beta_1 x_{1i} + \beta_2 x_{2ij} + \beta_3 x_{3ij} \\
&\qquad + \beta_4 x_{4ij} + \beta_5 x_{5ij} + \beta_6 x_{6ij} + b_{0i} \\
&= \boldsymbol{x}_{ij}^t \boldsymbol{\beta} + \boldsymbol{z}_{ij}^t \boldsymbol{b}_i \\
b_{0i} &\sim N(0, \sigma_{B0}^2)
\end{aligned}
$$

where $x_{3ij} = x_{1i} \times x_{2ij}$, and the other three variables $(x_{4ij}, x_{5ij}, x_{6ij})^t$ denote (centre, gender, and age), respectively. Furthermore, $\boldsymbol{\xi} = (\beta_4, \beta_5, \beta_6)^t$. Using the estimates of Model IV shown in Output 8.3, we set as follows:

1. Intercept: $\hat{\beta}_0 = -0.28$
2. treatment: $\hat{\beta}_1 = -0.18$
3. postc: $\hat{\beta}_2 = -0.10$
4. treatment*postc: $\hat{\beta}_3 = 2.07$
5. $\hat{\sigma}_{B0} = \sqrt{5.745}$

Then, consider the case where the ith subject's data in the placebo group has the following

1. centre $= 1$ ($\hat{\beta}_4 = 2.0(\text{centre} = 2); = 0(\text{centre} = 1)$)
2. gender $= 1$ ($\hat{\beta}_5 = -0.41$)
3. age $= 23$ ($\hat{\beta}_6 = -0.03$)
4. treatment $= 0$
5. $\boldsymbol{y}_i = (1, 0, 0, 1, 1,)^t$

First, let us compute J_{i0} (B.51) by employing the variable transformation $u = \sqrt{2}\hat{\sigma}x$,

$$J_{i0} = \int_{-\infty}^{\infty} e^{g_i(u|\hat{\boldsymbol{\beta}}, \hat{\sigma}_{B0}^2)} du = \sqrt{2}\hat{\sigma}_{B0} \int_{-\infty}^{\infty} e^{h_i(x)} dx,$$

where

$$h_i(x) = -\sum_{j=0}^{T} y_{ij}x + \sum_{j=0}^{T} \log[1 + \exp\{\boldsymbol{x}_{ij}^t\hat{\boldsymbol{\beta}} + \sqrt{2}\hat{\sigma}_{B0}x\}] - x^2.$$

But here, we do not include the constant $\sqrt{2}\hat{\sigma}_{B0}$ in the calculation that follows. In the above-stated ith subject's case, we have

$$\begin{aligned} \boldsymbol{x}_{i0}^t\hat{\boldsymbol{\beta}} &= \hat{\beta}_0 - 0.41 \times \text{gender} - 0.03 \times \text{age} = -1.38 \\ \boldsymbol{x}_{ij}^t\hat{\boldsymbol{\beta}} &= \hat{\beta}_0 + \hat{\beta}_2 - 0.41 \times \text{gender} - 0.03 \times \text{age} = -1.48, \ (j = 1, 2, 3, 4). \end{aligned}$$

Then, we have

$$\begin{aligned} h_i(x) &= 3x - \log[1 + \exp(-1.38 + \sqrt{2}\hat{\sigma}_{B0}x)] \\ &\quad -4\log[1 + \exp(-1.48 + \sqrt{2}\hat{\sigma}_{B0}x)] - x^2 \qquad \text{(B.77)} \\ h_i'(x) &= 3 - 2x - \sqrt{2} * \hat{\sigma}\frac{\exp(-1.38 + \sqrt{2}\hat{\sigma}_{B0}x)}{1 + \exp(-1.38 + \sqrt{2}\hat{\sigma}_{B0}x)} \\ &\quad -4\sqrt{2}\hat{\sigma}\frac{\exp(-1.48 + \sqrt{2}\hat{\sigma}_{B0}x)}{1 + \exp(-1.48 + \sqrt{2}\hat{\sigma}_{B0}x)} \\ h_i''(x) &= -2 - 2\hat{\sigma}^2\frac{\exp(-1.38 + \sqrt{2}\hat{\sigma}_{B0}x)}{[1 + \exp(-1.38 + \sqrt{2}\hat{\sigma}_{B0}x)]^2} \\ &\quad -8\hat{\sigma}^2\frac{\exp(-1.48 + \sqrt{2}\hat{\sigma}_{B0}x)}{[1 + \exp(-1.48 + \sqrt{2}\hat{\sigma}_{B0}x)]^2}. \end{aligned}$$

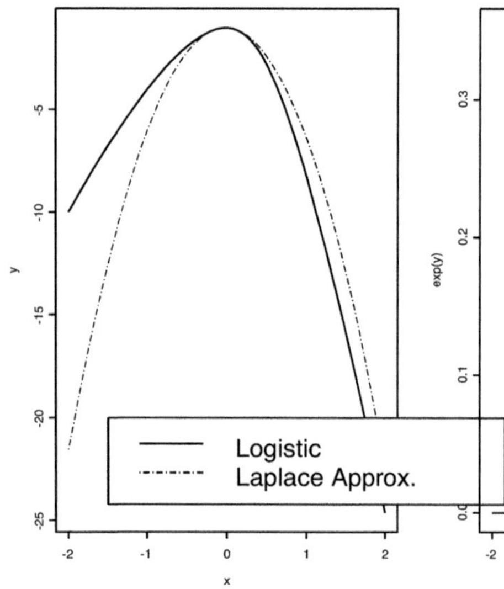

FIGURE B.3
The Laplace approximation of a logistic function $h_i(x)$ (B.77) (left) and of $e^{h_i(x)}$ (right).

First, let us apply the Laplace approximation with $x_{max} = -0.018416$, which yields $J_{i0} = 0.2732907$ and the comparison of $h_i(x)(e^{h_i(x)})$ and $\tilde{h}_i(x)(e^{\tilde{h}_i(x)})$ are shown in Figure B.3. From this figure, the LA approximation seems to be no good. So, we applied the Gauss–Hermite quadrature with $M = 15$ and the adaptive Gauss–Hermite quadrature with $M = 15$. The GH yields 0.2606460 and the adaptive GH yields 0.2849804. To obtain the true integral, we used the trapezoid formula (B.71) with $L = -4, U = 4$. For $K = 10, 50, 100$, the trapezoid formula yields $0.3198999, 0.2849809, 0.2849809$. In this case, the adaptive GH yields the approximate closest to the true value.

Second, let us compute a little bit more complicated integral J_{i3st} (B.54) including the second derivative with respect to sex ($s = 5$) and age ($t = 5$). In this case, as $x_{sij} = 1,\ x_{tij} = 23$ without reference to i, j, then we have

$$\frac{\partial^2 g_i}{\partial \beta_s \beta_t} = 23 \left\{ \frac{\exp(-1.38 + u)}{[1 + \exp(-1.38 + u)]^2} + 4 \cdot \frac{\exp(-1.48 + u)}{[1 + \exp(-1.48 + u)]^2} \right\}.$$

Therefore, we have

$$J_{i3st} = \int_{-\infty}^{\infty} \frac{\partial^2 g_i}{\partial \beta_s \beta_t} e^{g_i(u|\hat{\boldsymbol{\beta}}, \hat{\sigma}_{B0}^2)} du = \sqrt{2}\hat{\sigma}_{B0} \int_{-\infty}^{\infty} e^{h_i(x)} dx,$$

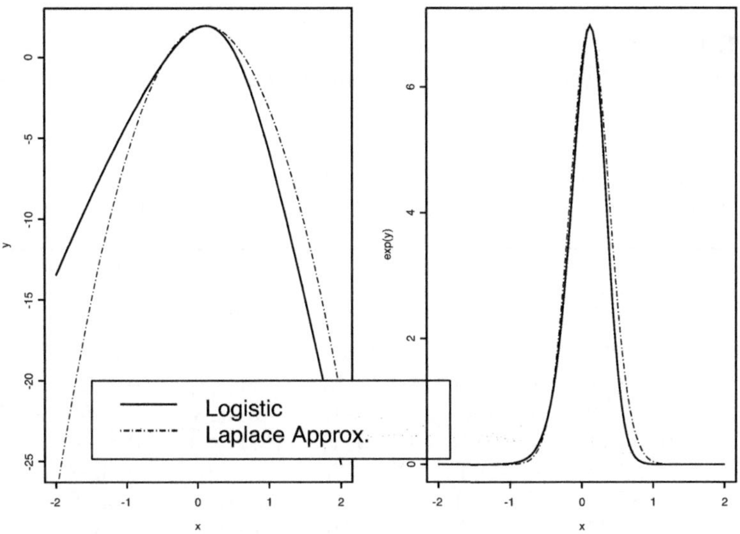

FIGURE B.4
The Laplace approximation of a logistic function $h_i(x)$ (B.78) (left) and of $e^{h_i(x)}$ (right).

where

$$\begin{aligned} h_i(x) &= \log\left(\frac{\exp(-1.38+\sqrt{2}\hat{\sigma}_{B0}x)}{[1+\exp(-1.38+\sqrt{2}\hat{\sigma}_{B0}x)]^2}\right. \\ &\qquad \left. + \frac{4\exp(-1.48+\sqrt{2}\hat{\sigma}_{B0}x)}{[1+\exp(-1.48+\sqrt{2}\hat{\sigma}_{B0}x)]^2}\right) \\ &\quad + \log 23 + 3x - \log[1+\exp(-1.38+\sqrt{2}\hat{\sigma}_{B0}x)] \\ &\quad -4\log[1+\exp(-1.48+\sqrt{2}\hat{\sigma}_{B0}x)] - x^2. \end{aligned} \tag{B.78}$$

Here, we omit the second derivatives. Here also we do not include the constant $\sqrt{2}\hat{\sigma}_{B0}$ in the evaluation of the integral. First, let us apply the Laplace approximation with $x_{max} = 0.1161$, which yields $J_{i3st} = 4.856587$ and the comparison of $h_i(x)(e^{h_i(x)})$ and $\tilde{h}_i(x)(e^{\tilde{h}_i(x)})$ are shown in Figure B.4. From this figure, here also, the LA approximation seems to be no good. So, we applied the Gauss–Hermite quadrature with $M = 15$ and the adaptive Gauss–Hermite quadrature with $M = 15$. The GH yields 4.053789 and the adaptive GH yields 4.331131. To obtain the true integral, we used the trapezoid formula (B.71) with $L = -4, U = 4$. For $K = 10, 50, 100$, the trapezoid formula yields $5.061485, 4.331131, 4.331131$. In this case, the adaptive GH yields the true value.

In a similar manner, we can calculate other derivatives (B.52)–(B.54) and finally, we can obtain the MLE using the Newton–Raphson algorithm.

TABLE B.2
Relationship between the number of nodes M for the adaptive Gauss–Hermite quadrature and the estimates (s.e.) of some selected variables in the mixed-effects logistic regression Model IV applied to the *Respiratory Data* using SAS `PROC GLIMMIX`. The number of nodes with the asterisk (*) implies that a greater number of nodes is unlikely to change the estimates.

M	intercept	age	treatment	post	treatment *post	$\hat{\sigma}^2_{B0}$
1	-0.2759	-0.03018	-0.1528	-0.1014	2.0458	5.1120
	(0.8182)	(0.0207)	(0.7110)	(0.4112)	(0.6209)	(1.3984)
3	-0.2612	-0.0290	-0.2066	-0.1023	2.0552	5.1260
	(0.8130)	(0.0205)	(0.7052)	(0.4129)	(0.6230)	(1.3952)
5	-0.2683	-0.0294	-0.1905	-0.1027	2.0657	5.4853
	(0.8326)	(0.0211)	(0.7174)	(0.4138)	(0.6248)	(1.4780)
7	-0.2747	-0.0297	-0.1759	-0.1028	2.0696	5.7018
	(0.8449)	(0.0215)	(0.7255)	(0.4139)	(0.6257)	(1.5688)
9	-0.2760	-0.0298	-0.1737	-0.1030	2.0716	5.7557
	(0.8479)	(0.0216)	(0.7276)	(0.4140)	(0.6263)	(1.6032)
11	-0.2758	-0.0298	-0.1748	-0.1030	2.0721	5.7537
	(0.8477)	(0.0216)	(0.7274)	(0.4140)	(0.6264)	(1.6054)
13*	-0.2755	-0.0298	-0.1756	-0.1030	2.0720	5.7470
	(0.8473)	(0.0216)	(0.7271)	(0.4141)	(0.6264)	(1.6014)
15	-0.2754	-0.0298	-0.1757	-0.1030	2.0719	5.7445
	(0.8471)	(0.0216)	(0.7270)	(0.4141)	(0.6263)	(1.5991)
20	-0.2755	-0.0298	-0.1756	-0.1030	2.0719	5.7453
	(0.8472)	(0.0216)	(0.7270)	(0.4141)	(0.6263)	(1.5994)

B.3.3.2 Determination of the number of nodes

To determine the number of nodes M in some applications, you should examine the *convergence* of the estimates as $M \to$ large and select M such that a greater number of nodes is unlikely to change the estimates.

In Tables B.2 and B.3, we showed the relationship between the number of nodes M for the adaptive Gauss–Hermite quadrature and the estimates (s.e.) of some selected variables in the mixed-effects logistic regression model IV and Va applied to the *Respiratory Data* (Table 8.1) using SAS `PROC GLIMMIX`, respectively. These tables show that we can select $M = 13$ or $M = 15$.

In a similar manner, we showed the relationship between the number of nodes M for the adaptive Gauss-Hermite quadrature and the estimates (s.e.) of all the variables included in the mixed-effects Poisson regression Model Va applied to the *Epilepsy Data* (Table 9.1) using SAS `PROC GLIMMIX`. This table shows that the adaptive Gauss–Hermite quadrature with $M = 1$ or the

TABLE B.3
Relationship between the number of nodes M for the adaptive Gauss–Hermite quadrature and the estimates (s.e.) of some selected variables in the mixed-effects logistic regression Model Va applied to the *Respiratory Data* using SAS `PROC GLIMMIX`. The number of nodes with the the asterisk (*) implies that a greater number of nodes is unlikely to change the estimates.

M	age	treatment	post	treatment *post	$\hat{\sigma}^2_{B0}$	$\hat{\sigma}^2_{B1}$
1	-0.0300	-0.1635	-0.1208	2.1092	4.9504	0.5298
	(0.0210)	(0.7071)	(0.4299)	(0.6562)	(1.4583)	(0.9843)
3	-0.0290	-0.1996	-0.1290	2.1534	5.0664	1.0809
	(0.0214)	(0.7060)	(0.4460)	(0.6744)	(1.5271)	(0.9066)
5	-0.0293	-0.1884	-0.1297	2.1659	5.3930	1.1330
	(0.0220)	(0.7176)	(0.4488)	(0.6816)	(1.6389)	(1.1323)
7	-0.0295	-0.1824	-0.1294	2.1653	5.5023	1.0706
	(0.0221)	(0.7215)	(0.4472)	(0.6807)	(1.6875)	(1.1860)
9	-0.0295	-0.1817	-0.1298	2.1663	5.5251	1.0630
	(0.0221)	(0.7223)	(0.4471)	(0.6809)	(1.7023)	(1.1976)
11	-0.0295	-0.1819	-0.1298	2.1666	5.5271	1.0636
	(0.0221)	(0.7223)	(0.4472)	(0.6810)	(1.7043)	(1.1985)
13*	-0.0295	-0.1820	-0.1298	2.1666	5.5265	1.0641
	(0.0221)	(0.7223)	(0.4472)	(0.6810)	(1.7040)	(1.1979)
15	-0.0295	-0.1820	-0.1298	2.1666	5.5261	1.0642
	(0.0221)	(0.7223)	(0.4472)	(0.6810)	(1.7036)	(1.1978)
20	-0.0295	-0.1820	-0.1298	2.1666	5.5260	1.0642
	(0.0221)	(0.7223)	(0.4472)	(0.6810)	(1.7035)	(1.1978)

Laplace approximation is sufficiently good, but we shall select $M = 5$ or more, taking account of the goodness of the estimation of the variance components.

B.3.3.3 Limitations

In the previous sections, the adaptive Gauss–Hermite quadrature (AGHQ) is shown to be very accurate even for a moderate number of nodes M. However, the dimension r of the random effects $\boldsymbol{b}_i$ included in the models was relatively small at 1 or 2. For example, in the mixed-effects Poisson regression Model Va ($r = 2$: random intercept and random slope) fitted to the *Epilepsy Data*, the AGHQ with $M = 1$, or the Laplace approximation, was shown to be surprisingly accurate compared with the AGHQ with $M = 20$, where the AGHQ needs numerical evaluations of integrals at a total of $20^2 = 400$ quadrature points. Obviously, the number of evaluation points increases exponentially with the number of random effects. In the mixed-effects Poisson

TABLE B.4
Relationship between the number of nodes M for the adaptive Gauss–Hermite quadrature and the estimates (s.e.) of some selected variables in the mixed-effects Poisson regression model Va applied to the *Epilepsy Data* using SAS `PROC GLIMMIX`. The number of nodes with the the asterisk (*) implies that a greater number of nodes is unlikely to change the estimates.

M	age	treatment	post	treatment *post	$\hat{\sigma}^2_{B0}$	$\hat{\sigma}^2_{B1}$
1	-0.0195	0.0272	0.0120	-0.3085	0.5004	0.2401
	(0.0154)	(0.1942)	(0.1099)	(0.1530)	(0.1000)	(0.0615)
3	-0.0195	0.0271	0.0121	-0.3084	0.5009	0.2397
	((0.0154)	(0.1943)	(0.1098)	(0.1529)	(0.1001)	(0.0614)
5*	-0.0192	0.0271	0.0120	-0.3087	0.5014	0.2414
	(0.0154)	(0.1944)	(0.1101)	(0.1533)	(0.1002)	(0.0619)
7	-0.0195	0.0271	0.0120	-0.3087	0.5014	0.2415
	(0.0154)	(0.1944)	(0.1101)	(0.1533)	(0.1002)	(0.0619)
9	-0.0195	0.0271	0.0120	-0.3087	0.5014	0.2415
	(0.0154)	(0.1944)	(0.1101)	(0.1533)	(0.1002)	(0.0619)
11	-0.0195	0.0271	0.0120	-0.3087	0.5014	0.2415
	(0.0154)	(0.1944)	(0.1101)	(0.1533)	(0.1002)	(0.0619)
13	-0.0195	0.0271	0.0120	-0.3087	0.5014	0.2415
	(0.0154)	(0.1944)	(0.1101)	(0.1533)	(0.1002)	(0.0619)
15	-0.0195	0.0271	0.0120	-0.3087	0.5014	0.2415
	(0.0154)	(0.1944)	(0.1101)	(0.1533)	(0.1002)	(0.0619)
20	-0.0195	0.0271	0.0120	-0.3087	0.5014	0.2415
	(0.0154)	(0.1944)	(0.1101)	(0.1533)	(0.1002)	(0.0619)

regression Model VIIQ ($r = 3$: random intercept, random slope on t_j and random slope on t_j^2) fitted to the *Epilepsy Data*, the AGHQ with $M = 1$ or the Laplace approximation was also shown to be surprisingly accurate compared with the AGHQ with $M = 20$, where the AGHQ needs numerical evaluations of integrals at a total of $20^3 = 8000$ quadrature points (Table B.5).

In the case of mixed-effects logistic regression models, on the other hand, the AGHQ sometimes face the convergence problem. For example, the mixed-effects logistic regression Model VIIQ with $r = 3$ fitted to the *Respiratory Data* faced the convergence problem with $M = 15$, where we need numerical evaluations of integrals at a total of $15^3 = 3375$ quadrature points. So, the alternative methods of approximations that require less computational load are needed for generalized (non-Gaussian) linear mixed-effects models with r greater than or equal to 3 for mixed-effects logistic regression models. SAS software provides two different approximate methods called penalized quasi-

TABLE B.5
Relationship between the number of nodes M for the adaptive Gauss–Hermite quadrature and the estimates (s.e.) of some selected variables in the mixed-effects Poisson regression model VIIQ ($r = 3$) applied to the *Epilepsy data* using SAS `PROC GLIMMIX`.

M	xvisit	xvisit2	treatment *xvisit	treatment *xvisit2	$\hat{\sigma}^2_{B0}$	$\hat{\sigma}^2_{B1}$
1	-0.00960	-0.00377	-0.1466	0.01739	0.5061	0.2318
	(0.1171)	(0.02745)	(0.1597)	(0.03714)	(0.1043)	(0.06777)
5	-0.00963	-0.00376	-0.1468	0.01743	0.5064	0.2334
	(0.1173)	(0.02750)	(0.1601)	(0.03722)	(0.1043)	(0.06830)
7	-0.00959	-0.00377	-0.1468	0.01744	0.5034	0.2334
	(0.1173)	(0.02750)	(0.1601)	(0.03722)	(0.1042)	(0.06828)
13	-0.00960	-0.00377	-0.1469	0.01744	0.5063	0.2333
	(0.1173)	(0.02750)	(0.1600)	(0.03722)	(0.1042)	(0.06826)
15	-0.00960	-0.00377	-0.1469	0.01744	0.5063	0.2334
	(0.1173)	(0.02750)	(0.1601)	(0.03722)	(0.1042)	(0.06828)
20	-0.00960	-0.00377	-0.1469	0.01744	0.5063	0.2334
	(0.1173)	(0.02750)	(0.1601)	(0.03722)	(0.1042)	(0.06828)

likelihood (PQL) and marginal quasi-likelihood (MQL). However, these two methods are known to be *less accurate* than the adaptive Gauss–Hermite quadrature and even more invalid when there is missing data. For details on these methods, see Diggle et al. (2002) and Fitzmaurice et al. (2011), for example.

However, in the case of binary repeated measures design, there is not so much information available regarding random effects beyond random intercept or, at most, random intercept plus slope with constant slope over time. Therefore, in the above example of the mixed-effects logistic regression, Model VIQ with random intercept only was selected as the best model among models with a quadratic term on time. Furthermore, most of the mixed-effects logistic regression models and Poisson regression models introduced for parallel group randomized controlled trials have one or two random effects, i.e., $r \leq 3$. Therefore, the adaptive Gauss–Hermite quadrature with a reasonable number of nodes could be the first-line method.

Bibliography

[1] Aitkin M, Anderson D, and Hinde J. Statistical modelling of data on teaching styles (with discussion). *Journal of Royal Statistical Society, Series A*, **144**: 419–461, 1981.

[2] Akaike H. A new look at the statistical model identification. *IEEE Transactions on Automatic Control*, **19**: 716–723, 1974.

[3] Allison PD. Handling Missing Data by Maximum Likelihood. *SAS Global Forum 2012*, Paper 312, 2012.

[4] Amatya A, Bhaumik DK, and Gibbons RD. Sample size determination for clustered count data. *Statistics in Medicine*, **32**: 4162–4179, 2013.

[5] Bhaumik D, Roy A, Aryal S, Hur K, Duan N, Normand SLT, Brown CH, and Gibbons RD. Sample size determination for studies with repeated continuous outcomes. *Psychiatr. Ann.* **38**: 765–771, 2008.

[6] Campbell MJ and Walters SJ. *How to Design, Analyse and Report Cluster Randomised Trials in Medicine and Health Related Research*, Wiley, 2014.

[7] Carpenter JR, Pocock S, and Lamm CJ. Coping with missing data in clinical trials: A model-based approach applied to asthma trials. *Statistics in Medicine*, **21**: 1043–1066, 2002.

[8] Carpenter JR and Kenward MG. *Multiple Imputation and Its Application*, John Wiley & Sons, 2013.

[9] Chen X. The adjustment of random baseline measurements in treatment effect estimation. *J. Stat. Plan. Inference*, **136**: 4161–4175, 2006.

[10] Cook RJ and Wei W. Selection effects in randomized trials with count data. *Statistics in Medicine*, **21**: 515–531, 2002.

[11] Cook RJ and Wei W. Conditional analysis of mixed Poisson processes with baseline counts: Implications for trial design and analysis. *Biostatistics*, **4**: 479–494, 2003.

[12] Crager MR. Analysis of covariance in parallel-group clinical trials with pretreatment baselines. *Biometrics*, **43**: 895–901, 1987.

[13] D'Agostino RB, Massaro JM, and Sullivan LM. Non-inferiority trials: Design concepts and issues – the encounters of academic consultants in statistics. *Statistics in Medicine*, **22**: 169–186, 2003.

[14] Daniels MJ and Hogan JW. *Missing Data in Longitudinal Studies: Strategies for Bayesian Modelling and Sensitivity Analysis*, Chapman & Hall/CRC, 2008.

[15] Davis CS. Semi-parametric and non-parametric methods for the analysis of repeated measurements with applications to clinical trials. *Statistics in Medicine*, **10**: 1959–1980, 1991.

[16] Demidenko E. *Mixed Models: Theory and Applications with R*. Second Edition, John Wiley & Sons, Inc., 2013.

[17] Dempster AP, Laird NM, and Rubin DB. Maximum likelihood from incomplete data via the EM algorithm. *Journal of the Royal Statistical Society, Series B*, **39**: 1–22, 1977.

[18] Diggle PJ, Heagerty P, Liang KY, and Zeger SL. *Analysis of Longitudinal Data*, 2nd ed, Oxford University Press, 2002.

[19] Diggle PJ and Kenward MG. Informative dropout in longitudinal data analysis. *Journal of the Royal Statistical Society, Series C*, **43**: 49–93, 1994.

[20] Donner A and Klar N. *Design and Analysis of Cluster Randomization Trials in Health Research*, Wiley, 2000.

[21] Efron B. *The Jackknife, the Bootstrap and Other Resampling Plans*. SIAM, Philadelphia, 1982.

[22] Eldridge S and Kerry S. *A Practical Guide to Cluster Randomised Trials in Health Services Research*, Wiley, 2012.

[23] European Agency for the Evaluation of Medicinal Products. *Points to Consider on Switching between Superiority and Non-inferiority* (CPMP/EWP/482/99), July 27, 2000.

[24] European Medicines Agency. *Guideline on the Choice of the Non-Inferiority Margin* (Doc. Ref. EMEA/CPMP/EWP/2158/99). `http://www.emea.europa.eu/pdfs/human/ewp/215899en.pdf`, July 14, 2009.

[25] Everitt BS. A Monte Carlo investigation of the likelihood ratio test for the number of components in a mixture of normal distributions. *Multi. Behav. Res.*, **16**: 171–180, 1981.

[26] Everitt BS and Hothorn T. *A Handbook of Statistical Analysis Using R*, 2nd ed, CRC Press, 2010.

[27] Everitt BS and Pickles A. Other methods for the analysis of longitudinal data, in *Statistical Aspects of the Design and Analysis of Clinical Trials* (Revised Edition), pp. 170-173, Imperial College Press, 2004.

[28] Fitzmaurice GM, Laird NM, and Ware JH. *Applied Longitudinal Analysis*, John Wiley & Sons, 2011.

[29] Greenhouse SW and Geisser S. On methods in the analysis of profile data. *Psychometrika*, **24**: 95–112, 1959.

[30] Hardin JW and Hilbe JM. *Generalized Estimating Equations*, Second Edition, CRC Press, 2013.

[31] Hayes RJ and Moulton LH. *Cluster Randomised Trials*, Chapman & Hall, 2009.

[32] Hedeker D, Gibbons RD, and Waternaux C. Sample size estimation for longitudinal designs with attrition: Comparing time-related contrasts between two groups. *Journal of Educational and Behavioral Statistics*, **24**: 70–93, 1999.

[33] Hedeker D and Gibbons RD. *Longitudinal Data Analysis*, John Wiley & Sons, New York, 2006.

[34] Hida E and Tango T. On the three-arm non-inferiority trial including a placebo with a prespecified margin. *Statistics in Medicine*, **30**: 224–231, 2011.

[35] Hida E and Tango T. Response to Joachim Röhmel and Iris Pigeot. *Statistics in Medicine*, **30**: 3165–3165, 2011.

[36] Hida E and Tango T. Three-arm noninferiority trials with a prespecified margin for inference of the difference in the proportions of binary endpoints. *Journal of Biopharmaceutical Statistics*, **23**: 774–789, 2013.

[37] Huynh H and Feldt LS. Estimation of the Box correction for degrees of freedom for sample data in randomized block and split-plot designs. *Journal of Education Statistics*, **1**: 69–82, 1976.

[38] ICH, Harmonised Tripartite Guideline. Statistical Principles for Clinical Trials, 1998.

[39] ICH, Harmonised Tripartite Guideline. Choice of Control Group and Related Issues in Clinical Trials, 2000.

[40] Kapur K, Bhaumik R, Tang XC, Hur K, Reda DJ, and Bhaumik DK. Sample size determination for longitudinal designs with binary response. *Statistics in Medicine*, **33**: 3781–3800, 2014.

[41] Kenward MG and Roger JH. Small sample inference for fixed effects from restricted maximum likelihood. *Biometrics*, **53**: 983–997, 1997.

[42] Koch GG and Tangen CM. Nonparametric analysis of covariance and its role in noninferiority clinical trials. *Drug Information Journal*, **33**: 1145–1159, 1999.

[43] Koch A and Röhmel J. Hypothesis testing in the "gold standard" design for proving the efficacy of an experimental treatment relative to placebo and a reference. *Journal of Biopharmaceutical Statistics*, **14**: 315–325, 2004.

[44] Kwong KS, Cheung SH, Hayter AJ, and Wen MJ. Extension of three-arm non-inferiority studies to trials with multiple new treatments. *Statistics in Medicine*, **31**: 2833–2843, 2012.

[45] Laird NM and Ware JH. Random-effects models for longitudinal data. *Biometrics*, **38**: 963–974, 1982.

[46] Lee Y, Nelder JA, and Pawitan Y. *Generalized Linear Models with Random Effects: Unified Analysis via H-Likelihood*, Chapman & Hall/CRC, 2006.

[47] Liang KY and Zeger SL. Longitudinal data analysis of continuous and discrete responses for pre-post designs. *Sankhya: The Indian Journal of Statistics, Series B*, **62**: 134–148, 2000.

[48] Lin H, McCulloch CE, Turnbull BW, Slate EH, and Clark LC. A latent class mixed model for analysing biomarker trajectories with irregularly scheduled observations. *Statistics in Medicine*, **19**: 1303–1318, 2000.

[49] Lin H, Turnbull BW, McCulloch CE, and Slate EH. Latent class models for joint analysis of longitudinal; biomarker and event process data: Application to longitudinal prostate-specific antigen readings and prostate cancer. *Journal of the American Statistical Association*, **97**: 53–65, 2002.

[50] Little RJA. Pattern-mixture models for multivariate incomplete data. *Journal of the American Statistical Association*, **88**: 125–134, 1993.

[51] Little, RJA and Rubin DB. *Statistical Analysis with Missing Data* (2nd edition). Wiley, New York, 2002.

[52] Little RC, Milliken GA, Stroup WW, Wolfinger RD, and Shabenberger O. *SAS for Mixed Models*, second edition, SAS Institute Inc., Cary, NC. USA, 2006.

[53] Mallinckrodt CH, Lane PW, Schnell D, Peng Y, Mancuso JP. Recommendations for the primary analysis of continuous endpoints in longitudinal clinical trials. *Therapeutic Innovation & Regulatory Science*, **42**: 303–319, 2008.

[54] Marcus R, Peritz E, and Gabriel KR. On closed testing procedures with special reference to ordered analysis of variance. *Biometrika*, **67**: 655–660, 1976.

[55] McLachlan GJ. On bootstrapping the likelihood ratio test statistics for the number of components in a normal mixture. *Applied Statistics*, **36**, 318–324, 1987.

[56] McLachlan GJ and Peel D. *Finite Mixture Models.* John Wiley & Sons, Inc., 2000.

[57] Molenberghs G. and Kenward MG. *Missing Data in Clinical Studies*, New York: John Wiley & Sons, 2007.

[58] Muthen B. and Shedden K. Finite mixture modeling with mixture outcomes using the EM algorithm. *Biometrics*, **55**: 463–469, 1999.

[59] Nakamura, R, Tango, T, Taguchi, N, and Hida E. A mixture model combined with proportional odds model for longitudinal measurement data in randomized controlled trials. *The 28th International Biometric Conference*, Kobe, 2012.

[60] National Research Council. *The Prevention and Treatment of Missing Data in Clinical Trials*, Panel on Handling Missing Data in Clinical Trials, Committee on National Statistics, Division of Behavioral and Social Sciences and Education, Washington, DC: National Academies Press, 2010.

[61] Pigeot I, Schäfer J, Röhmel J, and Hauschke D. Assessing non-inferiority of a new treatment in a three-arm clinical trial including a placebo. *Statistics in Medicine*, **22**: 883–899, 2003.

[62] Pinheiro JC and Bates DM. *Mixed-Effects Models in S and S-PLUS* Springer Verlag, New York, 2000.

[63] Press WH, Teukolsky SA, Vetterling WT, and Flannery BP. *Numerical Recipes, the Art of Scientific Computing*, Third Edition, Cambridge University Press, 2007.

[64] Proudfoot J, Goldberg D, Mann A, Everitt BS, Marks I, and Gray JA. Computerized, interactive multimedia cognitive-behavioural program for anxiety and depression in general practice. *Psychological Medicine*, **33**: 217–227, 2003.

[65] Röhmel J and Pigeot I. A comparison of multiple testing procedures for the gold standard non-inferiority trial. *Journal of Biopharmaceutical Statistics*, **20**: 911–926, 2010.

[66] Röhmel J and Pigeot I. Statistical strategies for the analysis of clinical trials with an experimental treatment, an active control and placebo, and a prespecified fixed non-inferiority margin for the difference in means. *Statistics in Medicine*, **30**: 3162–3164, 2011.

[67] Roy A, Bhaumik DK, Aryal S, and Gibbons RD. Sample size determination for hierarchical longitudinal designs with differential attrition rates. *Biometrics*, **63**: 699–707, 2007.

[68] Rubin, DB. Inference and missing data. *Biometrika*, **63**: 581–592, 1976.

[69] Rubin, DB. *Multiple Imputation for Nonresponse in Surveys*, New York, John Wiley & Sons, 1987.

[70] SAS Institute Inc. *SAS/STAT User's Guide*, Version 9.3, Cary, NC, USA, 2013.

[71] Schafer, JL. *Analysis of Incomplete Multivariate Data*, New York: Chapman & Hall, 1997.

[72] Schwartz G. Estimating the dimension of a model. *The Annals of Statistics*, **6**: 461–464, 1978.

[73] Schwartz S, et al. Effects of troglitazone in insulin-treated patients with type II diabetes mellitus. Troglitazon and Exogenous Insulin Study Group. *New. Engl. J. Med.*, **338**: 861–866, 1998.

[74] Self SG and Liang KY. Asymptotic properties of maximum likelihood estimates and likelihood ratio tests under nonstandard conditions. *Journal of American Statistical Association*, **82**: 605–610, 1987.

[75] Siddiqui O, Hung HMJ, and O'Neill R. MMRM versus LOCF: A comprehensive comparison based on simulation study and 25 NDA data sets. *Journal of Biopharmaceutical Statistics* **19**: 227–246, 2009.

[76] Siddiqui O. MMRM versus MI in dealing with missing data: A comparison based on 25 NDA data sets. *Journal of Biopharmaceutical Statistics* **21**: 423–436, 2011.

[77] Skene AM and White SA. A latent class model for repeated measurements experiments. *Statistics in Medicine*, **11**: 2111–2122, 1992.

[78] Spiegelhalter DJ, Best NG, Carlin BP, and van der Linde A. Bayesian measures of model complexity and fit (with discussion). *J. Roy. Statist. Soc. B.*, **64**: 583–640, 2002.

[79] Stanek EJ. Choosing a pretest-postest analysis. *American Statistician*, **42**: 178–183.

[80] Stucke K and Kieser M. A general approach for sample size calculation for the three-arm "gold standard" non-inferiority design. *Statistics in Medicine*, **31**: 3579–3596, 2012.

[81] Takada M and Tango T. Statistical models for estimating the treatment effect of eliminating symptom based on the patient's daily symptom diary in the area of gastrointestinal disease (in Japanese). *Japanese Joint Statistical Meeting*, Tokyo, November 14, 2014.

[82] Taguchi N and Tango T. A latent class mixture model combined with proportional odds model for repeated measurements in clinical trials. *The 24th International Biometric Conference*, Dublin, 2008.

[83] Tango T. Mixture models for the analysis of repeated measurements in clinical trials. *Japanese Journal of Applied Statistics*, **18**:143–161, 1989.

[84] Tango T. A mixture model to classify individual profiles of repeated measurements. In *Data Science, Classification and Related Methods*, Hayashi et al. (eds.). Springer-Verlag, Tokyo, pp 247–254, 1998.

[85] Tango T. *Randomized Controlled Trial* (in Japanese). Asakura Publishing Co. Ltd, 2003.

[86] Tango T. Sample size formula for randomized controlled trials with counts of recurrent events. *Statistics and Probability Letters*, **79**: 466–472, 2009.

[87] Tango T. On the repeated measures designs and sample sizes for randomized controlled trials. *Biostatistics*, **17**: 334–349, 2016a.

[88] Tango T. New repeated measures design and sample size for randomized controlled trials. *XXVIIIth International Biometric Conference*, Victoria, Canada, 10–15 July, 2016b.

[89] Tango T. Power and sample size for the S:T repeated measures design combined with a linear mixed-effects model allowing for missing data. *Journal of Biopharmaceutical Statistics*, in press, 2017.

[90] Thall P and Vail SC. Some covariance models for longitudinal count data with overdispersion. *Biometrics*, **46**: 657–671, 1990.

[91] The R for Statistical Computing. `http://www.r-project.org`.

[92] Thode Jr. HC, Finch SJ, and Mendell NR. Simulated percentage points for the null distribution of the likelihood ratio test for a mixture of two normals. *Biometrics*, **44**: 1195–1201, 1988.

[93] US Food and Drug Association (FDA). *FDA Guidance for Industry Non-Inferiority Clinical Trials.* `http://www.fda.gov/downloads/Drugs/GuidanceComplianceRegulatoryInformation/Guidances/UCM202140.pdf`, August, 31, 2011.

[94] van Buuren S. *Flexible Imputation of Missing Data*, Boca Raton, Chapman & Hall/CRC, 2012.

[95] Verbeke G and Lesaffre E. A linear mixed-effects model with heterogeneity in the random-effects population. *Journal of the American Statistical Association*, **91**: 217–221, 1996.

[96] Verbeke G and Lesaffre E. The effect of misspecifying the random effects distribution in linear mixed models for longitudinal data. *Computational Statistics and Data Analysis*, **23**: 541–556, 1997.

[97] Verbeke G and Molenberghs G. *Linear Mixed Models for Longitudinal Data*, Springer, 2001.

[98] White IR, Royston P, and Wood AM. Multiple imputation using chained equations: Issues and guidance for practice. *Statistics in Medicine*, **30**: 377–399, 2011.

[99] Winkens B, van Breukelen GJP, Schouten HJA, and Berger MPF. Randomized clinical trials with a pre- and a post-treatment measurement: Repeated measures versus ANCOVA models. *Contemporary Clinical Trials*, **28**: 713–719, 2007.

[100] Yano Y, Suzuki H, Kumada H, Shimizu K, Hayashi N, and Tango T. Double-blinded placebo-controlled randomized trial of Gritiron for patients with chronic hepatitis. *Clinical Medicine and Research*, **66**: 2629–2644, 1989.

Index

For Product Safety Concerns and Information please contact our EU representative GPSR@taylorandfrancis.com Taylor & Francis Verlag GmbH, Kaufingerstraße 24, 80331 München, Germany

Batch number: 10725800

Printed by Printforce, the Netherlands